Managing the Spino-Pelvic-Hip Complex

An integrated approach

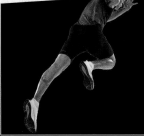

Carl Todd

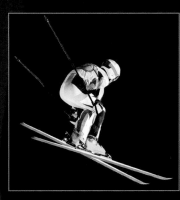

Assistant Editor Suzanne Scott

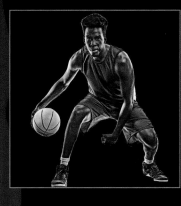

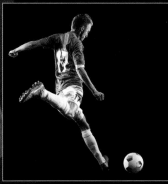

Foreword by Jorge Esteves

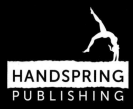

Managing the
Spino-Pelvic-Hip
Complex

First published in Great Britain in 2023 by Handspring Publishing, an imprint of
Jessica Kingsley Publishers
An imprint of Hodder & Stoughton Ltd
An Hachette UK Company

1

A CIP catalogue record for this title is available from the British Library and the Library of Congress

ISBN 978 1 91342 629 3
eISBN 978 1 91342 630 9

Printed and bound in China by C & C Offset Printing Co Ltd

Jessica Kingsley Publishers' policy is to use papers that are natural, renewable and recyclable products and made from wood grown in sustainable forests. The logging and manufacturing processes are expected to conform to the environmental regulations of the country of origin.

Handspring Publishing
Carmelite House
50 Victoria Embankment
London EC4Y 0DZ

www.handspringpublishing.com

CONTENTS

About the author   vii
Foreword by Jorge Esteves   ix
Acknowledgments   xi
Abbreviations   xii

CHAPTER 1   Introduction   3

CHAPTER 2   Integrating the "five 'ATEs" into clinical practice   23

CHAPTER 3   Applied anatomy   53

CHAPTER 4   Pain, pathology and dysfunction   87

CHAPTER 5   EvaluATE   123

CHAPTER 6   ManipulATE   169

CHAPTER 7   ActivATE   211

CHAPTER 8   IntegrATE   253

Appendix 1   276
Appendix 2   278
Appendix 3   280
Index   287

ABOUT THE AUTHOR

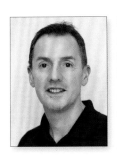 **Carl Todd** PhD MSc (Sports Med) BSc (Hons) Ost DO CSCS Cert Ed is a registered osteopath, qualified lecturer, published author and a certified strength and conditioning specialist. His academic qualifications include a PhD in orthopedics and clinical science and a master's degree in sport injury medicine.

Carl is consultant osteopath to the Football Association. In 2005 he became the first osteopath to be appointed by the FA to work with the England Football team. To date he has worked over 200 international games and with them has attended four FIFA World Cup tournaments and three UEFA European Championships. Since 2009 Carl has acted as consultant osteopath to Chelsea Football Club and to Team GB male and female Basketball at the London 2012 Olympics, and for Athletics at the Tokyo 2020 Olympics. He has previously consulted for many other soccer clubs, as well as for Honda UK and the England Cricket Board.

His academic appointments include 10 years (2005–2015) as associate lecturer at the School of Healthcare, Oxford Brookes University, UK. At the time of publication, he is Visiting Fellow, Cranfield University; Honorary Lecturer, Swansea University; and Researcher, University of Gothenburg.

Carl has a keen interest in sports medicine and a wealth of experience in the treatment and management of both elite and amateur-level athletes. He is an active practitioner and has designed and delivers his own courses on functional integrated approaches to managing the athlete. He has published papers in peer-reviewed journals and lectures regularly at medical conferences, both nationally and internationally.

About the Assistant Editor

Suzanne Scott PhD is a movement coach with a professional focus on the role of specific movement training in athlete rehabilitation and performance optimization. She has worked extensively in team sport, particularly soccer, and has a research background in exercise physiology, anatomy and bone health.

FOREWORD by Jorge Esteves

It is a true honor to be asked to write a foreword for Dr Carl Todd's book on a highly relevant topic to clinicians in the fields of sports and musculoskeletal care. I have known Dr Todd for over 20 years as a tutor, colleague and friend. I have had the privilege to witness his personal and professional development, from his undergraduate education in osteopathy to completing his doctoral research degree and as a leading clinician in the field of elite sport. Carl is someone I truly admire for his constant striving for excellence in person-centered care.

Managing the Spino-Pelvic-Hip Complex: An integrated approach is a well-conceived and well-written book informed by Dr Todd's clinical reasoning strategies that stem from many years working across a range of sports from amateur to elite level, but crucially, the book is also informed by relevant clinical research. It is not a book on technique or protocol-based clinical interventions, but importantly a tool that enables sports and musculoskeletal practitioners to critically reflect on their current practice and develop evidence-informed clinical interventions centered on the person seeking care.

The book is centered around the concept of the "five 'ATEs" – EvaluATE, EducATE, ManipulATE, ActivATE, IntegrATE. The "five 'ATEs" is a well-conceived conceptual model, which provides clinicians with the required knowledge, skills and competencies to provide person-centered care by emphasizing the role of education, exercise and return to play – or simply to activities of daily living. Although manual therapy still plays a vital role in patient care, in this book clinicians are provided with the tools to shift from passive and low-value care to an integrated approach where education, exercise, and physical and emotional well-being are central to high-value person-centered clinical care.

As the carefully crafted content of this book unfolds, sports and musculoskeletal practitioners are presented with evidence-informed therapeutic strategies that can be easily implemented in their daily clinical practice. Notably, the reader is presented with a range of clinical evaluation, treatment and management strategies that are strongly underpinned by a strong focus on a well-developed clinical reasoning. The focus on clinical reasoning is particularly relevant because it de-emphasizes the role of therapeutic techniques or clinical "recipes," emphasizing critically informed clinical reasoning. As such, the book enables the reader to critically consider the role of the proposed strategies not only in the field of sports care but in a wide range of musculoskeletal pain and dysfunction, and arguably health problems where through chronicity, individuals have lost their sense of agency and consequently their ability to undergo their activities of daily living.

I commend Dr Todd for his ability to present complex issues in a user-friendly framework, which enables clinicians to develop their clinical competence profile in a critically informed way. I highly recommend the book to any sports or musculoskeletal practitioner – it is an excellent resource for continued professional development.

Jorge Esteves
Gzira, Malta
March 2022

ACKNOWLEDGMENTS

The initial concept for this book began as an idea that was seeded and nurtured in my mind and encouraged by students over many years of teaching. Although the beginning of this project pre-dates 2019, the book quickly became a product of the many lockdowns that we had to endure as a direct result of the Covid pandemic. Throughout these periods, I tried to be productive with my time as clinical and professional work in sport throughout the United Kingdom and the rest of the world was put on hold.

There are many individuals without whose support this book would never have been possible, and to each and every one of you I am extremely grateful. Although it is impossible to mention everyone personally, I would like to acknowledge and thank all those from Handspring Publishing, especially Mary Law and Andrew Stevenson, from meeting initially in 2019 to supporting the project to completion. I am grateful to Kerry Parkinson Day for her assistance in my early days with writing, guidance and positive encouragement. Dr Suzanne Scott, my Associate Editor and good friend, took on considerably more work than she initially anticipated; for this I will be forever grateful. I am extremely humbled by her drive and passion for excellence, and the final version reads so much better for her contribution.

I am eternally grateful to my wife, Mel, for her continual patience and unconditional support – without you by my side, I would never have achieved anything in my professional career; to my boys, Max, Callum and Will – perhaps in some small way this book might help you all to dream big; to my parents for their support in life, especially for giving me the ambition to succeed and for my father's words, "Always strive to do the best"; finally, to the many clinicians, patients, athletes and students that I have had the privilege to meet – I thank you all for sharing your experiences and you have all truly inspired me to write this book.

ABBREVIATIONS

ADLs	Activities of daily living		**GTO**	Golgi tendon organ
AS	Ankylosing spondylitis		**HAGOS**	Hip and Groin Outcome Score
ASIS	Anterior superior iliac spine		**HHD**	Handheld dynamometer
ASLR	Active straight leg raise		**HVLA**	High-velocity, low-amplitude
Ax	Assessment		**ICC**	Intra-class correlation
BK	Bent knee		**ILA**	Inferior lateral angle
BPFS	Back Pain Functional Scale		**IO**	Internal oblique
BPS	Bio-psychosocial		**ITB**	Iliotibial band
CFT	Cognitive functional therapy		**IVD**	Intervertebral disk
CI	Confidence interval		**LBP**	Low back pain
CNS	Central nervous system		**LSJ**	Lumbosacral junction
CT	Computed tomography		**MET**	Muscle energy technique
DL	Double-leg		**MRI**	Magnetic resonance imaging
DOMS	Delayed-onset muscle soreness		**MSK**	Musculoskeletal
ECM	Extra-cellular matrix		**MU**	Motor unit
EO	External oblique		**MVC**	Maximum voluntary contraction
EMG	Electromyographic, electromyography		**NSAID**	Non-steroidal anti-inflammatory drug
FABER	Flexion, abduction, external rotation		**OA**	Osteoarthritis
FADIR	Flexion, adduction, internal rotation		**PAG**	Periaqueductal gray
FAI	Femoroacetabular impingement		**PAIVM**	Passive accessory intervertebral motion
FSU	Functional spinal unit		**PAP**	Post-activation potentiation
GHJ	Glenohumeral joint		**PBU**	Pressure biofeedback unit
GMed	Gluteus medius		**PI**	Pelvic incidence
GMin	Gluteus minimus		**PKB**	Prone knee bend
GMx	Gluteus maximus		**PNF**	Proprioceptive neuromuscular facilitation

PNS	Peripheral nervous system	**SKB**	Small knee bend
PPIVM	Passive physiological intervertebral motion	**SL**	Single-leg
		SLR	Straight leg raise
PRP	Protein-rich plasma	**SMT**	Symptom modification technique
PSIS	Posterior superior iliac spine	**SS**	Sacral slope
PT	Pelvic tilt	**STM**	Soft tissue manipulation
PTu	Pubic tubercle	**TA**	Transversus abdominis
QL	Quadratus lumborum	**TB**	Theraband®
RA	Rectus abdominis	**TFL**	Tensor fasciae latae
RDL	Romanian deadlift	**TLF**	Thoracolumbar fascia
RFD	Rate of force development	**TnP**	Tender point
ROM	Range of movement	**TrP**	Trigger point
RTP	Return to play	**VAS**	Visual analogue scale
SIJ	Sacroiliac joint		

Chapter 1 structure

Framework: "five 'ATEs"   3

Clinical reasoning   5

Bio-psychosocial model   8

Functional evaluation   9

Optimal alignment   13

Movement   15

Clinical evaluation   16

Conclusion   19

Framework: "five 'ATEs"

This book has been written to provide a framework to help clinicians make informed decisions for the effective management of the many complex presentations related to the spine, pelvis, hip and groin. I am not suggesting that this framework will provide the perfect solution. It will not be the complete answer for every situation that might be encountered; nor should it replace your own individual ideas and approaches. Instead, I will tell you a story, using the many case studies embedded throughout this book. I hope these will help to refine and integrate current concepts into a framework, one that has proved to be extremely useful for me throughout my years of working in both elite sport and clinical practice.

What makes this book unique or different from other published resources that are readily available to the world of physical and manipulative therapy? Well, the answer to this lies in words of the famous American football coach, Vince Lombardi: "Excellence is mastery of the fundamentals." This statement reflects my working practice because the framework that I propose in this book has become fundamental to my principles and way of working as an osteopath and rehabilitation specialist. I constantly challenge myself to master it through continual reflection and refinement, always striving to achieve excellence in clinical practice. While some may view me as a research-based clinician, this book is a compilation of my clinical experience, based on current scientific evidence and written from a clinical standpoint. The information that I present in these pages is intended to challenge current thought processes and previous education and training experiences. I hope that reading this book will broaden minds and begin to stretch beliefs.

The approach presented here will help clinicians to integrate current biomedical and bio-psychosocial approaches into a successful management plan. I will refer to this integrated framework as the "five 'ATEs."

Figure 1.1 provides an overview and Table 1.1, later on, provides more specificity. The diagram illustrating the framework depicts a continuous circle; however, as a deeper understanding of this approach is developed, it will become clearer that the "five 'ATEs" are interchangeable, indicating the importance of the potential for flexibility, depending on the presenting complaint or the situation under observation.

This chapter lays the foundations for what I believe should form the principles of biomedical and bio-psychosocial healthcare models that can be used side by side in elite sport. Specifically, it shows how to adopt functional and clinical approaches and how to position and evaluate these approaches, using clinical reasoning skills, within the context of the "five 'ATEs" framework I propose.

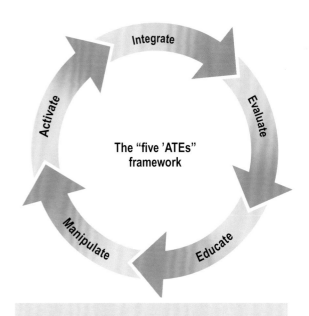

Figure 1.1
The "five 'ATEs" framework.

Table 1.1 Management strategy based on the "five 'ATEs" framework

ATE	FUNCTION
EvaluATE	<ul><li>Collate a case history, gather information and identify the likelihood of red flags</li><li>Establish whether this is an acute or a chronic issue</li><li>Perform a biomedical evaluation (functional and clinical)</li><li>Perform a bio-psychosocial (BPS) evaluation</li><li>Use questionnaires including STarT Back Screening Tool, Back Pain Function Scale (BPFS), Copenhagen Hip and Groin Outcome Score (HAGOS) – see Appendices at the end of the book</li><li>Engage in the decision-making process, develop hypotheses, establish goals or refer for further investigations</li><li>Use symptom modification techniques to reduce biomechanical strain and help *educATE*</li><li>Clinician *re-evaluATE*</li></ul>
EducATE	<ul><li>Reassure the patient through a clearer understanding</li><li>Help to dispel beliefs about previous or past experiences</li><li>Empower the patient and develop self-confidence through cognitive tuition</li><li>Clinician *re-evaluATE*</li></ul>
ManipulATE	<ul><li>Address soft tissue, articular and neural tissue dysfunction with appropriate manipulative therapy</li><li>Help with pain modulation</li><li>Improve function by reducing biomechanical strain</li><li>Improve joint range of movement (ROM) and muscle flexibility</li><li>Clinician *re-evaluATE*</li></ul>
ActivATE	<ul><li>Facilitate motor control patterns</li><li>Use symptom modification techniques to reduce biomechanical strain</li><li>Retrain motor control through ROM</li><li>Clinician *re-evaluATE*</li></ul>
IntegrATE	<ul><li>Perform objective strength and capacity measurements</li><li>Encourage gradual exposure and return to functional activity</li><li>Encourage gradual exposure and return to sporting activity</li><li>Clinician *re-evaluATE*</li></ul>

There are three goals for this chapter:

1. To use the "five 'ATEs" to develop reasoning skills to apply the key principles of biomedical and bio-psychosocial models, in a system-based, integrated approach that may be used in a clinical, sporting or gym-based environment.

2. To help develop a deeper understanding and appreciation of the concept of applying a functional and clinical approach to enable successful treatment outcomes.

3. To provide a knowledge base of the terminology and background literature that will be of use for reading this book.

So, what constitutes a framework? The following definition reflects my interpretation of what a framework is:

The framework is the supporting structure based on a system of concepts, which are the "five 'ATEs," and is founded on my clinical experience and reflection on patient outcomes across the course of my professional practice. It may be used to decide a plan of action for approaching or managing complex musculoskeletal issues.

Four of the aspects of this integrated framework will have a chapter specifically dedicated to them, while the underlying theme of *educATE* will run throughout this book. For ease of understanding, I will use the following icons when discussing specific aspects of the "five 'ATEs." What follows is a brief explanation of my understanding of each aspect.

EvaluATE

 This refers to the process of judging or calculating the quality, importance, amount or value of something. In the context of this book, this will involve the therapeutic relationship developed through patient–clinician interactions aimed at collating a story, to inform clinical reasoning and drive the evaluation process. This may involve functional, clinical and bio-psychosocial approaches.

EducATE

 This refers to the process of providing information or training for an individual on a particular subject. This may involve topics that include intellectual, moral and social aspects. Within the context of musculoskeletal medicine, education provides a deeper understanding between patient and clinician with the purpose of helping to reassure, support and nurture during the management of musculoskeletal issues.

ManipulATE

 This refers to the process of applying a hands-on skill that is a form of treatment that may directly influence an individual's symptoms or function. The term "manipulation" in the context of this book will be used in relation to any technique (joint, soft tissue or muscle activation technique) that can be used to affect the articular, myofascial and nervous systems.

ActivATE

 This refers to the process of encouraging an individual to be active, "switch on" or become more operative. In the context of this book, activation denotes progression from a passive to an active treatment approach. This involves up-regulation of the nervous system, therefore targeting motor control, muscle capacity and strength.

IntegrATE

 This refers to the ability to restore an individual to a functional state by integrating the "ATEs" approach. In the context of musculoskeletal medicine, integration may involve taking into consideration an individual's specific requirement: for example, their tissue response to treatment and exercise response. *IntegrATE* helps develop a clearer understanding through education, movement and functional exercise.

Clinical reasoning

 Clinical reasoning is the process that encompasses critical thinking, judgment, problem-solving and decision-making (Levett-Jones et al., 2010; Tanner, 2006). It can be viewed as the cognitive process that incorporates inferential thinking skills and knowledge to make clinical decisions (Jones, 1992). Developing a level of proficiency in our clinical skills is extremely important and knowing when and how to apply these skills effectively is crucial. Effective clinical reasoning does not happen by coincidence; nor can it be developed by reading this book or through observing other clinicians in practice. In my opinion, it requires a structured framework that can be developed only through exposure to continual clinical practice, with the reflective thinking required to contemplate and evaluate outcomes.

There are many clinical reasoning approaches that can be used in practice. What follows is an overview of the more common approaches: pattern recognition,

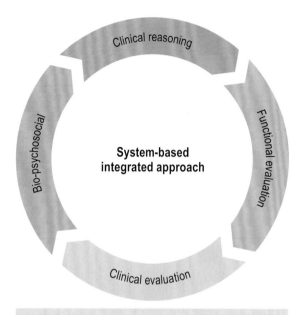

Figure 1.2
System-based integrated approach.
Note it is possible to initiate this approach from any part of the circle.

prior clinical knowledge and experience, interpretative reasoning, hypothetical deductive reasoning and diagnostic reasoning (McCarthy, 2010).

Pattern recognition

Some clinicians can reach a swift and successful resolution with patients, and because of this they are often classified as expert clinicians. At this point, I would like to make it absolutely clear that I do not view myself as an expert clinician. While I may have developed a great deal of experience and knowledge around this subject, I am only too aware that there is still much to learn. It has been suggested that expert clinicians can achieve high levels of success with difficult patients, where other clinicians fail. An expert clinician will rely heavily on pattern recognition, based on clinical experience (and intuition),

to deal with problems efficiently and effectively (Rivett and Jones, 2004).

It has been stated that it takes 10 years' experience to become "expert" in a particular field (Gobet and Wood, 1999). It may be true that some clinicians do not succeed because they do not have enough clinical experience, or perhaps they fail to pick up on patient cues during the process of collating a case history. Inexperienced clinicians may lack confidence in their ability, which can be inadvertently communicated to the patient or athlete during the evaluation. Gaining experience and becoming expert in a discipline should not necessarily be measured by time (Rivett and Jones, 2004). For example, I have come across many clinicians who have been qualified for 10 or more years, but over this period have used the same treatment approach with every patient. This, in my opinion, could have a detrimental effect on their clinical practice. While they may have achieved reasonable clinical outcomes by doing the same thing day in, day out, this clinical reasoning approach will have its drawbacks if they have failed to read widely within their chosen field, consider other approaches and reflect on their particular style. The expert clinician may become biased towards their own treatment approach. For example, they may draw on past experiences and prejudices, or form assumptions that could impede the collection of information. These preconceptions can cause the misinterpretation of information and perhaps even a failure to recognize potential signs of serious pathology. It has previously been shown that family doctors (general practitioners) who rely on pattern recognition will reach the correct diagnosis, despite frequent failures to identify the most critical features of a problem (Groves et al., 2003), and many clinicians use pattern recognition for routine and familiar problems. However, when the problem is not routine, pattern recognition is not an optimal strategy.

Hypothetical deductive reasoning

The second approach to clinical reasoning involves using the hypothetical deductive model. This model is more rational and involves the processes of data collection, hypothesis generation and hypothesis testing. More than one hypothesis should be generated because the best evaluation of a hypothesis is gained only by testing it against others. Consistent use of the hypothetical deductive model enables a clinician to build knowledge from past experiences and repeated exposure to clinical presentations and facilitates the structured retrieval of information from their long-term memory. The process by which information is structured and retrieved from our long-term memory is called an illness script. Illness scripts are the result of applying three components: the problem in relation to a pathological mechanism, the condition in relation to the patient's contextual features and the consequences of their signs and symptoms (Feltovich and Barrows, 1984).

Hypotheses are developed from the observation and acquisition of cues the patient offers to a clinician during the evaluation. The clinician applies that information to test the hypotheses, to decide whether these should be included or excluded. Hypotheses are generated and subsequently tested for their validity. This process makes the hypothetical deductive approach much more robust than pattern recognition.

Initially this process can be time-consuming, as it involves combining many other factors, such as:

- mechanism of injury: traumatic, repetitive, dynamic or static loading
- components of pattern recognition in relation to the clinical presentation
- the biomedical model using functional and clinical evaluation to examine biomechanics, soft tissue, articular and neural-related signs and symptoms, alongside the bio-psychosocial model that considers the individual and their emotions, beliefs, past experiences and social environments
- the functional impact on movement in relation to consequences of the clinical picture or the physical activity.

Knowledge and practitioner insight

The well-known phrase "Knowledge is power" is commonly attributed to Sir Francis Bacon. In this context, sources of knowledge can influence our reasoning processes and may directly affect how accurate our clinical decisions may be. Higgs et al. (2004) suggest that knowledge should be classified into two distinct categories, propositional and non-propositional. Propositional knowledge may be gained through scientific research study; this can be easily accessed through online resources, textbooks and peer-reviewed papers. Non-propositional knowledge refers to professional craft and personal knowledge. Professional craft knowledge can relate to clinical competences that we acquire or that develop through clinical experience. Personal knowledge is also gained through clinical experiences, developed through active engagement in reflective practice. The benefit of non-propositional knowledge lies in the ability of the clinician to evaluate accurately and make a decision. It may be that expert clinicians have developed a greater level of knowledge, helping them to understand and make judgments based on the quality of their knowledge, compared with less experienced clinicians (Gobet and Wood, 1999).

Diagnostic reasoning

Once a case history has been completed and clinical reasoning approaches have been reviewed, the objective examination may be used to gather more accurate information. The purpose of performing both functional and clinical evaluations is to test the hypotheses that have been generated, by using the hypothetical deductive approach. Some clinical evaluations have previously been validated against a gold standard and are more accurate and reliable compared with others. Similarly, other evaluations have higher levels of sensitivity and specificity compared with others (Magee, 2014). Knowledge of these evaluations and their subsequent inclusion to help inform an evidence-based decision may increase the probability of a more accurate diagnostic process.

Symptom modification techniques

It must be stressed that there is never 100 percent certainty with any clinical evaluation and that no diagnostic test is 100 percent valid (McCarthy, 2010). However, diagnostic reasoning can be especially effective in the validation of hypothesis testing and this is precisely what symptom modification techniques (SMTs) provide.

 The process of using SMTs helps to validate hypotheses and may also prove to be tremendously effective within patient or athlete education. For this reason, using this clinical reasoning approach starts to integrate the second part of the "five 'ATEs" framework and begins to *educATE*.

Lewis (2009) first described SMTs for use in shoulder assessment. Evidence suggests low specificity for orthopedic tests commonly employed to evaluate shoulder pathology (Magee, 2014), which can impair diagnostic outcomes. The aim of SMTs is to identify one or more methods that may reduce symptoms and/or increase movement and function. It places less emphasis on diagnosis and more on attempting to provide pain modulation and encourage function. SMTs within diagnostic reasoning offer a way to assess the shoulder objectively, by identifying movements or positions that may be contributing to the patient's symptoms, rather than a pathoanatomical structure. Movement and manual manipulative therapy techniques are then used as a means to guide the treatment.

I have found using the SMT approach to be extremely beneficial for evaluation of the spine, pelvis, hip and groin. Compared with the shoulder, it is much more difficult to reposition the spine, pelvic girdle, hip and groin manually. This is due to the complexity of the many articular and myofascial structures that cross these regions. However, I have found manual manipulative therapy, with and without neuromuscular activation exercises, equally efficient and effective for addressing pain, inducing neuromodulation of symptoms and improving movement and function.

Generally, I perform a short series of passive or active manipulative techniques, or I might coach the patient through a short series of controlled activation exercises, involving a particular region of the body that I feel may be influencing their symptoms. I then re-evaluate their initial presentation. Using SMTs appropriately can have an immediate effect on function and can be viewed as a mini-treatment. Although complex in nature, symptoms are often mechanically induced, but are generally consistent with maladaptive and cognitive compensations that may become a mechanism for underlying pain (O'Sullivan, 2000). In my opinion, for SMTs to be used effectively, a thorough understanding of movement and control issues is essential before applying an SMT approach, and this will be discussed in greater detail later.

Interpretative reasoning

This process of clinical reasoning runs in conjunction with the other reasoning processes that I have highlighted within this section. The benefit of interpretative reasoning is that it involves the patient or athlete in the decision-making process. Adopting this strategy allows the patient to narrate their interpretation of their story, raising their concerns and queries through unfolding the chain of events that has led to their issue, much like a novel. This starts to bring in the bio-psychosocial model, and what factors may be playing a role in determining a patient's understanding of their issue, which the clinician will aim to interpret to grasp the problems more effectively (Jones and Edwards, 2006). This two-way approach helps the patient play a significant part in the reasoning process and assists the clinician in challenging the patient's understanding and beliefs.

Bio-psychosocial model

 In recent years, the bio-psychosocial (BPS) model has gained significant recognition in the management of chronic pain with increasing evidence that cognitive, emotional and social factors can influence pain perceptions, levels of distress and coping strategies (O'Sullivan et al., 2018). There has been criticism of the biomedical model for a lack of evidence base, especially around the challenge of identifying a pathoanatomical cause of pain (Maher et al., 2017), combined with the biomedical model's failure to reduce the growing healthcare costs for disability and chronicity with musculoskeletal pain (O'Sullivan et al., 2018). Furthermore, findings from investigations on magnetic resonance imaging (MRI) have highlighted only a weak correlation with patient-reported low back pain (LBP). In addition, incidental findings such as intervertebral disk degeneration appear to be increasingly prevalent in individuals that are asymptomatic (Brinjikji et al., 2015).

However, it is important to stress that, in my experience of working in elite sport, the biomedical model still has significant relevance. The sporting environment creates situations where athletes suffer from both acute and chronic bouts of pain. Therefore, to implement a specific management plan, clinicians should have a clear understanding of what tissues or structures they are rehabilitating. MRI investigations can be extremely useful as they can serve as a reference point to confirm and evaluate the extent and severity of injury and to differentiate between edema and tissue damage (Connell et al., 2004). MRI can also help with the return-to-play timeframe, especially if a target is set for a particular competition or game (Comin et al., 2013; Ekstrand et al., 2012). Having a fundamental understanding of healing processes, such as scar tissue formation (Crema et al., 2015), allows for anatomical structures to be loaded appropriately throughout the rehabilitation process and reduces the risk of re-injury (Ekstrand et al., 2012; Askling et al., 2007).

I have heard some clinicians remark that the BPS model has no place in sport and that everything should be biomedical and biomechanical. I would argue that this is not the case and, in my opinion, being open-minded to both models has enabled me to develop into a more rounded clinician. Both biomedical and BPS models have value; a recent study combining these approaches has highlighted their effectiveness for short- and medium-term improvements for back performance, pain reduction, disability and kinesiophobia (Saracoglu et al., 2020).

Functional evaluation

 Functional evaluation should encompass a combination of tests that include functional movement evaluations and assessments, to determine the ability of an athlete or patient to maintain optimal alignment and demonstrate the coordinated movement and mobility requirements necessary to perform static and/or dynamic tasks.

Functional evaluation can therefore be viewed as an integrated assessment of multiple body regions and systems, which may be required to perform a movement pattern (Kivlan and Martin, 2012). This might provide an advantage over more traditional clinical evaluations because components of joint mobility, muscle flexibility, motor control, coordination and balance, and endurance may be evaluated simultaneously across multiple regions, such as the spino-pelvic-hip complex, by observing the movement patterns of how an athlete or patient should normally function (Okada et al., 2011; Cook et al., 2006; Mills et al., 2005).

Figure 1.3 highlights the fundamental principles that I consider should be taken into account to determine the functional evaluation of an athlete or patient.

If, on observation, an athlete demonstrated lack of coordinated ability or impaired movement, resulting in them failing to reach the full ROMs required to perform a task, I would classify them as dysfunctional. Dysfunction is defined as pain, asymmetry or injury that impairs normal movement and the performance of a functional activity (Kivlan and Martin, 2012). In sport, for example, an athlete might demonstrate a lack of frontal (side to side), transverse (rotation left or right) and sagittal (forwards and backwards) plane mobility, specifically around the hip joint. These are fundamental movements that are required in preparation to perform a task such as kicking a ball. In this instance, the athlete

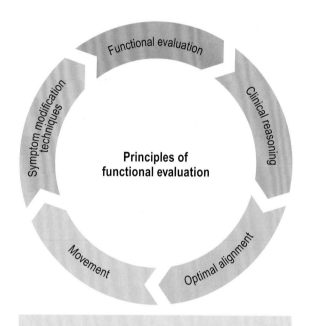

Figure 1.3
Principles of functional evaluation.

structure and function. They control and transfer forces through the pelvic girdle, between the upper and lower body, during normal movement and sporting actions (Robertson et al., 2009).

Theoretical models have historically inspired new musculoskeletal approaches for applying the concept of function and movement. Panjabi (1992) initially proposed the idea that, for optimal spinal stability to be successful, the body requires three systems (Figure 1.5).

Control system

The control system includes both the central nervous system (CNS) and the peripheral nervous system (PNS). These systems together ensure optimal regulation of both motor control and sensory motor feedback. This includes, for example, stabilizing the body prior to a predicted challenge (Hodges and Mosley, 2003) or increasing neural activity proportionally to the increased demands of performing a functional task (van Dieën and de Looze, 1999).

Passive system

Panjabi's theory (1992) suggests that the bones, joint capsules, ligaments and fascia are all inherent in the passive system. Some might question the role of fascia as a passive structure, as recent explanations suggest that fascia is capable of performing a functional role, contributes to the proprioceptive system and may help with myofascial force transmission (Stecco et al., 2009; van der Wal, 2009). The passive system consists of joints and their ligaments, and physiological movement occurs by neural feedback through joint proprioception and mechanoreceptors, especially when the ligaments and joint capsules are subjected to tension forces at their end of range. As a result, the passive system will assist the neural system by translating and relaying information to the spinal cord and the brain, from the deep pressure, position and movement of limbs, which is mediated through their respective joint receptors and has been shown to influence motor feedback and muscle function (Umphred, 2007).

may start to develop coping strategies within their musculoskeletal system to overcome the distinct lack of hip joint mobility; this eventually leads to over-compensation and maladaptive, abnormal or non-functional movement patterns (Sahrmann, 2002).

When starting to understand the principles of functional evaluation, it is important to grasp the fundamental role that the kinetic chain plays in allowing an athlete to perform functional movement (Figure 1.4). Essentially, the body can be viewed as a chain of segments or links, formed from joints and ligaments and influenced by numerous myofascial connections, with each component affecting every segment during movement. If one part of the chain is in motion, it will affect the movement in the links in other chains (Myers, 2009). The connections that affect movement are the soft tissues and their related components. Soft tissues distribute strain; transmit force, torque and load; and affect

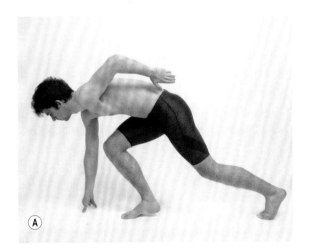

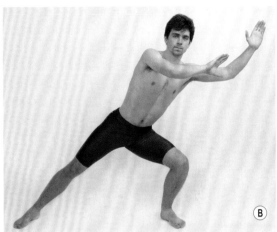

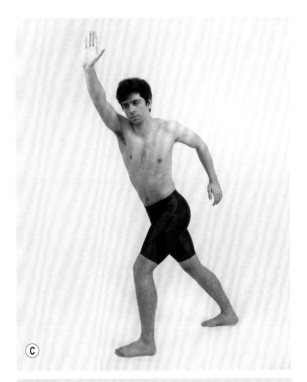

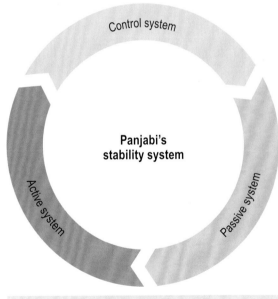

Figure 1.5
Panjabi's stability system.

Figure 1.4
Kinetic chain and functional movement.

A: In the sagittal plane. B: In the frontal plane. C: In the transverse plane.

Active system

Understanding the active system requires an awareness of the physiology of muscle fibers, motor units and muscle stiffness. Force and stability are provided through the muscles and tendons of the active system. This system works particularly closely with the neural system, ensuring feedback through muscle spindles and Golgi tendon organs (GTOs). Muscle spindles are located in the muscle belly and GTOs are located within the musculotendinous junctions. GTOs respond to increases in tension within the muscle and function to help protect the muscle from further damage by creating "autogenic inhibition" (Guyton, 1991). Muscle spindle activity can instigate a chain reaction that is often referred to as the "stretch reflex" or "myotactic reflex" (Guyton, 1991).

Muscle fibers

Skeletal muscle fibers are generally classified as either type 1 – slow-twitch – or type 2 – fast-twitch. There is a further classification of type 2 fast-twitch fibers, consisting of three subtypes: 2A, 2X and 2B. These are differentiated by expression of their myosin heavy chain gene (Talbot and Maves, 2016). Types 1 and 2A rely on oxidative metabolism, compared with types 2X and 2B, which rely on glycolytic metabolism. It is important to note that humans do not appear to have any 2B fibers (Schiaffino and Reggiani, 2011). Human muscles contain varying degrees of type 1 and 2 fibers, but different muscle groups are shown to have varying degrees of fiber types. For example, the human soleus is predominantly type 1, compared with the triceps brachii muscle, which is predominantly type 2 (Schiaffino and Reggiani, 2011; Bassel-Duby and Olsen, 2006; Guyton, 1991; Johnson et al., 1973). Skeletal muscle fibers and the motor neuron that is responsible for innervating these fibers make up a motor unit.

Motor units

The motor unit (MU) consists of the alpha motor neuron and the muscle fibers it innervates. It is the basic functional unit in the active system, allowing production of force and movement (Hunter et al., 2016; Duchateau and Enoka, 2011). The number of fibers contained within a single MU may vary, depending on the task they perform. For example, the hand and eye may contain no more than 100 muscle fibers within a single MU, compared with the 1,000 muscle fibers within a single MU in the leg (Buchthal and Schmalbruch, 1970).

The total number of motor units that are recruited and the discharge rate of the action potentials that innervate each MU control the production of the force that is generated within skeletal muscles (Hunter et al., 2016; Enoka et al., 2003). Essentially, two main types of MU exist: slow low-threshold units and fast high-threshold units (Lieber, 2009). Slow motor units are fatigue-resistant, have more type 1 fibers and are likely to contain greater concentrations of proprioceptors, capable of performing low-threshold postural control tasks. Fast motor units contain more type 2 fibers, fatigue quickly and are predominantly recruited for high-threshold tasks, specifically when increases in load are required to perform the activity.

Muscle stiffness

Muscle spindles not only play a huge contributory role in joint proprioception but also are responsible for generating muscle stiffness. Clinical experience has led to me to believe that muscle stiffness is often misinterpreted. Patients may refer to their loss of mobility as a result of muscle stiffness or their association of muscle stiffness with pain. Muscle stiffness provides strength and support to the musculoskeletal system and consists of two components: intrinsic muscle stiffness and reflex-mediated stiffness.

Intrinsic muscle stiffness

Intrinsic muscle stiffness is dependent on the viscoelastic properties of the muscle and relies on the actin and myosin cross-bridges. It can be influenced through strength training, which results in muscle hypertrophy and a subsequent increase in muscle stiffness. Primarily seen as a passive mechanism, intrinsic muscle stiffness may not contribute to the dynamic response of movement (Johansson et al., 1991).

An example of the clinical relevance of this type of stiffness relates to the deep muscular system of the spinal column. This has been shown to contain 4–7 times more muscle spindles than the superficial muscular system of the spinal column (McGill, 2007). An increased concentration of muscle spindles in the deeper muscular system may increase muscle stiffness. Not only does this influence posture and alignment when performing low-threshold activities, but it will assist with proprioceptive awareness.

Reflex-mediated muscle stiffness

Reflex-mediated stiffness is controlled by the excitation of the alpha motor neuron, which depends on the reflexes associated with muscle spindle activity (Johansson et al., 1991). This system is dynamic in nature, with reflex muscle activation increasing stiffness to help provide a neurological response to postural displacement.

A clinical example of this can be observed when a patient is asked to perform a lumbar flexion movement. An increased activation or an up-regulation of the lumbar multifidus muscles occurs as a result of the forward postural displacement and increase in lumbar flexion loading. Similarly, when the patient is asked to come back to a normal aligned standing posture, the activity of the lumbar multifidus muscles becomes reduced or down-regulated as less spinal loading is required (Comerford and Mottram, 2012).

Optimal alignment

 Functional alignment, relating specifically to the spine, pelvis and hip, may be viewed as the integration of these three anatomical regions that provides shape, position, form and function. Alignment, which allows us to keep the body upright and to function, and which lets us move efficiently while conserving our energy, ensures we can walk on two legs: in other words, maintain our bipedalism (Roussouly and Pinheiro-Franco, 2011; Roussouly and Nnadi, 2010).

Every patient or athlete has what I describe as a functional alignment that is unique to them. I believe this will have developed over time, maybe in response to sports-specific training and loading. For example, young elite skiers have been shown to have reduced spinal and hip mobility, compared to non-athletes of a similar age (Todd et al., 2015; 2016). As a result, it is important for clinicians to attempt to develop a clearer understanding of the biomechanics related to the particular sporting environment in which they want to work. Athletes who compete in a rotational or asymmetric sport, such as tennis or golf, may have a very different alignment to those who compete in a predominantly sagittal sport such as athletics. In addition, athletes who compete in the same sport may also have very different alignments: for example, a soccer player who plays on the right side and kicks with the right foot, compared to one who plays on the left side and kicks with the left foot. If optimal functional alignment is to be achieved, two important components are required. These are called form closure and force closure (Figure 1.6).

Form closure

In general terms, form closure relates to how well the articular surfaces of two joints fit together, requiring no extra forces to maintain the stability of the articular system. Optimal function requires the articular system to maintain alignment between the joint surfaces and their ligamentous supports. In general, every joint has the freedom to move in many directions. The direction of movement can be divided into either a neutral zone or an elastic zone (Panjabi, 1992). When a joint is put in a neutral zone, the joint surfaces can translate, relative to each other and the joint capsule, with their ligamentous attachments, offering no resistance to movement. In contrast, the elastic zone is where the joint capsule and ligamentous attachments do provide resistance to movement. This is dependent on the congruity and architecture of the joint surfaces and the compliance of the joint capsule and ligamentous structures.

Force closure

Force closure is described as the extra forces needed to keep an object in place (Snijders et al., 1993) and to

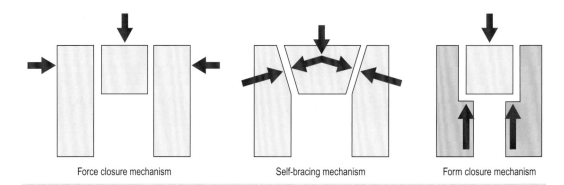

Force closure mechanism   Self-bracing mechanism   Form closure mechanism

Figure 1.6
Form closure and force closure.

increase articular compression between joint surfaces (Vleeming et al., 1990ab), facilitating stabilization. Essentially, force closure operates as a self-locking mechanism. It is not clear to what degree a group of muscles may have to contract around a joint to perform optimal force closure. However, the ability to evaluate this becomes clinically relevant when patients are asked to perform specific tasks. This will be more apparent in the discussion of functional movement.

Figure 1.7 provides an overview of what I would expect to see when an athlete or patient is standing in optimal functional alignment. To maintain this, they require both form and force closure throughout their musculoskeletal system. Note how the body weight is evenly distributed through the lower limbs. Generally, I start at the pelvis and scan visually upwards or downwards, observing and palpating for any significant asymmetries or biomechanical or alignment issues. These may include scoliosis and/or increased or decreased lordosis and kyphosis curvatures, pelvic tilt, femoral head position and femoral anteversion or retroversion, leg length inequalities, which may be structural or functional, knee joint valgus or varus, and foot biomechanics, such as the position of talus, pes planus or pes cavus.

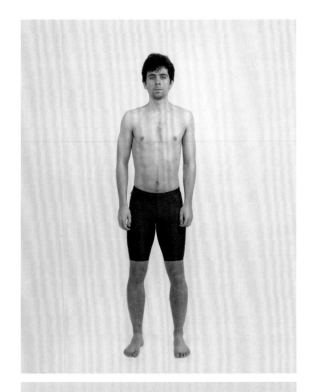

Figure 1.7
Optimal functional alignment.

Movement

Optimal dynamic activity requires two elements to be present within the movement systems: mobility and stability (Hoffman and Gabel 2013). Functional movement requires both the mobility and stability systems to work in unison. If, as clinicians, we have a thorough understanding of the biomechanics of a particular sport, we can hypothesize the ratio of mobility to stability that an athlete may require to perform a given task. For example, let's consider an Olympic archer compared to an Olympic gymnast. The archer may incline more towards the stability system at the expense of the mobility system, whereas the gymnast, while still requiring stability, may place a greater emphasis on the mobility system.

To relate the evaluation of functional movement to clinical practice, it is important to understand the concepts of motor control, joint centration and joint dissociation that occur within the complexity of human movement, and also to analyze the interaction between all the environments in which an individual may be placed, to complete a desired task (Dingenen et al., 2018). Impaired or non-functional (dysfunction) movement may occur if there is a loss of synergy between the mobility and stability systems (Hodges et al., 2002). Pain has also been shown to disrupt the synergy between the two systems (Hodges et al., 2003).

Motor control

Motor control can be viewed as the process that maintains optimal alignment and initiates, directs and grades purposeful movement for performing a skilled task. It depends on the capacity of the muscle to perform the task and also on processing sensory input, interpreting both stability and dynamic activity, and establishing strategies that overcome predictable and unexpected movement challenges (Hodges and Mosley, 2003). Panjabi's control system relates to the CNS, determining motor control requirements through contraction of the deep and superficial muscles for stability and coordinated dynamic mobility through feedback and feedforward control mechanisms (Diedrichsen et al., 2010). For an athlete to perform efficiently, the level of stability and the degree of dynamic mobility will become task-specific and be determined by the nature of the intended movement, the load demands required for the performance of that movement, and perception of the risks that may be associated with that activity (van Dieën and de Looze, 1999).

Joint centration and dissociation

Joint centration is the ability to hold a joint in its ideal position, allowing for maximum load uptake with minimum strain. This creates the greatest articular contact between two joint surfaces, accommodating optimal load transfer by neuromuscular control. The length–tension relationship between the functional antagonists of a joint is then directly able to influence the muscle synergy needed to stabilize and transmit loads across the joint surfaces (Kolar et al., 2009).

An awareness of stabilization/control and dissociation will allow full understanding of this process. An individual must have the ability to stabilize or control one segment of an articulation as they dissociate the other segment of that articulation. This causes the dissociation to become the neuromuscular-controlled movement of a particular segment of an articulation. In order to perform optimal movement, coordinated neuromuscular control of joint stabilization and dissociation is required.

Figure 1.8A highlights the length–tension relationship of the hip musculature to maintain joint centration. An example of this in action is provided by the deep fibers of the psoas major and gluteus maximus muscles acting as functional antagonists to help maintain joint centration of the femoral head in the acetabulum and allow optimal hip joint ROM around the axis of rotation (Gibbons, 2007). Inhibition of the functional antagonists results in up-regulation of other muscle synergists, to help achieve joint centration. An example of this in action is when an athlete develops inhibition of the psoas muscle as a result of surgery for femoroacetabular impingement (FAI), or the

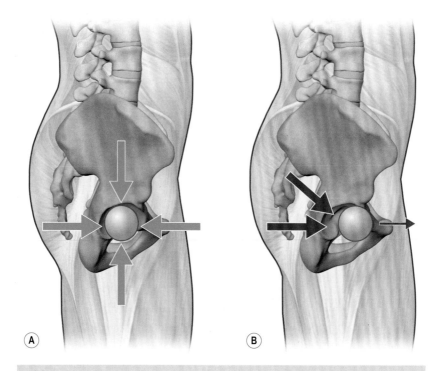

Figure 1.8
Joint centration.

A Length–tension relationship of the hip musculature to maintain joint centration. **B** Loss of joint centration.

inhibition may have developed prior to the initial surgery as a compensatory mechanism. Other hip flexors, like the tensor fasciae latae (TFL), may have become over-recruited or more dominant, and this may require further investigation, using a reliable clinical tool such as the adapted Ober's test (Reese and Bandy, 2003). The distal positioning of the TFL's anatomical attachment relative to the axis of hip joint rotation means it simply cannot provide optimal joint centration and allows the femoral head to translate forward and medially (Figure 1.8B) when the action of hip flexion is performed (Sahrmann, 2002; Lee, 2011).

It is much easier to relate the concept of joint centration to the pelvis and hip complex. I believe this may be due to a combination of the joint architecture and the associated muscles and soft tissue components that connect or cross the pelvis and hip complex. It might be more difficult to apply this concept to individual or smaller joints, such as the costovertebral articulations that help to form the ribcage. Stabilization and dissociation, including the length–tension relationship of the functional antagonists, is more difficult to conceptualize in this particular region of the body.

Clinical evaluation

Clinical evaluation should involve subjective and objective examination processes (Dutton, 2004; Magee, 2014) and may include muscular, articular and neural testing alongside strength and capacity measurements. Clinical evaluation

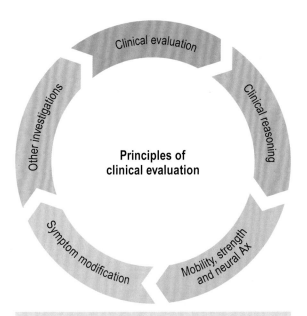

Figure 1.9
Principles of clinical evaluation.
Ax = Assessment.

Table 1.2 Potential red flags in the case history	
Condition	**Symptoms**
Cancer	• Persistent night pain • Fever, night sweats • Unexplained weight loss • Loss of appetite • Fatigue • Lumps or growths
Cardiovascular	• Shortness of breath on physical exertion • Dizziness • Pain or feeling of heaviness in chest • Pulsating pain • Constant, severe pain in calf or arm • Swelling or discoloration in extremities
Gastrointestinal/ Genitourinary	• Frequent or severe abdominal pain • Frequent heartburn or indigestion • Frequent nausea or vomiting • Change in bowel or bladder function • Menstrual irregularities
Neurological	• Frequent or severe headaches • Difficulty swallowing or changes in speech • Visual disturbances • Balance, coordination • Fainting, drop attacks

might also include other diagnostic investigations such as structured questionnaires, radiology or specific blood tests.

According to this definition, clinical evaluation (Figure 1.9) involves performing a biomedical examination that may include ROM, strength, and special tests that are all intended to identify specific pathologies or impairments (Martin et al., 2010).

Clinicians may also request specific diagnostic evaluations from other healthcare practitioners, as signs and symptoms related to potential red flags (Table 1.2) may be highlighted during the subjective history (Adams and Leveson, 2012).

Similarly, yellow flags (Table 1.3) may also be an indication that the signs and symptoms should be viewed with caution or that a particular treatment or exercise technique may be contraindicated. They may also suggest that an underlying psychosocial issue may be present that requires further cognitive testing (Stewart et al., 2011).

Table 1.3 Potential yellow flags in the case history: symptoms that may require investigation

- Bilateral symptoms
- Neurological symptoms related to nerve root or peripheral nerve
- Multiple nerve root involvement
- Abnormal sensation patterns such as dermatome spread and peripheral nerve patterns
- Progressive weakness, gait disturbances
- Multiple inflamed joints
- Psychosocial issues such as pain beliefs, expectations, fear, anxiety, activity avoidance, personality traits, perceptions of work, relationships, contextual issues relating to job requirements, family pressure and injury claims

Structured questionnaires can be useful here; for example, STarT Back is a validated screening tool (see Appendix 1 at the end of this book) to match patients to the particular style of treatment that is most suitable to their specific needs (Hill et al., 2008; 2011). For example, when underlying bio-psychosocial aspects are highlighted, exploring these may the most appropriate treatment approach. The Back Pain Functional Scale (BPFS) is another validated questionnaire (Appendix 2) and is useful for comparing the functional ability outcome of patients (Stratford et al., 2000). The benefit is that it provides information to the clinician about how an individual may or may not be improving with treatment over a specific timeframe. The Copenhagen Hip and Groin Outcome Score (HAGOS) is a third validated questionnaire (Appendix 3), designed to quantitatively measure young to middle-aged, physically active patients with hip and groin disability (Thorborg et al., 2011). It is thus a questionnaire that is extremely suitable for the athletic population.

Reliability, validity and accuracy

Evaluations need to be reliable, valid and accurate. For example, when choosing a particular evaluation or when combining a cluster of evaluations, it is important for the test or tests to be consistent. This not only will depend on the individuals performing the test and what it is they are attempting to evaluate, but also will take into consideration whether the evaluation is accurate for managing outcomes (Cleland and Koppenhaver, 2010; Cipriani and Noftz, 2007). A widely used index for test–retest, intra-tester and inter-tester reliability analysis is the intra-class correlation coefficient (ICC). The ICC reliability value ranges from 0 to 1, values closer to 1 representing higher reliability. When reliability values are shown to be less than 0.5, they are indicative of being poor; between 0.5 and 0.75, moderate; between 0.75 and 0.9, good; greater than 0.9, excellent (Koo and Li, 2016).

Throughout this book, I will refer to the reliability and validity values for each clinical evaluation where appropriate. Awareness of the usefulness of every test is always important and clinicians should understand that one test in isolation should never be interpreted as the single greatest deciding factor for making a diagnosis. Furthermore, when the literature for one test performed by different authors is analyzed, wide variability is often shown in the outcomes (Cleland and Koppenhaver, 2011; Fritz and Wainner, 2001). There may be many reasons for this: for example, reliability may be affected by the cooperation of the patient, their ability to relax and to tolerate pain, the skill and experience of the clinician performing the test, or the calibration of any equipment that may have been used to perform the test (Cipriani and Noftz, 2007).

Sensitivity and specificity

Another useful way to determine whether an evaluation is beneficial for diagnostic purposes relates to how sensitive and how specific it may be. Evidence-based studies relating to the sensitivity and specificity of clinical tests have been shown to vary significantly. Sensitivity relates to the ability of a test to detect correctly whether a patient may have a particular problem. Specificity, on the other hand, relates to the ability of a test to detect if a patient may *not* have a particular problem (Sackett et al., 2000). A highly sensitive test is extremely useful for identifying patients who are likely to have the condition being tested for, and a highly specific test for identifying those who are likely *not* to have the condition being tested for.

Examples in clinical practice might include a situation where I might be uncertain whether a patient is presenting with a particular condition. I could use an evaluation with a high level of sensitivity to try to detect if they have the injury. For example, the quadrant test is a highly sensitive tool that assesses lumbar extension and rotation (Laslett et al., 2006). If this test reproduces low back pain symptoms, I can be highly confident that the athlete may have lumbar facet joint pain. Compare this with a situation when I use a highly specific test, such as the straight leg raise (SLR), to measure whether a patient might not have a particular condition (Majlesi et al., 2008). In this instance, if the test fails to reproduce neural symptoms, then I can be highly confident that the athlete may not have sciatica. No test is capable of being 100 percent sensitive or 100 percent specific. Generally, the rule for a good test value is 80 percent but this leaves 20 percent of patients incorrectly identified, leading to an interpretation of the results as false positives or false negatives. In addition, some tests may be shown to be more sensitive or specific than others. This does not necessarily mean they should be rejected, but it is important to understand that a single evaluative test should never be used in isolation under any circumstances (Magee, 2014). Instead, using a cluster of three or more positive pain provocation evaluations results in much greater sensitivity and specificity values (Laslett et al., 2005).

Conclusion

To summarize, the purpose of this chapter was to provide an overview of the framework for effective management of the complex presentations that relate to the spine, pelvis, hip and groin. Integrating the "five 'ATEs" approach within this framework offers flexibility for clinicians to combine their clinical reasoning skills with bio-psychological, functional and clinical evaluations. Furthermore, this will ensure there is sufficient evidence and understanding for both clinicians and patients to make informed decisions regarding the management of musculoskeletal issues.

References

Adams, S. and Leveson, S., 2012. Clinical prediction rules. *British Medical Journal*, 344, pp. 8312–8322.

Askling, CM., Tengvar, M., Saartok, T. et al., 2007. Acute first-time hamstring strains during high-speed running: a longitudinal study including clinical and magnetic resonance imaging findings. *American Journal Sports Medicine*, 35, pp. 197–206.

Bassel-Duby, R. and Olson, E., 2006. Signaling pathways in skeletal muscle remodeling. *Annual Review Biochemistry*, 75(1), pp. 19–37.

Brinjikji, W., Luetmer, P., Comstock, B. et al., 2015. Systematic literature review of imaging features of spinal degeneration in asymptomatic populations. *American Journal Neuro-radiology*, 36, pp. 818–816.

Buchthal, F. and Schmalbruch, H., 1970. Contraction times and fiber types in intact human muscle. *Acta Physiologica Scandinavica*, 79(4), pp. 435–452.

Cipriani, DJ. and Noftz, JB. 2007. The utility of orthopedic clinical tests for diagnosis. In: *Scientific Foundations and Principles of Practice in Musculoskeletal Rehabilitation*. Saunders/Elsevier, pp. 557–565.

Cleland, J., Koppenhaver, S., Su, J. et al., 2010. *Netter's Orthopaedic Clinical Examination*. 2nd ed. Philadelphia: Saunders/Elsevier.

Comerford, M., and Mottram, S., 2012. The management of uncontrolled movement. In: *Kinetic Control*. Melbourne: Churchill Livingstone.

Comin, J., Malliaras, P., Naquie, P. et al., 2013. Return to competitive play after hamstring injuries involving disruption of the central tendon. *American Journal Sports Medicine*, 41, pp. 111–115.

Connell, DA., Schneider-Kolsky, ME., Hoving, JL. et al., 2004. Longitudinal study comparing sonographic and MRI assessments of acute and healing hamstring injuries. *AJR American Journal Roentgenology*, 183, pp. 975–984.

Cook, G., Burton, L. and Hoogenboom, B., 2006. Pre-participation screening: the use of fundamental movements as an assessment of function – part 1. *North American Journal Sports Physical Therapy*, 1(2), pp. 62–72.

Crema, MD., Yamada, AF., Guermazi, A. et al., 2015. Imaging techniques for muscle injury in sports medicine and clinical relevance. *Current Reviews in Musculoskeletal Medicine*, 8(2), pp. 154–161.

Diedrichsen, J., Shadmehr, R. and Ivry, R., 2010. The coordination of movement: optimal feedback control and beyond. *Trends in Cognitive Sciences*, 14(1), pp. 31–39.

Dingenen, B., Blandford, L., Comerford, M. et al., 2018. The assessment of movement health in clinical practice: a multidimensional perspective. *Physical Therapy in Sport*, 32, pp. 282–292.

Duchateau, J. and Enoka, R., 2011. Human motor unit recordings: origins and insight into the integrated motor system. *Brain Research*, 1409, pp. 42–61.

Dutton, M., 2004. *Orthopaedic Examination, Evaluation and Intervention*. 2nd ed. New York: McGraw-Hill.

Ekstrand, J., Healy, JC., Walden, M. et al., 2012. Hamstring muscle injuries in professional football: the correlation of MRI findings with return to play. *British Journal Sports Medicine*, 46, pp. 112–117.

Enoka, R., Christou, E., Hunter, S. et al., 2003. Mechanisms that contribute to differences in motor performance between young and old adults. *Journal Electromyography and Kinesiology*, 13(1), pp. 1–12.

Feltovich, PJ. and Barrows, HS., 1984. Issues of generality in medical based problem solving. In: H. Schmidt and ML. De Volder, eds. *Tutorials in Problem-based Learning: A*

New Direction in Teaching the Health Professions. Assen, Netherlands: Van Gorcum, pp. 128–142.

Fritz, J. and Wainner, R., 2001. Examining diagnostic tests: an evidence-based perspective. *Physical Therapy*, 81(9), pp. 1546–1564.

Gibbons, S., 2007. Assessment and rehabilitation of the stability function of psoas major. *Manuelletherapie*, 11, pp. 177–187.

Gobet, F. and Wood, D., 1999. Expertise, models of learning and computer-based tutoring. *Computers & Education*, 33(2–3), pp. 189–207.

Groves, M., O'Rourke, P. and Alexander, H., 2003. The clinical reasoning characteristics of diagnostic experts. *Medical Teacher*, 25(3), pp. 308–313.

Guyton, A., 1991. *Textbook of Medical Physiology*. 8th ed. Philadelphia: W. B. Saunders.

Higgs, J., Richardson, B. and Dahlgren, M., 2004. *Developing Practice Knowledge for Health Professionals*. Edinburgh: Butterworth-Heinemann.

Hill, JC., Dunn, KM., Lewis, M. et al., 2008. A primary care back pain screening tool: identifying patient subgroups for initial treatment. *Arthritis Care and Research*, 59, pp. 632–641.

Hill, JC., Whitehurst, DG., Lewis, M. et al., 2011. Comparison of stratified management for low back pain with current best practice (STarT Back): a randomised controlled trial. *Lancet*, 378, pp. 1560–1571.

Hodges, P. and Moseley, G., 2003. Pain and motor control of the lumbopelvic region: effect and possible mechanisms. *Journal Electromyography Kinesiology*, 13(4), pp. 361–370.

Hodges, P., Gurfinkel, V., Brumagne, S. et al., 2002. Coexistence of stability and mobility in postural control: evidence from postural compensation for respiration. *Experimental Brain Research*, 144(3), pp. 293–302.

Hodges, P., Moseley, G., Gabrielsson, A. et al., 2003. Experimental muscle pain changes feedforward postural responses of the trunk muscles. *Experimental Brain Research*, 151(2), pp. 262–271.

Hoffman, J. and Gabel, P., 2013. Expanding Panjabi's stability model to express movement: a theoretical model. *Medical Hypotheses*, 80(6), pp. 692–697.

Hunter, S., Pereira, H. and Keenan, K., 2016. The aging neuromuscular system and motor performance. *Journal Applied Physiology*, 121(4), pp. 982–995.

Johansson, H., Sjölander, P. and Sojka, P., 1991. Receptors in the knee joint ligaments and their role in the biomechanics of the joint. *Critical Reviews in Biomedical Engineering*, 18(5), pp. 341–368.

Johnson, M., Polgar, J., Weightman, D. et al., 1973. Data on the distribution of fiber types in thirty-six human muscles. *Journal Neurological Sciences*, 18(1), pp. 111–129.

Jones, M., 1992. Clinical reasoning in manual therapy. *Physical Therapy*, 72(12), pp. 875–884.

Jones, MA., and Edwards, I., 2006. Learning to facilitate change in cognition and behaviour. In: Gifford, L. (ed.), *Topical Issues in Pain*. 5th ed. Falmouth: CNS Press.

Kivlan, BR. and Martin, RL., 2012. Functional performance testing of the hip in athletes: a systematic review for reliability and validity. *International Journal Sports Physical Therapy*, 7(4), pp. 402–412.

Kolar, P., Neuwirth, J., Sanda, J. et al., 2009. Analysis of diaphragm movement during tidal breathing and during its activation while breath holding using MRI synchronized with spirometry. *Physiology Research*, 58(3), pp. 383–392.

Koo, T. and Li, M., 2016. A guideline of selecting and reporting intraclass correlation coefficients for reliability research. *Journal Chiropractic Medicine*, 15(2), pp. 155–163.

Laslett, M., Aprill, C., McDonald, B. et al., 2005. Diagnosis of sacroiliac joint pain: validity of individual provocation tests and composites of tests. *Manual Therapy*, 10(3), pp. 207–218.

Laslett, M., McDonald, B., April, C., et al., 2006. Clinical predictors of screening zygapophyseal joint blocks: development of clinical prediction rules. *Spine Journal*, 6, pp. 370–379.

Lee, D. 2011. *The Pelvic Girdle: An Integration of Clinical Expertise and Research*. 4th ed. Edinburgh: Churchill Livingstone/ Elsevier.

Levett-Jones, T., Hoffman, K., Dempsey, J. et al., 2010. The 'five rights' of clinical reasoning: an educational model to enhance nursing students' ability to identify and manage clinically 'at risk' patients. *Nurse Education Today*, 30(6), pp. 515–520.

Lewis, J., 2009. Rotator cuff tendinopathy/subacromial impingement syndrome: is it time for a new method of assessment? *British Journal Sports Medicine*, 43(4), pp. 259–264.

Lieber, R., 2009. *Skeletal Muscle Structure, Function, and Plasticity*. Baltimore: Lippincott Williams & Wilkins.

Magee, D., 2014. *Orthopedic Physical Assessment*. 6th ed. St Louis: Saunders/Elsevier.

Maher, C., Underwood, M., Buchbinder, R., 2017. Non-specific low back pain. *Lancet*, 389, pp. 736–747.

Majlesi, J., Togay, H., Unalan, H. et al., 2008. The sensitivity and specificity of the slump and straight leg raise tests in patients with lumbar disc herniation. *Journal Clinical Rheumatology*, 14(2), pp. 87–91.

Martin, H., Kelly, B., Leunig, M. et al., 2010. The pattern and technique in the clinical evaluation of the adult hip: the common physical examination tests of hip specialists. *Arthroscopy: Journal Arthroscopic Related Surgery*, 26(2), pp. 161–172.

McCarthy, C. 2010. *Combined Movement Theory: Rational Mobilization and Manipulation of the Vertebral Column.* Edinburgh: Churchill Livingstone/Elsevier.

McGill, S., 2007. *Low Back Disorders.* 2nd ed. Leeds: Human Kinetics.

Mills, J., Taunton, J. and Mills, W., 2005. The effect of a 10-week training regimen on lumbo-pelvic stability and athletic performance in female athletes: a randomized-controlled trial. *Physical Therapy in Sport*, 6(2), pp. 60–66.

Myers, T., 2009. *Anatomy Trains.* 2nd ed. Edinburgh: Churchill Livingstone/Elsevier.

Okada, T., Huxel, K. and Nesser, T., 2011. Relationship between core stability, functional movement, and performance. *Journal Strength Conditioning Research*, 25(1), pp. 252–261.

O'Sullivan, P., 2000. Masterclass. Lumbar segmental 'instability': clinical presentation and specific stabilizing exercise management. *Manual Therapy*, 5(1), pp. 2–12.

O'Sullivan, P., Caneiro, JP., O'Keefe, M. et al., 2018. Cognitive functional therapy: an integrated behavioral approach with articular exercises for the targeted management of disabling low back pain. *Physical Therapy*, 98, pp. 408–423.

Panjabi, M., 1992. The stabilizing system of the spine. Part I. Function, dysfunction, adaptation, and enhancement. *Journal Spinal Disorders*, 5(4), pp. 383–389.

Reese, N. and Bandy, W., 2003. Use of an inclinometer to measure flexibility of the iliotibial band using the Ober test and the modified Ober test: differences in magnitude and reliability of measurements. *Journal Orthopaedic Sports Physical Therapy*, 33(6), pp. 326–330.

Jones, M. and Rivett, D., 2004. *Clinical Reasoning for Manual Therapists.* Edinburgh: Butterworth Heinemann.

Robertson, B., Barker, P., Fahrer, M. et al., 2009. The anatomy of the pubic region revisited. *Sports Medicine*, 39(3), pp. 225–234.

Roussouly, P. and Nnadi, C., 2010. Sagittal plane deformity: an overview of interpretation and management. *European Spine Journal*, 19(11), pp. 1824–1836.

Roussouly, P. and Pinheiro-Franco, J., 2011. Biomechanical analysis of the spino-pelvic organization and adaptation in pathology. *European Spine Journal*, 20(S5), pp. 609–618.

Sackett, D., Richardson, W. and Straws, S., 2000. *Evidence-Based Medicine: How to Practice and Teach.* 2nd ed. London: Harcourt.

Sahrmann, S., 2002. *Diagnosis and Treatment of Movement Impairment Syndromes.* Philadelphia: Mosby, p. 63.

Saracoglu, I., Arik, MI., Afsar, E. et al., 2020. The effectiveness of pain neuroscience education combined with manual therapy and home exercise for chronic low back pain: a single-blind randomized controlled trial. *Physiotherapy Theory and Practice.* DOI: 10.108/09593985.2020.1809046.

Schiaffino, S. and Reggiani, C., 2011. Fiber types in mammalian skeletal muscles. *Physiological Reviews*, 91(4), pp. 1447–1531.

Snijders, C., Vleeming, A. and Stoeckart, R., 1993. Transfer of lumbosacral load to iliac bones and legs. *Clinical Biomechanics*, 8(6), pp. 285–294.

Stecco, A., Macchi, V., Stecco, C. et al., 2009. Anatomical study of myofascial continuity in the anterior region of the upper limb. *Journal Bodywork Movement Therapies*, 13(1), pp. 53–62.

Stewart, J., Kempenaar, L. and Lauchlan, D., 2011. Rethinking yellow flags. *Manual Therapy*, 16(2), pp. 196–198.

Stratford, PW., Binkley, JM. and Riddle, DL., 2000. Development and initial validation of the Back Pain Function Scale. *Spine*, 25, pp. 2095–2102.

Talbot, J. and Maves, L., 2016. Skeletal muscle fiber type: using insights from muscle developmental biology to dissect targets for susceptibility and resistance to muscle disease. *Wiley Interdisciplinary Reviews: Developmental Biology*, 5(4), pp. 518–534.

Tanner, C., 2006. Thinking like a nurse: a research-based model of clinical judgement in nursing. *Journal Nursing Education*, 45(6), pp. 204–211.

Thorborg, K., Hölmich, P., Christensen, R. et al., 2011. The Copenhagen Hip and Groin Outcome Score (HAGOS): development and validation according to the COSMIN checklist. *British Journal Sports Medicine*, 45(6), pp. 478–491.

Todd, C., Kovac, P., Swärd, A. et al., 2015. Comparison of radiological spino-pelvic sagittal parameters in skiers and non-athletes. *Journal Orthopaedic Surgery and Research*, 10(1), p. 162.

Todd, C., Swärd, A. and Agnvall, C., 2016. Clinical spino-pelvic parameters in skiers and non-athletes. *Journal Sports Medicine*, 3(3), p. 22.

Umphred, H. 2007. *Neurological Rehabilitation.* 5th ed. St Louis: Mosby/Elsevier.

Van der Wal, J., 2009. The architecture of the connective tissue in the musculoskeletal system – an often-overlooked functional parameter as to proprioception in the locomotor apparatus. *International Journal Therapeutic Massage & Bodywork*, 2(4), pp. 9–23.

van Dieën, J. and de Looze, M., 1999. Directionality of anticipatory activation of trunk muscles in a lifting task depends on load knowledge. *Experimental Brain Research*, 128(3), pp. 397–404.

Vleeming, A., Stoeckart, R., Volkers, A. et al., 1990a. Relation between form and function in the sacroiliac joint. *Spine*, 15(2), pp. 130–132.

Vleeming, A., Volkers, A., Snijders, C. et al., 1990b. Relation between form and function in the sacroiliac joint. *Spine*, 15(2), pp. 133–136.

Chapter 2 structure

Introduction	23
Functional evaluation of the spine	25
Functional evaluation of the pelvis and hip	27
Positional alignment	31
Clinical evaluation	33
Clinical reasoning	43
Conclusion	48

Introduction

I will use many case studies in this book, which will help to provide a foundation for reflective thinking and demonstrate the value of a structural framework in clinical practice. In this chapter, we will follow one particular case study from presentation to completion, when a resolution is reached. This case is an example that will explain the fundamentals of the "five 'ATEs" framework and how to integrate the principles of functional and clinical evaluation into a system-based approach.

Case study: Patient A

So, let's begin to apply the "five 'ATEs" within the context of a clinical case. Patient A is 24-year-old male professional goalkeeper (soccer), presenting with right-sided low back pain (LBP) that referred into his right lower abdominal and anterior hip region. He reported that an acute increase in symptoms became progressively worse after a training session that morning. When he was getting off the coach at the team hotel, he twisted on his right leg while weight-bearing and he found this to be excruciatingly painful. The team physician had examined him and decided that he would wait 24 hours before deciding whether to investigate further with a magnetic resonance imaging (MRI) scan. In the meantime, I was asked if I could help.

EvaluATE: initial hypotheses

As a goalkeeper, Patient A needs to perform specific tasks, such as taking long kicks. He requires greater mobility through his right side to execute the many phases related to kicking a ball. For example, in the backswing phase, the spine and kicking leg are maximally rotated and

extended. This creates a tension arc that pre-stretches the adductor and abdominal lines, stores potential energy and assists with the explosive contraction of the hip flexor muscles to perform the activity of kicking (Brophey et al., 2007). At the same time, his standing left leg requires greater stability to allow for the high-speed movements performed by the kicking leg. By understanding the clinical picture and mechanism of injury and gaining a knowledge of Patient A's regular regimen, which includes field and gym-based training, I can form an initial hypothesis. The specific movement demands involved in taking long kicks might have led to reactive overload and fatigue within Patient A's soft tissues, resulting in compensatory, non-functional alignment. However, before I can make this assumption, I have to consider all my initial hypotheses. These include:

- An articular issue affecting the hip joint: perhaps the combined mechanism of flexion, adduction and internal rotation involved in kicking may have compressed or impinged the hip joint (Reiman et al., 2015). For example, it could be femoroacetabular impingement syndrome, which is commonly seen in rotational sports (Harris-Hayes et al., 2009). I will discuss the pathomechanism of this condition in Chapter 4.

- A muscular injury: perhaps intrinsic in nature and insidious, and more likely stemming from overload rather than a specific incident. It could, for example, be related to the oblique muscles, the deep hip flexors and the adductor muscles. Soft tissue injuries may occur in isolation or may involve multiple entities (Morelli and Smith, 2001). Alternatively, an acute incident, such as twisting on his weight-bearing leg when he stepped off the coach, may have involved an intrinsic hip joint stabilizer such as the obturator muscles.

- A spinal restriction: perhaps lack of dynamic mobility in the spinal column affecting the soft tissue structures that cross the anterior pelvis and hip joint. Increased soft tissue strain can arise from the development of spinal asymmetry, which may have stemmed from Patient A repeatedly kicking with his right foot. Furthermore, perhaps the symptoms are a result of nerve root irritation causing radicular pain or radiculopathy (Furman and Johnson, 2019). Alternatively, neural tissues may have become trapped between the many interfaces that cross the anterior pelvis and hip and have become inflamed (Macintyre et al., 2006).

- Impaired respiratory function: loss of respiratory function or altered respiratory mechanics (Lewit, 1999), affecting diaphragm function and the length–tension relationship of the abdominals, particularly the oblique muscles. The length–tension relationship of these muscles has an effect on spino-pelvic alignment and optimal function of the spino-pelvic canister. Therefore, dysfunction in these muscles can give rise to global muscle over-recruitment, and subsequent compensatory mechanisms throughout the body.

Using the system-based integrated framework, I am now currently at the *evaluATE* stage. Having considered my initial hypotheses, I now need to think about them in the context of a functional evaluation. Generally, I begin with evaluation of standing functional alignment, paying attention to palpation of the bony alignment and resting tone of the soft tissues in this position, before progressing to evaluate functional movement. In my opinion, both hands should be used for palpation. The entire hand, rather than just the fingers or thumbs, should remain relaxed and mold itself around the bony landmarks and soft tissues, in order to gain as much information as possible. Later in this chapter, I will introduce evaluation of positional alignment while the patient is lying on the couch, which is performed similarly to

when the patient is standing. This has clinical relevance because of the possibility of highlighting a correlation between the findings of both functional and positional evaluations. For example, if I were to observe that a patient in standing was demonstrating an anterior pelvic tilt on one side relative to the other, I would also expect to see a difference in the height of the pelvic crests, anterior superior iliac spines (ASISs) and pubic tubercles when evaluating the positional alignment. Observation during this process supplies information relating to the bony alignment and soft tissue tone, and in addition will provide an impression of the joint mobility that may be readily available.

High-performance sport, or any exercises that require repetitive axial and or rotational movements, will place higher loads on the spine, pelvis, hip and groin. This leads to changes in the length–tension relationships of the musculoskeletal system and in turn can result in an altered functional alignment and posture (such as that discernible in sitting and lying). Athletes have been shown to have a different spino-pelvic alignment in standing, compared to non-athletes (Todd et al., 2015; 2016). For example, there is an increase in anterior pelvic tilt, an increase in anterior thigh and erector spinae muscle tone, and a greater angle of lumbar lordosis. There is no such thing as perfect alignment or posture, or, indeed, an ideal way to move. The human body has an incredible ability to adapt and cope, to overcome postural challenges and muscle dysfunction as it attempts to develop new movement strategies.

All individuals are able to optimize their performance of tasks and activities by using a variety of strategies. With this in mind, compare the standing posture in Figure 2.1. Note how the spino-pelvic complex has rotated into anterior pelvic tilt over the right hip joint and observe how the body alignment has attempted to correct itself further up the kinetic chain, through contralateral thoracolumbar rotation, to bring the eyes level, ensuring that a forward gaze is maintained.

In this particular example, the right leg is held in relative internal rotation compared with the left leg and this produces a shortening effect, with over-activity in the rectus femoris, tensor fasciae latae (TFL) and adductor muscles, alongside relative lengthening and inhibition of gluteus medius and gluteus minimus. This means that this individual, while capable of demonstrating an ability to compensate around the right hip, has clearly started to develop reduced form and force closure (see Chapter 1), specifically around the spine, pelvis and hip complex.

Case study: more on Patient A

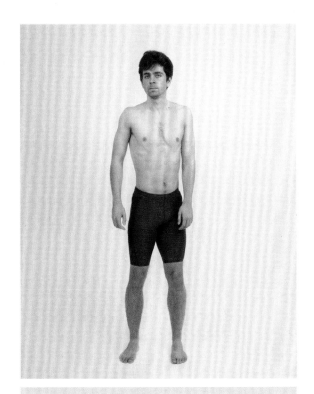

Figure 2.1
Standing compensatory non-functional alignment.

 Patient A, similar to the person in Figure 2.1, demonstrated a compensatory non-functional alignment in standing, with his spine and pelvic complex rotating around his right hip joint. On palpation, it was evident that the right hip was exhibiting increased muscular tone in the TFL, anterior thigh and adductors. Right-sided anterior pelvic tilt was noted, with subsequent increased thoracolumbar paraspinal activity. Respiratory mechanics appeared to be compromised, with the right lower ribs demonstrating reduced rib expansion on inhalation. In cases like this I would expect to observe, on movement testing, a loss of relative hip joint internal rotation and flexion. Similarly, the spinal column would demonstrate a loss of thoracolumbar rotation to the right.

This presentation results in a non-optimal compensatory alignment. Patient A might, as a consequence, demonstrate reduced form and force closure around the pelvic girdle, specifically in functional activities such as the single-leg (SL) stance test, which will be evaluated shortly. Positional alignment palpation might highlight asymmetries in muscle tone and bony landmarks, and provide some level of appreciation of the quality and resting tone of the soft tissues that cross this region. Let's explore these thoughts further.

Functional evaluation of the spine

 Evaluating the spinal column as a functional unit provides an opportunity for the clinician to observe the interdependence and integration of the three spinal curvatures: lumbar, thoracic and cervical. These curvatures are often described independently in anatomical studies but common sense indicates that they are functionally dependent on each other. Given the interdependence of the spinal regions, functional evaluation of the spine should include a combination of movement tests to determine if an individual has the ability to maintain optimal alignment, such as remaining stable in the neutral zone (Panjabi, 1992), and to demonstrate the coordinated movement and mobility requirements necessary to perform a dynamic task (Lee, 2011). The spinal column moves through ranges of flexion, extension, lateral flexion and rotation, and although I will attempt to describe each region separately, describing specific functional evaluation of the spine is challenging, as both static and dynamic movement would clearly include the pelvic girdle and hip joint.

Spinal functional evaluation in the sagittal plane, which involves flexion and extension, is highlighted in Figures 2.2 and 2.3. Special attention should be directed to the movement and timing of flexion that occurs in the thoracic and lumbar regions. There should be no rotation or lateral flexion within these parts of the spine during sagittal movement. The muscles should work synergistically, to allow for controlled and balanced movement to take place within the kinetic chain, demonstrating no restriction or loss of segmental or multi-segmental motion in the lumbar spine. During flexion of the spine (Figure 2.2), the femoral heads should remain centered in the acetabulum and the innominates should

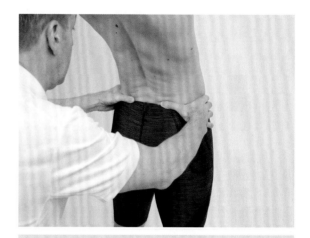

Figure 2.3
Optimal spinal extension.

move equally, as anterior tilt of the pelvic girdle occurs over the femoral heads. With extension of the spine too (Figure 2.3), the femoral heads should remain centered in the acetabulum and the innominates should move equally as the pelvis tilts posteriorly over the femoral heads.

Spinal functional evaluation in the frontal plane, involving lateral flexion or side bending of the spinal column to the right, is shown in Figure 2.4. At the end of range, a spinal curve should be formed with each segment contributing equally to the range of motion. The muscles should work synergistically to allow for controlled and balanced movement to occur within the kinetic chain, demonstrating no restriction or loss of segmental or multi-segmental motion or translation in the lumbar spine. Palpation of both the posterior superior iliac spines (PSISs) on spinal lateral flexion to the right will highlight a left posterior innominate rotation relative to the right, which should also be similar for the sacrum. Equally, specific attention should be paid to the lateral tilt that occurs within the pelvic girdle, resulting in abduction of the right femur and adduction of the left femur.

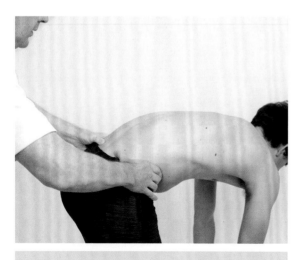

Figure 2.2
Optimal spinal flexion.

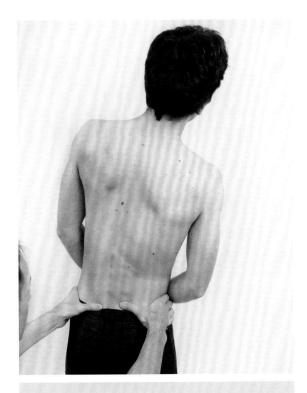

Figure 2.4
Optimal spinal lateral flexion.

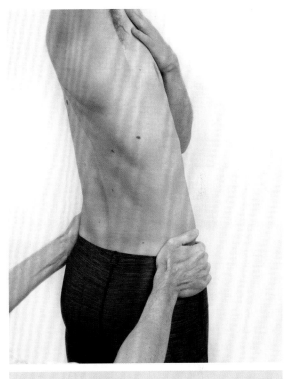

Figure 2.5
Optimal spinal rotation.

Spinal functional evaluation in the transverse plane, which involves rotation to the right, is highlighted in Figure 2.5. As shown, stabilizing the pelvis helps ensure that the range of spinal rotation occurs independently of hip or pelvic motion. Close attention should be paid to the movement and timing of the rotation that occurs in the thoracic and lumbar spine. The muscles should work synergistically, to allow for controlled and balanced movement to take place within the kinetic chain, demonstrating no restriction or loss of segmental or multi-segmental motion or translation in the lumbar spine. Spinal rotation to the right should highlight a posterior rotation of the right innominate, relative to the left.

Functional evaluation of the pelvis and hip

The pelvis is considered to be one of the central segments that assists with the proximal to distal sequencing of high-speed body movements (Shan and Westerhoff, 2005). The pelvic girdle consists of the two sacroiliac joints (SIJs), which are designed to provide stability through form and force closure and to counterbalance the load of the upper and lower extremities, and the pubic symphysis (Vleeming et al., 1990ab). The range of movement (ROM) in the SIJs is estimated to be approximately 0.4–4.3° of rotation and 0.7 mm translation (Jacob and Kissling, 1995). The pubic symphysis is a secondary cartilaginous joint located between the two pubic bones. Similarly to the SIJ, a small ROM occurs in the pubic symphysis. It is estimated that 2 mm of vertical motion and 3° in the coronal axis are available (Walheim and Selvik, 1984).

A small ROM can occur in the pelvic girdle in three planes of motion: anterior and posterior pelvic tilt in the sagittal plane, lateral tilt in the coronal plane, and rotation in the transverse plane (Greenman, 1996; Vleeming et al., 1990ab; Vleeming et al., 2007). Viewed as a mobile platform, the pelvic girdle facilitates the balance of lumbar lordosis and hip joint extension, to maintain human standing upright posture. Any impairment of pelvic movement may reduce an athlete's performance and induce a higher risk of recurrence and chronicity of groin injury (Walden et al., 2015). As a consequence, the pelvic girdle becomes a mechanism through which the spinal column communicates with the lower extremity. Restoration of active pelvic tilt should always be considered for the management of injured athletes, as this will allow for efficient mechanical energy transfer during sports actions (Naito et al., 2012). Therefore, the pelvic girdle becomes an integral component of the human body by providing form and force closure for alignment (stability) with both the static and dynamic requirements of functional movement (Naito et al., 2012; Vleeming et al., 1990ab).

Functional evaluation of the hip joint involves assessing its capacity to provide dynamic movement and alignment through stability. The architecture of this joint allows for the round femoral head to articulate with the concave acetabulum of the pelvis. Tri-planar motion is available through this joint:

- In the sagittal plane: flexion 100° and extension 20°
- In the frontal plane: abduction 45° and adduction 30°
- In the transverse plane: internal rotation 30–40° and external rotation 60°.

These are similar movements to those of the glenohumeral joint but there is a greater demand for stability,

due to the larger loads imposed on the hip joint; shearing in any direction is prevented but motion is allowed. When a person is standing erect with optimal alignment, the body weight is distributed evenly through the pelvic girdle to the femoral head and neck, with each hip joint supporting approximately 33 percent of body weight.

The squat is a functional movement test (Figure 2.6), and squatting is essential for performing the task of standing from sitting, or vice versa. Patients with intra-articular hip pain have been shown to demonstrate reduced squat depth, compared to those without pain who were able to demonstrate an increased squat depth (Lamontagne et al., 2009). To perform this

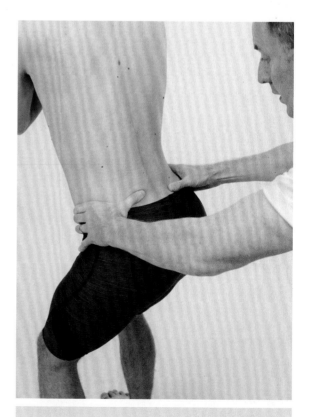

Figure 2.6
Functional squat.

evaluation, I begin by observing the patient anteriorly. Each knee should remain aligned over each foot, reducing the occurrence of any rotational knee joint valgus or varus components. Careful attention should be paid to the degree of flexion that occurs in the knees and hips as the ankles perform the motion of dorsiflexion. Standing posteriorly and palpating the pelvic girdle, I ask the patient to repeat the squat, noting how the pelvis performs an anterior active tilt on the femoral heads and observing whether the thoracic girdle remains aligned over the pelvic girdle, with a small degree of forward movement observed as the hips and pelvis move posteriorly. Patients with intra-articular hip joint pathology will demonstrate altered spino-pelvic motion when evaluated with this test (Lamontagne et al., 2009). Throughout the squat, the muscles should work synergistically, to allow for controlled and balanced movement to occur within the kinetic chain, demonstrating no restriction or loss of segmental or multi-segmental motion or translation in the lumbar spine.

Single-leg stance test

Spinal stabilization, while demonstrating hip joint dissociation with the single-leg (SL) stance test, is illustrated in Figure 2.7. This test evaluates the ability to maintain form and force closure by stabilizing and transferring load through one leg, while demonstrating mobility through dissociation with the other leg. The test is performed similarly to the stork/Gillet test for the SIJ, but puts more emphasis on observing whether the spinal column and pelvis remain in alignment (neutral zone) when the patient is asked to lift one leg off the floor and hold the position for 30 seconds. Specific attention must be paid to observing whether the spine deviates or shifts away from the aligned vertical position, whether the pelvic crests deviate or shift away from the horizontal plane,

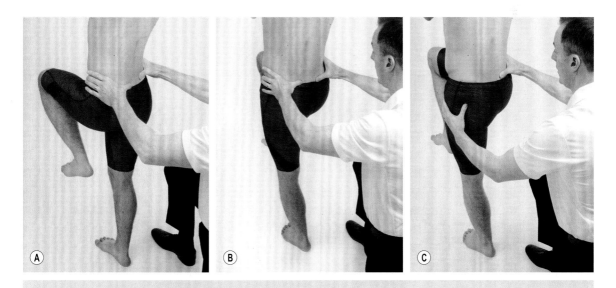

Figure 2.7
Single-leg stance test.

A With the pelvis positioned over the weight-bearing leg. **B** For movement of the innominate on the non-weight-bearing leg. **C** For femoral centration on the weight-bearing leg.

and whether compensatory movements are made with the contralateral leg or arms. This evaluation has been shown to have very good inter- and intra-rater reliability: 1.0 and 0.88, respectively (Tidstrand and Horneji, 2009).

The diagnostic accuracy of this test in detecting pain that could be related to lateral gluteal tendinopathy, sacroiliac pain and/or LBP, or hip joint intra-articular pain, during a 30-second hold in SL stance, is high, with a sensitivity of 100 percent and specificity of 97 percent (Lequesne et al., 2008). Examination is undertaken through palpation of the PSIS and pelvic girdle (Figure 2.7A), and observation.

1. There should be no pelvic anterior, posterior or lateral tilt, or rotation motion, when the pelvis is positioned over the weight-bearing leg. Hip abduction function is normal and should maintain the pelvis almost perpendicular to the femur in the SL stance position (Youdas et al., 2007).

2. Movement of the innominate relative to the sacrum on the non-weight-bearing leg should highlight only a small degree of posterior pelvic rotation when the hip is actively flexed (Figure 2.7B), and this should be similar on the contralateral side. The innominate should remain posteriorly rotated, relative to the sacrum, when an SL stance test is performed. This evaluation has been shown to have moderate (left 0.59, right 0.59) to good (left 0.67, right 0.77) levels of inter-tester reliability, depending on which measuring scales are used (Hungerford et al., 2007).

3. The femoral head should remain centered in the acetabulum (Figure 2.7C) when load is transferred through the hip, as in the SL stance, and when the hip is in non-weight-bearing, performing active hip flexion.

Case study: more on Patient A

 Functional evaluation of Patient A highlighted reduced ROM with spinal rotation to the right. Segmental and myofascial restrictions were noted in the lower thoracic and thoracolumbar regions. Spinal flexion (see Figure 2.2) was pain-free and shown to be within normal parameters for this athlete. Similarly, spinal extension (see Figure 2.3) was shown to be pain-free. However, when performing a quadrant test by combining active spinal extension and rotation (right and left), Patient A demonstrated reduced ROM to the right, although he was pain-free bilaterally (Figure 2.8). The quadrant test is used to evaluate the possibility of facet joint pain; it has a high sensitivity (100 percent) but low specificity (22 percent). As a result, because Patient A reported no pain when performing this test, I could rule out lower lumbar

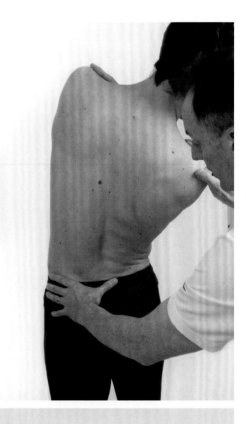

Figure 2.8
Standing extension quadrant test.

facet joint pain as a potential hypothesis (Stuber et al., 2014; Laslett et al., 2006). With the right leg in weight-bearing (see Figure 2.7A), an anterior translation of the innominate occurred, relative to the sacrum, when the contralateral hip was flexed, highlighting a loss of stability through the pelvic girdle (Hungerford et al., 2007). However, no pain was reported after 30 seconds in this position, which effectively rules out lateral gluteal tendinopathy, SIJ pain and LBP (Lequesne et al., 2008). In non-weight-bearing (see Figure 2.7B), anterior translation of the innominate was noted, relative to the sacrum, and pain was reported when the right hip was actively flexed.

At this point, I have ascertained that Patient A is unlikely to have lower lumbar facet joint pain but he is clearly demonstrating an inability to perform optimal spinal rotation. He has pain and awareness on active hip flexion and is failing to transfer optimal load effectively through the pelvic girdle in SL stance. Therefore, the evaluation outcome suggests that it is unlikely that his symptoms are related to SIJ pain, LBP or lateral hip tendinopathy.

It is clear that functional evaluation has its limitations when providing the information that the clinician requires to begin resolving a clinical puzzle. Functional evaluation is much more holistic in nature, requiring an understanding of regional interdependence and the possibility that distal unrelated impairments may contribute to a patient's primary complaint (Wainner et al., 2007). There are problems in relying solely on this model: for example, being worried about the lack of a pathoanatomical diagnosis as to what exactly the pain-provoking structure may be. It is important for clinicians not to become obsessed with or dependent on pathoanatomical diagnoses. In a significant percentage of patients, LBP is diagnosed as non-specific, there being no known pathoanatomical cause for the symptoms, as will be discussed in later chapters.

Positional alignment

After performing functional evaluation and prior to performing a clinical evaluation, the clinician can employ positional alignment palpation to observe whether bony alignment and soft tissue tension (or tone) correlate with the functional and clinical findings. It can be argued that this particular type of evaluation is neither functional nor clinical, as it involves a structural assessment of the patient, either supine or prone. In spite of this, I find this approach particularly useful to help integrate the outcomes of both functional and clinical evaluation. Palpation should be performed with the entire hand, paying particular attention to the levels of the bony prominences and the symmetry of soft tissue tone and tension. Particular care should be taken with any lack of motion, if detected; conversely, any increased translatory motion exhibited between sides should be explored. The benefit of evaluating positional alignment is that it helps to form an impression of why an individual may demonstrate reduced levels of mobility. For example, if the innominate was observed to be rotated more anteriorly, relative to the sacrum, prior to testing hip flexion ROM, and if loss of hip flexion ROM is subsequently detected, this might actually be a result of the positional alignment of the innominate, rather than the hip joint. In my clinical experience, I have often come across differences in interpretation of hip flexion ROM between clinicians arising as a result of this misinterpretation. In this instance, an increased anterior pelvic tilt may be reducing the available free space for hip joint to perform adequate flexion (Swärd Aminoff et al., 2018).

Figure 2.9A highlights how to perform a positional evaluation with the patient supine. Note how I start with the patient in supine and compare, using palpation, the levels of the medial malleoli with the heights of the ASIS and the iliac crests (Figure 2.9B). Gentle compression is applied through the anterior innominates and any loss of spring or tension noted. The pubic tubercles (Figure 2.9C) are palpated for symmetry, tension or pain, as is the ribcage (Figure

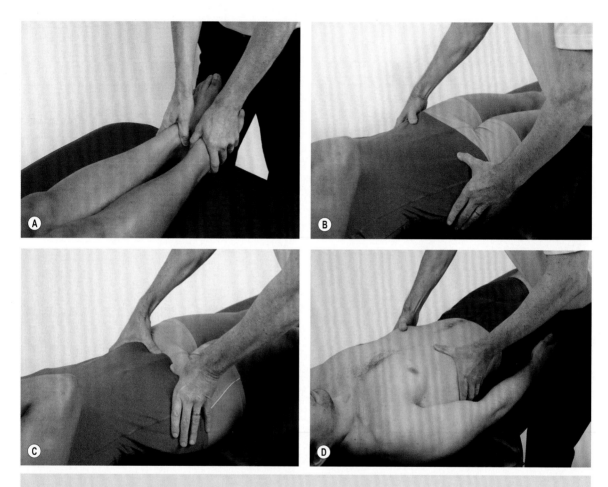

Figure 2.9
Supine positional alignment evaluation.
A Medial malleoli. **B** Anterior superior iliac spine and iliac crests. **C** Pubic tubercles. **D** Ribcage and abdominal musculature.

2.9D), applying gentle compression and translation to observe for any loss of motion or signs of pain. After this, soft tissue tension is palpated and compared across the lower rectus abdominis and oblique muscles and the inguinal region.

The process is repeated to assess the patient in prone (Figure 2.10A) with palpation of the PSIS, the inferior lateral angle of the sacrum and the depth of the sacral base (Figure 2.10B). The degree of spring in the L5 spinous process is noted; a negative spring test is dictated by a freely moving lumbar spine and is indicative of an anterior sacral torsion (Figure 2.10C). A positive spring test is dictated by a rigid lumbar spine and is indicative of a posterior sacral torsion. Palpation of the sacral sulcus can be achieved by applying a gentle springing motion on the opposite ilium. Soft tissue tension and tone can be palpated and compared across the multifidus and paraspinal muscles and the gluteal muscle complex.

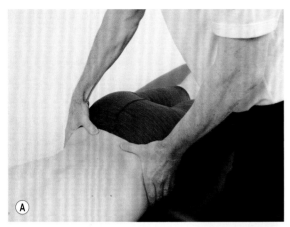

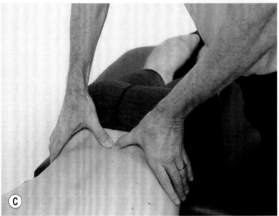

Figure 2.10

Prone positional alignment evaluation.

A Posterior superior iliac spine. **B** Sacral sulcus.
C L5 spinous process.

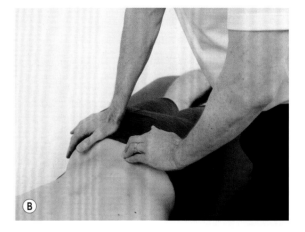

left. Assessment of joint play (anterior/posterior compression of the ASIS) highlighted restriction in motion; however, the end-feel was soft. Palpation highlighted increased tone in the adductors, TFL and abdominals, particularly the obliques on the right side relative to the left. These findings appeared to be consistent when Patient A was evaluated in prone (see Figure 2.10A–C), with the heights of the PSIS, inferior lateral angle and ischial tuberosity being higher on the right relative to the left, and an increased resting tone being noted on palpation of the multifidus, gluteus maximus and gluteus medius, and hamstrings.

While the findings from the functional and positional evaluations appear to correlate, at this stage they are meaningless, as I have not sufficiently tested my initial hypotheses. It is time to introduce the clinical evaluation.

Case study: more on Patient A

In supine (see Figure 2.9A–D), Patient A demonstrated a positional alignment similar to that in standing. His right medial malleolus appeared to be lower, relative to the left, with the height of his ASIS, iliac crest and pubic tubercle also appearing lower, relative to the

Clinical evaluation

In Chapter 1, I outlined the role of clinical evaluation within this integrated approach. Figure 2.11 highlights the factors that should be considered for an appropriate investigation. These include subjective and objective examination processes, muscular, articular and neural testing, and strength and capacity measurements,

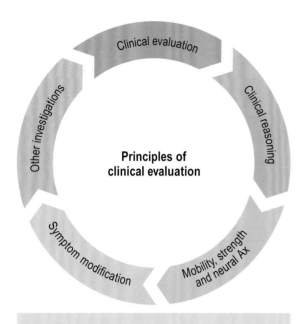

Figure 2.11
Clinical evaluation considerations.
Ax = Assessment.

but might also involve other diagnostic investigations, such as radiology or specific blood tests (Dutton, 2004; Magee, 2014).

The value of many of the clinical tests proposed in orthopedic texts is often questioned, given their relatively poor levels of reproducibility and validity (Hegedus et al., 2008; Rubinstein and van Tulder, 2008). Sadly, in my opinion, this has led to a decline in the capability of some clinicians to perform effective clinical evaluations (Feddock, 2007), as they prefer to rely instead on laboratory tests and clinical imaging. It is important to emphasize that the subtleness, precision and palpatory awareness required to perform any clinical test accurately must be of the highest caliber. "Attention to detail" is a phrase I use regularly when educating patients and lecturing to students. I will cover the clinical evaluations that I use predominantly in detail throughout this book, but in this chapter I will explain the clinical evaluations

that I consider to be most appropriate and relevant for Patient A.

Case study: more on Patient A

 At this stage, with Patient A, I need to integrate what I have already ascertained through functional and positional evaluations, alongside using the relevant clinical evaluations either to confirm or to challenge my findings and to test my hypothesis with greater confidence.

Here is a recap of my findings so far:

- An articular hip joint issue: perhaps resulting from the combination of flexion, adduction and internal rotation involved in kicking, which may have compressed or impinged the joint.

- A muscular injury: as a consequence of a specific incident to the intrinsic stabilizer muscles of the hip or as a result of repetitive overload to the oblique muscles, the deep hip flexors and the adductor muscles. This can occur with an isolated muscle specifically or involve several muscle groups.

- A spinal restriction: lack of dynamic mobility in the spinal column affecting the soft tissue structures that cross the anterior pelvis and hip joint. Spinal asymmetry may have developed from Patient A constantly kicking with his right foot. There may be referral from nerve root irritation or from nerve tissue that may have become inflamed as the nerves cross over the anterior pelvis and hip.

- Impaired respiratory function: loss of respiratory function or altered respiratory mechanics affecting the diaphragm and the abdominal muscles. There may be a reduced/increased length–tension relationship of these muscles affecting spino-pelvic alignment and optimal function of the spino-pelvic canister, resulting in global muscle over-recruitment and subsequent compensatory mechanisms.

Now, let's relate this information to our case. Patient A presented with a reactive tissue overload, caused by repetitive overuse from taking long kicks from the goal line. All the soft tissue structures that are recruited to perform the mechanism of kicking would be involved and, as a direct result of repetitive overload, this would have led to a reaction in these tissues. In my experience, this can indicate multiple structures and typically presents as highly sensitized tissues. For example, muscles such as the hip flexors, the adductors and the abdominals, which are all required for kicking, directly affect the mechanics of the spino-pelvic-hip complex. When a patient presents as highly sensitized around reactive tissues that have become inflamed or strained, it is much more difficult to test with high specificity. So, what do we do? It is fundamental to this case that we perform the appropriate clinical evaluations to test specifically:

- the hip joints
- the pelvic girdle
- the lumbar and thoracic spine
- the neural system
- the respiratory system.

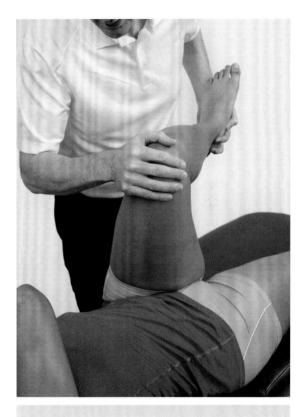

Figure 2.12
Hip joint passive flexion, adduction and internal rotation.

Hip joint: passive flexion, adduction and internal rotation (FADIR)

Figure 2.12 highlights the FADIR test, which is used to evaluate if there may be an articular component to an individual's anterior hip and groin pain. The patient should be in supine lying, while the clinician encourages passive hip joint flexion to 90°, followed by adduction and then internal rotation. Reproduction of symptoms may suggest a positive test: this would be reported as discomfort or pain in the groin region when the hip is passively taken to the end of range. This test has been shown to be highly sensitive (94 percent) but low in specificity (11 percent) for investigating intra-articular hip joint pathology (Ranawatt et al., 2017; Reiman et al., 2015).

Case study: more on Patient A

Patient A, similar to the person in Figure 2.12, demonstrated loss of active and passive right hip joint flexion and internal rotation in supine, with the hip and knee flexed at 90°. Anterior groin pain was reported when the hip was placed at 90° flexion and taken passively to the limit of internal rotation. This suggests that there may be an articular component to our case. However, it is important to stress that this test has a poor level of specificity and should be used as a screening tool, rather than a diagnostic one (Reiman and Thorborg, 2014). As a consequence, I need to keep an open mind with regard to the possibility that Patient A has potential intra-articular pathology.

Adductor evaluation

Figure 2.13A highlights adductor flexibility. With one hand, the tested leg is placed in neutral, avoiding hip joint lateral rotation; the other hand is placed on the non-tested ASIS. I then begin to abduct the tested leg, noting any movement inferiorly of the ASIS on the non-tested side before the abducted leg reaches 45°, as this may indicate hypertonic adductors. If the abducted leg is flexed at the knee and further abduction is achieved, then the short adductors are eliminated. Reliability for this test is shown to be moderate to good (intra-tester intra-class coefficient (ICC) 0.67 and inter-tester ICC 0.74) (Hölmich et al., 2004) for evaluating adductor pain on flexibility testing.

Palpation of the adductor muscles in supine or side lying (Figure 2.13B) can be performed and has been shown to have high sensitivity for predicting muscle injuries. The intra-tester (ICC 0.89) and inter-tester (ICC 0.94) reliability have been shown to be good to excellent for evaluating adductor pain on palpation (Hölmich et al., 2004). Furthermore, the absence of pain on adductor palpation has also been shown to be effective for predicting a negative MRI result (Serner et al., 2016).

Adductor strength can be evaluated clinically using manual resistance. A straight leg position is better for eliciting a pelvic girdle pain response (Figure 2.13C). The test's intra-tester (ICC 0.79) and inter-tester (ICC 0.79) reliability have both been shown to be good for evaluating adductor strength (Mens et al., 2002).

For bent knee evaluation, the patient is supine with their knees at 60° and feet placed on the couch, although it has been suggested that this emphasizes adductor longus and this test still requires external validation (Figure 2.13D). I generally place my elbow or fist between the patient's knees and instruct them to squeeze. In terms of diagnostic accuracy, reproduction of pain with this evaluation has moderate sensitivity (43 percent) and high specificity (91 percent) (Verrall et al., 2005).

With the single-leg adductor test (Figure 2.13E), the patient is supine, with the tested leg taken into slight abduction and internal rotation, and is asked to contract against my resistance. Moving the tested leg into an outer-range or inner-range position can modify the evaluation; care must therefore be taken to avoid misinterpreting which position (inner, mid, outer range) may be symptomatic. The diagnostic accuracy for this evaluation rests on a low sensitivity (30 percent) but excellent specificity (91 percent) (Verrall et al., 2005). Special attention should be paid to which position reproduces the most information about sensitivity, as this may give an indication of the specific structures involved in this presentation.

Case study: more on Patient A

 Patient A was able to perform all the adductor evaluations and demonstrated good power on resisted muscle testing, according to the Oxford Manual Muscle Grading Scale (Naqvi and Sherman, 2021; Table 2.1). These specific adductor tests have all been shown to be reliable and to have moderate to high levels of sensitivity and specificity (Mens et al., 2002; Hölmich et al., 2004; Verrall et al., 2005). In addition, adductor inhibition was highlighted on resisted adductor testing in single-leg, outer-range evaluation (see Figure 2.13E), with trigger points and tenderness apparent on palpation. Both single-leg adductor evaluation and palpation have been shown to have high levels of accuracy for diagnostic testing (Serner et al., 2016; Verrall et al., 2005). Patient A was already demonstrating a

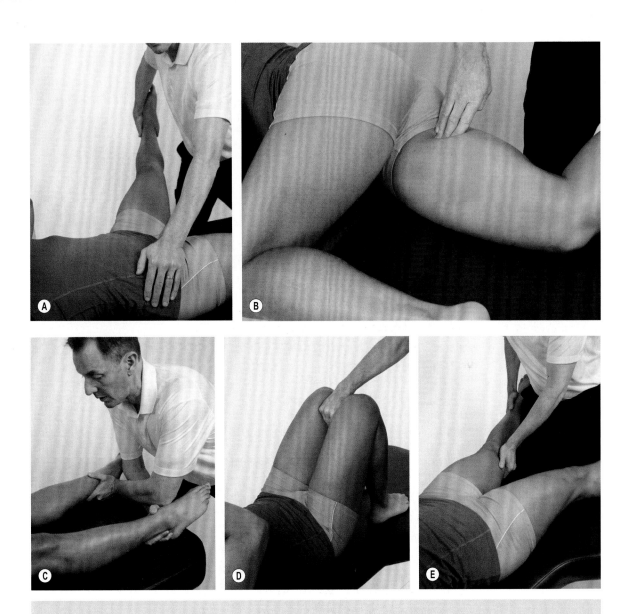

Figure 2.13

Adductor evaluation.

A Adductor flexibility. **B** Adductor side-lying palpation. **C** Adductor strength testing in straight leg, emphasizing the pelvic girdle.
D Adductor strength testing with knees bent at 60°, emphasizing adductor longus. **E** Adductor strength testing, single-leg outer range.

Table 2.1 Oxford Manual Muscle Grading Scale	
Grade	**Description**
0 **None**	No visible or palpable contraction
1 **Trace**	Visible or palpable contraction
2 **Poor**	Full range of movement (ROM) gravity eliminated
3 **Fair**	Full ROM against gravity
4 **Good**	Full ROM against gravity, moderate resistance
5 **Normal**	Full ROM against gravity, maximal resistance

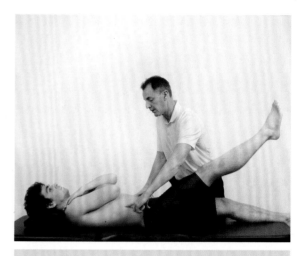

Figure 2.14
Active straight leg raise.

non-functional standing alignment, as he had developed relative hip joint internal rotation on his kicking leg. This may have altered his adductor flexibility, reducing frontal plane ROM, and it could therefore be hypothesized that he was overloading his adductor tissues in this reduced range when he attempted to open up his hip and take his kicking leg into an outer-range position.

Active straight leg raise (ASLR)

Figure 2.14 highlights the ASLR. This test has been shown to be extremely useful for evaluating pelvic function (Mens et al., 2006) and has demonstrated good intra-tester (ICC 0.83) and inter-tester (ICC 0.87) reliability. In terms of diagnostic accuracy, high levels of both sensitivity (87 percent) and specificity (94 percent) are shown.

The patient lies supine and is instructed to perform an ASLR, to evaluate for any reproduction of pain or discomfort over the pubic region and/or the lower abdominals. I would normally associate this with reduced levels of force closure around the pelvic girdle (Vleeming et al., 1990ab). Special attention should be paid to any hip flexor inhibition and/or over-activity of the oblique muscles. This is often observed, with increased translatory motion around the thoracolumbar junction, on the contralateral side to the leg that is being raised, and the two should be compared.

Case study: more on Patient A

 On performing the ASLR evaluation (see Figure 2.14), Patient A reported discomfort across the right anterior hip, with pain and discomfort on palpation over the right lower abdominal wall and into the iliac fossa. Inhibition of his right hip flexors during execution of the ASLR was also observed. Although the ASLR, according to Mens et al. (2006), has been shown to have high levels of sensitivity and specificity for accurately diagnosing pelvic-related pain, there are many soft tissues located within this region. Classification of the clinical signs and symptoms associated with groin pain, in relation to a specific anatomical structure, was first proposed by Hölmich (2007). In recent years, the Doha Agreement has attempted to standardize the currently used definitions and terminology between healthcare professions and countries worldwide (Weir et al., 2015).

As I mentioned previously, the mobility and stability systems of movement can be examined separately but are functionally dependent on each other. To illustrate this, when an ASLR test is performed, the hip joint and hip flexor muscles can be viewed as the mobility system (Beales et al., 2010), while the structures around the SIJ and pelvic girdle could be viewed as the stability system (Mens et al., 2006). In this case, Patient A was demonstrating that he had lost the synergy between these systems, and as a result his deep muscular system, involving the deep fibers of his psoas muscle, may have become inhibited due to pain and tissue fatigue, with a resultant over-recruitment of the superficial muscular system (Hodges et al., 2003; 2002).

Abdominal muscles

Evaluation of rectus abdominis (Figure 2.15A) and the oblique muscles (Figure 2.15B) is performed with the patient in supine, the arms crossed over the chest. I normally instruct the patient to perform a sit-up and I observe the quality of movement and listen to the patient's report of any symptoms. Manual resistance is then applied centrally against the patient's chest, to emphasize the rectus abdominis muscle. The intra-tester ICC (0.63) and inter-tester ICC (0.57) for reliability have been shown to be moderate for evaluating rectus abdominis using this test (Hölmich et al., 2004).

Alternatively, manual resistance can be applied through the contralateral shoulder as the patient performs an oblique crunch to generate more activity in

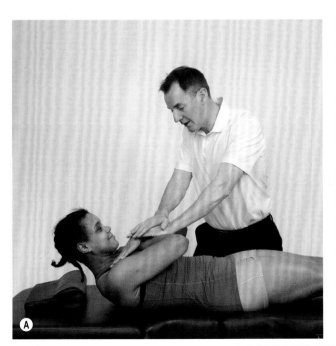
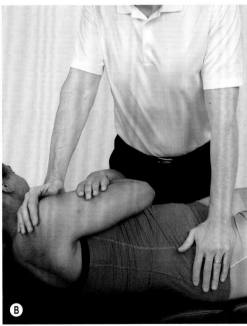

Figure 2.15

Evaluation of the abdominal muscles.

A Resisted rectus abdominis sit-up. **B** Resisted oblique sit-up.

the oblique muscles. The intra-tester ICC (0.51) and the inter-tester ICC (0.41) for this test as an evaluation of the oblique muscles have demonstrated poor to moderate reliability (Hölmich et al., 2004).

Case study: more on Patient A

Abdominal testing of Patient A, similar to that shown in Figures 2.15A and 2.15B, highlighted nothing abnormal, other than inhibition with resisted rotation to the right. Of clinical relevance in this case, this highlights that there is a lesser likelihood of an intrinsic abdominal muscle injury. The inhibition associated with rotation to the right could therefore be hypothesized to result from soft tissue overload caused by a repetitive functional movement (long kicking). Such an interpretation is similar to the hypothesis and evaluation scenario of the single-leg adductor inhibition that was previously described. The presence of pain has been shown to disrupt muscle recruitment, which would affect the relationship between stability and dynamic mobility, making it difficult for an individual to perform a task efficiently (van Dieën et al., 2003). In Patient A, pain inhibition, due to an inflammatory response in the soft tissues, may be affecting his ability to perform long kicks.

Adapted Thomas test

Figure 2.16 highlights the evaluation of structures that cross the anterior hip and thigh. The patient is supine at the end of the couch, bringing the non-tested leg into hip flexion and holding it at the knee. I support the limb and passively lower the tested leg into extension, while stabilizing the ipsilateral side of the pelvis with my hand and monitoring for the following signs:

1. reproduction of groin pain or reproduction of a click (inflamed psoas "clicking" over the anterior pelvic eminence)

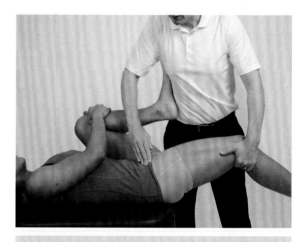

Figure 2.16
Adapted Thomas test.

2. inability of the tested thigh to remain flat on the couch (hypertonic hip flexors)

3. inability of the tested leg to reach 90° knee flexion (hypertonic rectus femoris)

4. reports of lower lumbar spine arching or reproduction of LBP

5. abduction or external rotation of the hip (hypertonic TFL)

6. an anterior translation of the ASIS, indicating a lengthened state of the hip flexors, often associated with inhibition on contraction in this position.

In terms of diagnostic accuracy, this test has high sensitivity (89 percent) and specificity (92 percent) (Reiman et al., 2015).

Case study: more on Patient A

Patient A demonstrated an increased abduction and external rotation of his right hip and an increased translation of his right ASIS when he performed the adapted Thomas test (see Figure 2.16). This indicated shortening of his TFL muscle and lengthening of his deep hip flexor architecture. The adapted Thomas test has a high level of accuracy from a clinical standpoint, which gives this evaluation real diagnostic value (Reiman et al., 2015).

Now let's put all this information together. Remember that, in standing, Patient A demonstrated a non-functional alignment, and that palpation of his TFL appeared to be more toned on the right, relative to the left. Furthermore, anterior pelvic tilt was also more evident on the right side in weight-bearing. So, having previously noted this information during the functional evaluation, I see exactly what I would expect to see, using the adapted Thomas test to perform the clinical evaluation.

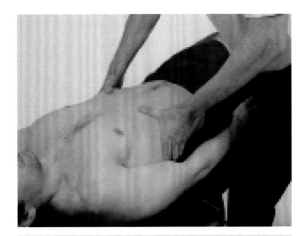

Figure 2.17
Respiratory control.

Respiratory control

Figure 2.17 shows evaluation of the lower ribcage and diaphragmatic breathing through palpation. If dysfunction occurs within the thoracolumbar canister, then compensation patterns may follow (Lewit, 1999). A loss of ribcage translation on one side may be an indication of poor respiratory mechanics. Respiratory motor control is observed by instructing the patient to perform deep inhalation and exhalation while I place my hands over the lower ribs and palpate, observing for any loss of rib expansion (bucket handle and pincer mechanism), or tenderness around the diaphragm and oblique attachments.

Case study: more on Patient A

 Respiratory mechanics, as shown in Figure 2.17, appeared to demonstrate a reduction in mobility that was evident on palpation over the lower ribcage, specifically on the right. Tender points could be palpated around the attachments of the oblique muscles across the lower right ribcage. Additionally, reduced rib expansion was noted on the right when Patient A was instructed to perform deep inhalation. Respiratory dysfunction, although frequently painless, can lead to musculoskeletal dysfunction that contributes to persisting and recurring issues within the thoracic spine (Greenman, 1996). The diaphragm, due to its extensive muscular and fascial attachments, has a huge effect on respiration, spinal stabilization, active pelvic tilt and fluid dynamics (Lewit, 1999). However, it is unlikely that Patient A would have developed respiratory dysfunction from the training session the previous morning. What if Patient A, through the very nature of his sports-specific training, had developed faulty movement patterns and postural changes that had eventually increased stiffness in both the thoracic spine and the ribcage, reducing respiratory muscle activation (Jung and Kim, 2018)? The implications could be far-reaching, having an impact on the interdependence of the regions of the lower extremity and the spino-pelvic-hip complex, increasing vulnerability of the hip joint during dynamic actions.

Lumbar segmental passive evaluation

Segmental passive evaluation is more difficult to carry out in the lumbar and thoracolumbar spine, as clinicians may find it difficult to passively move heavier or larger patients. However, the benefit of performing this evaluation appropriately is that it enables the clinician to assess for any segmental changes in ROM, pain or the joints' end-feel (Haneline et al., 2008). The patient is placed in a side-lying position with spine in neutral and knees bent (Figure 2.18). The passive physiological intervertebral motion (PPIVM) is performed in flexion, lateral flexion and rotation, and then in extension, lateral flexion and rotation, to evaluate vertebral movement in physiological ranges compared with the adjacent joint(s) (Inscoe et al., 1995). With practice, we should be able to palpate the segmental motion (gapping) between the spinous processes and to note any specific restrictions in motion that would result in less "gapping" or, alternatively, increased translation between the segments; these would indicate hypomobility or hypermobility, respectively, and are often associated with pain or tenderness. The results of this type of passive evaluation appear to be heavily dependent on the skill and expertise of the clinician, as the inter-rater reliability has previously demonstrated relatively poor agreement (Panzer, 1992; Inscoe et al., 1995).

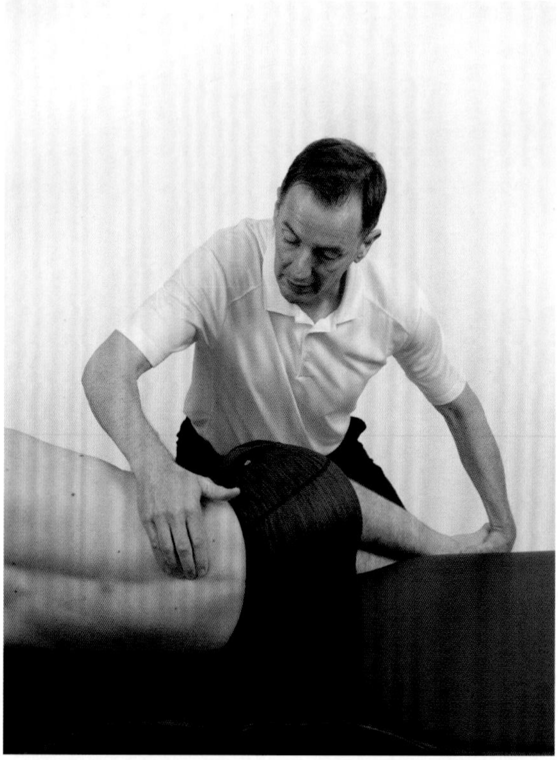

Figure 2.18
Lumbar segmental passive lateral flexion evaluation.

Case study: more on Patient A

It was evident on segmental mobility evaluation (see Figure 2.18) that Patient A demonstrated a reduction in spinal extension, lateral flexion right and rotation right, with palpable segmental restrictions in his lower thoracic and thoracolumbar spine (T8–10 and T12–L1). Tenderness was also reported on palpation over the right-sided thoracolumbar junction and thoracolumbar erector spinae muscles. Evidence of poor reliability between clinicians has led to some practitioners questioning the relevance of performing passive spinal evaluations, as shown in Figure 2.18 (Inscoe et al., 1995; Panzer, 1992). However, in my opinion, if this clinical evaluation is practiced enough, it will be mastered. Its relevance should be considered alongside the standing functional evaluations described earlier, with findings from both these approaches being reflected on as the clinician integrates all the information gathered.

By this stage, I am beginning to build a picture of this clinical puzzle from the information I have collated by integrating functional and clinical evaluations. Some of this may seem a little confusing. For example:

1. A positive test using hip joint FADIR evaluation implies that I could be dealing with an articular issue.

2. The deep hip flexors appear to be lengthened and inhibited, as do the oblique muscles and the adductor muscles, specifically on outer-range testing. So, which muscle group is predominantly the pain generator? This raises the question: could this be a hip joint-related or a muscle-related issue?

3. Spinal ROM appears restricted as well as rotation right, with thoracolumbar segmental restrictions noted on active/passive evaluation. However, it appears that lumbar extension is pain-free; I can therefore conclude from this part of the evaluation that a lower lumbar facet joint restriction is unlikely to be a source of symptoms.

4. Could segmental restrictions further up the spinal column be affecting the length–tension relationship of the musculature across the pelvic girdle?

5. Due to the anatomical closeness and neural innervation of these structures, would this have resulted in altered respiratory mechanics, or vice versa? For example, altered respiratory mechanics could have been the initiating event in the development of symptoms or could have altered muscle length–tension relationships across the spino-pelvic complex.

To evaluate these hypotheses further and bring a level of clarity to this case, I need to incorporate the diverse approaches of clinical reasoning to help collect and process the information gathered from Patient A, so that I can plan and implement an intervention and re-evaluate the outcome.

 Clinical reasoning

Case study: more on Patient A

Pattern recognition

I have often come across clinicians performing deep hip flexor myofascial release work, to help with LBP or anterior hip and groin pain. Perhaps the anatomical closeness of the deep hip flexors, such as psoas major and psoas minor (if present), and their connections, from the anterior aspect of the lumbar spine L1–4 to the lesser trochanter of the femur, makes them an ideal candidate for the use of pattern recognition and subsequent manipulative soft tissue therapy. In this instance, pattern recognition may have led the clinician to assume that releasing the deep hip flexor structures might help to alleviate LBP and/or anterior hip and groin pain. Perhaps past experiences have shown that this particular technique has helped with similar cases. Imagine what would have happened if this approach had been used for Patient A? The next time he was reviewed, he might have reported that his symptoms had improved and that he was confident to train. However, what if his symptoms improved for only a short period and returned later in the day? Alternatively, suppose that the symptoms initially felt better during the warm-up, but as the intensity of the training session increased, they returned with a vengeance. Is it safe to assume that Patient A simply needs more deep myofascial release work? There are many who practice this particular approach, with a tendency to release structures as a first line of treatment. However, the danger here lies with the possibility of misdiagnosis and results in chasing pain around the patient's body. So, what can we do? Let's find out.

Hypothetical deductive reasoning

Let's put the hypothetical deductive approach into context. Patient A reported with right-sided LBP that referred into the right lower abdominal and anterior hip region, after a training session. We have already hypothesized that this may have been the result of excessive kicking practice in training, which could have overloaded the soft tissues and resulted in fatigue and a reactive inflammatory component. But can those tissues actually be "tight"? Either from further questioning and picking up on cues that Patient A offered, or from paying attention to his reporting that symptoms came on gradually, it is evident that lack of tissue tolerance to load is being highlighted. Therefore, it is this issue that I would be inclined to suspect had led to his present reactive state. Additionally, on questioning, Patient A could not recall any specific instance, such as taking a long, powerful kick, that would have suggested that a particular incident contributed to his issues. This makes it less likely that Patient A may have developed a specific muscle strain.

Knowledge and practitioner insight

Propositional, professional craft and personal knowledge are powerful reasoning tools (McCarthy, 2010). This particular reasoning approach may give clinicians an almost "guru-like" persona. Some patients or athletes may, in fact, feel comfortable with this, as it takes the decision-making process out of their own hands, the clinician essentially making all the calls. Consider Patient A: imagine if I told him that I see conditions like this regularly and have published papers, written textbooks and lectured on courses around this particular issue. In addition, I tell him that I recall a similar incident involving another senior player of great standing, many years ago (before Patient A had turned professional) in a previous competition, and that I was able to manage it successfully. Patient A may be impressed with this knowledge and put his trust in me to solve his problems. From my clinical experience, I see danger here in the possibility of being able to steamroll Patient A and failing to include or involve him in the reasoning processes.

Diagnostic reasoning

A neurophysiological effect of pain modulation, increased tissue extensibility and improved fluid dynamics has been shown to occur following soft tissue manipulation (Loghmani and Whitted, 2016). Additionally, improved motor programming and motor control may also result from muscle energy techniques (Fryer, 2011), and a reduction in muscle tone from articular manipulation (Michael et al., 2017). The neurophysiological effect of performing a mini-treatment, such as a short series of symptom modification techniques (SMTs), may have helped to reduce the biomechanical strain across the spinal column and pelvic girdle, helping to begin to restore function. With this case, I performed SMT using manipulative therapy techniques to restore spinal rotation. Figures 2.19A and 2.19B highlight thoracic and lumbar segmental motion evaluation, palpated through the range. Note: if the range is restricted at any particular level, soft tissue, articular or muscle energy techniques can be applied. Then re-evaluate the influence that thoracolumbar mobility may have had on the initial presentation.

Figure 2.19C shows the SMT approach to assist with restoring hip flexion. The clinical reasoning behind using this technique is based on anterior chain over-activity in muscles such as the TFL, increasing anterior pelvic tilt. Anterior pelvic tilt will limit the available free range for the hip joint to perform flexion.

 Note that the patient is side-lying. I generally perform a short series of manipulative techniques actively or passively to the TFL muscle. This approach may also be combined with neural dynamic techniques for the femoral or obturator nerves (Shacklock, 2014).

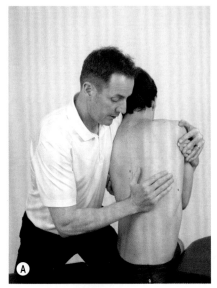

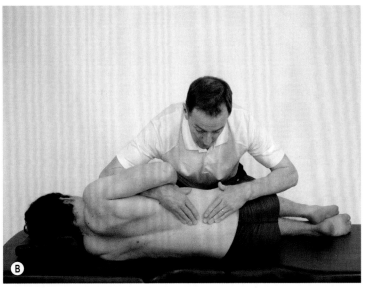

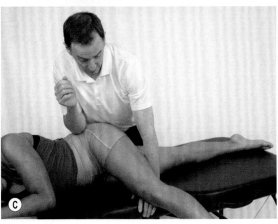

Figure 2.19
Symptom modification techniques to evaluate the influence of restriction of thoracic mobility on symptoms.
A Thoracic. **B** Lumbar. **C** Hip.

Re-evaluation should be carried out to ascertain what influence a lack of hip flexion might have on the initial presentation.

Re-evaluation of Patient A, after SMT to his thoracolumbar spine, highlighted an improvement in both spinal and hip ROM (see Figures 2.19A and 2.19B). It is highly likely that reduced spinal ROM may have influenced hip ROM. Spinal treatment has previously been shown to reduce hip pain (Cibulka and Delitto, 1993). Perhaps this may have improved through reflex relaxation of the soft tissues, changing the resting tone across the lower abdomen, pelvis and anterior thigh. This may have assisted in regaining active pelvic tilt, but similarly, an improvement in hip flexion ROM was also noted after performing SMT techniques (see Figure 2.19C) to Patient A's TFL muscle. Active pelvic tilt has been shown to influence hip joint mobility (Swärd Aminoff et al., 2018). Improving flexibility in the TFL and rectus femoris may have also influenced active pelvic tilt. For example, if the anterior chain musculature were hypertonic, this might have increased anterior pelvic tilt and thus increased the acetabular over-coverage, which would have resulted in limited active and passive hip flexion ROM. This might explain why Patient

A was symptomatic on clinical evaluation for hip joint FADIR testing.

Normalizing respiratory function, diaphragm and pelvic floor alignment may have helped to restore the length–tension relationship across the abdominal musculature, improving active pelvic tilt and hip flexion ROM (Jung and Kim, 2018). The pelvic floor (discussed in Chapter 3) forms the base of the thoracolumbar canister, and altered isometric tension could affect the resting tone of the pelvic floor and have an impact on breathing mechanics. It is quite possible that normalizing respiratory function helped improve optimal function for generating intra-abdominal pressure, which has been shown to be extremely important for spinal stabilization (Lewit, 1999).

Using this hypothetical deductive model to validate our hypotheses, both spinal and hip mobility were shown to improve; however, ASLR evaluation still highlighted inhibition of the deep hip flexors. Consequently, the final stage of the SMT approach would be to attempt to restore function to these structures.

 Figure 2.20 highlights activation of the deep hip flexors (psoas muscle). I perform a short series of activation techniques by applying manual resistance with the hip in external rotation to distract the leg, while instructing the patient to visualize "drawing" or "sucking" their hip into its socket (Gibbons, 2007). This technique is repeated 6–8 times and then the ASLR is re-evaluated.

Re-evaluation of Patient A, after performing SMT (see Figure 2.20) to evaluate whether activation techniques would help deep hip flexor function, highlighted a significant improvement in ASLR and a reduction in symptoms. It could then be concluded, through clinical reasoning and the use of SMT, that the deep hip flexor tissues may actually

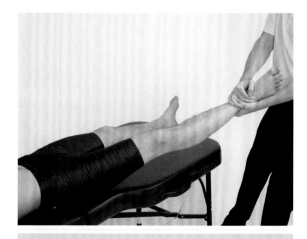

Figure 2.20
SMT to evaluate the influence of deep hip flexor activation on symptoms.

have been in a reactive state – inflamed, inhibited and susceptible to fatigue – from repeated kicking. If we consider the function of the deep hip flexors across the hip joint, pelvic girdle and lumbar spine, this may help to create a working hypothesis. Loss of acetabular compression and axial spinal stabilization may have worked in tandem to increase levels of LBP and anterior hip and groin pain. For example, the deep fibers of psoas will assist with stabilizing and centering the femoral head in the acetabulum, to allow optimal hip joint ROM around the axis of rotation (Gibbons, 2007). Inhibition of the psoas muscle, as a result of pain or fatigue, will encourage the up-regulation of other muscle synergists to help achieve this stabilization role. For example, other hip flexors, such as the TFL, may become over-recruited or more dominant. The distal positioning of the TFL's anatomical attachment, relative to the axis of hip joint rotation, means that it simply cannot provide optimal joint stability and thus allows the femoral head to translate forward and medially when the action of hip flexion is performed (Lee, 2011; Sahrmann, 2002). When this occurs, the hip may be held in relative internal rotation and, as a direct result, no further internal rotation would be available; the range would be significantly reduced, causing the spine and pelvic complex to rotate further around the symptomatic hip, the end result being a loss of both hip and spinal rotation. At the same time, the soft tissues crossing the pelvic girdle from the trunk to the lower extremity would become "wound up" or put under increased strain, causing a greater susceptibility to fatigue from overload, such as would be the case with prolonged kicking. As nerve innervation to the deep hip flexors originates from the upper lumbar spine (L1–2), it could be hypothesized that loss of axial spinal control and reduced rotation in the thoracolumbar spine might have caused segmental restrictions and influenced the neural drive to the deep hip flexors, resulting in muscle inhibition.

Interpretative reasoning

Consider how alignment and the subsequent standing posture and movements that are often adopted by athletes or patients might change in the presence of pain or over-arousal of their psychosocial status. Identifying an athlete or patient that may be at risk, or delayed in their recovery from injury, may be highly influenced by the presence of internal or external factors, including changes in behavioral patterns, increased anxiety, fear, avoidance, depression and lack of education, all leading to abnormal pain presentations and beliefs (O'Sullivan, 2000).

After reviewing Patient A, it became apparent that, as a result of the severity of his initial symptoms, he was particularly worried that he had ruptured a muscle in his pelvis or hip joint. He was also concerned that, if he was to train the next day, he might create further damage, which might even rule him out for the remainder of the competition. He said that he had had a similar episode once before, back at his club, and the treatment he was given had not helped. He also mentioned that another of his goalkeeper colleagues had a similar issue, which was resolved only by undergoing surgery. He asked me why I thought that previous treatments had not worked. At that point, I asked him if he could recall what had been the mechanism of the previous injury, what the previous symptoms were like and what type of treatment he had been given. I told him that these were really important factors, as all of them could be having a significant impact on his perception of his current issue. I proposed to Patient A that we should attempt to work together to try to change his perceptions. This was clearly a young man who was concerned about continuing to train and about the possibility that he might sustain a significant injury by carrying on.

 Sometimes, it does not matter what we do as clinicians, unless we have the ability to "click" with our patients and really get to know them, by showing affective and cognitive reassurance (Pincus et al., 2013). Patient A was not in a chronic state of pain but he did have his own preconceived ideas and beliefs around his injury. What if none of the back-room staff realized that he was in the middle of contract talks to move to another club? Patient A had previously mentioned to me in our initial discussions the possibility of his dream transfer, to play for a team that he had always supported as a boy. Can we blame him for being overly cautious and protective of himself? These are all significant factors in managing this particular case, and it really does not matter how good our clinical skills are if we cannot integrate psychology-informed practice into a successful management plan (Main and George, 2011). Perhaps the outcome of this case may be dependent on our ability as clinicians to reflect in action (Schon, 1983) and to think on our feet, but to be empathetic and genuine, to provide reassurance and clear explanations, and above all to *educATE*.

Case study: more on Patient A

Considering the bio-psychosocial model creates a completely different impression of this case. Patient A was in the later stages of a major competition, during which all athletes are under enormous pressure. This in itself may be enough to amplify a nervous system response, but although I do bear it in mind, it does not rank high in my order of hypothesis testing. My reasons are straightforward. Patient A presented with a reactive issue that had only recently occurred, associated with a clear biomechanical process earlier in the day. While I can sympathize with the patient's concerns, and the "external noise" that may influence the behavior of many athletes, it is less likely that the bio-psychosocial aspect, related to current environmental factors, is the main source of pain or having an impact on his symptoms.

Should we consider the bio-psychosocial aspect of pain? In my opinion: absolutely, yes! Perhaps the biomedical model, which uses functional and clinical evaluations, should not necessarily be viewed as being made up of purely physical or biomechanical entities. Although in sport the biomedical model is possibly the easiest way to conceptualize human movement, it is more likely a consequence of the interactions of stability and alignment, resulting from form and force closure, and dynamic activity, resulting from optimal movement through efficient motor control, *in addition* to an athlete or patient's bio-psychological status.

Conclusion

By using clinical reasoning to generate and test my hypotheses, I am now able to formulate a working hypothesis to plan the appropriate management strategy for this patient.

Case study: more on Patient A

 The working hypothesis for this case relates to Patient A developing an overload issue that had been caused by taking repetitive long kicks. As a result of reactive tissue overload to the deep fibers of his psoas, he developed anterior hip and groin pain, and a loss of hip joint ROM and pelvic and axial spine stability (Gibbons, 2007). Over-recruitment of the superficial muscular system may have increased relative hip joint internal rotation and anterior pelvic tilt and led to increased thoracolumbar rotation. The clinical relevance of this state of affairs is that it would result in loss of both stability and dynamic mobility, which may have disrupted the interaction among task, mobility and load, leading to a delay in muscle reflex activation (Van Dieën et al., 2003).

 In this scenario, the aim is to restore function to the spine, pelvic girdle, and hip and groin complex, through specific manipulative techniques, and to address restrictions in the thoracolumbar region and anterior hip joint.

 Alongside these interventions, neuromuscular activation techniques would be utilized to improve deep hip flexor muscle recruitment, in order to prepare Patient A for appropriate on-field loading. Clinical reasoning, used within the fundamental framework approach, helps with validating or rejecting hypotheses. In turn, this makes treatment and management around this particular case quite straightforward.

The management plan, leading to recovery for Patient A, is highlighted in Table 2.2. Ultimately, to maintain a lasting, positive outcome, the aggravating activity would have to be stopped or, at the very least, modified: for example, by reducing the volume (or amount) of kicking. However, in Patient A's case, he was able to train fully the next day, did not require any further investigations,

Table 2.2 Management plan for recovery

Evaluation	Action
1. *Re-evaluATE* thoracolumbar rotation	*ManipulATE* T12–L1 • High-velocity, low-amplitude thrust • Articular • Muscle energy technique • Soft tissue manipulation
2. *Re-evaluATE* anterior hip for muscular tightness	*ManipulATE* • Tensor fasciae latae • Rectus femoris • Adductors
3. *Re-evaluATE* active straight leg raise	*ActivATE* • Deep hip flexors (psoas major)
4. *Re-evaluATE* respiratory function	*Inhibit* • Diaphragm and obliques trigger points *ActivATE* • Respiratory function

such as an MRI scan, and did not miss a training session for the remainder of the competition.

The integrated approach, used in this case to *evaluATE*, became part of Patient A's daily pre- and post-training evaluation, and over the following few days he was taught how to observe for any deficits in hip joint ROM, thoracolumbar rotation and neuromuscular motor control. He learned how to address these himself, pre- and post-training, using specific exercise techniques that included a combination of mobility and neuromuscular motor control to enhance movement restoration.

In conclusion, an integrated approach, based on a sound clinical reasoning process, helped to restore function and reduce pain in the spine, hip and groin. This was achieved through manipulative therapy and neuromuscular activation techniques. Using a blend of techniques within the "five 'ATEs" approach to resolve Patient A's issues demonstrates that this is an effective and efficient framework. It enables the principles of functional and clinical evaluations to be integrated and informs sound clinical reasoning. This helped Patient A recover from his issue and ensured that he was fully available for subsequent training sessions and matches.

References

Beales, D., O'Sullivan, P. and Briffa, N., 2010. The effects of manual pelvic compression on trunk motor control during an active straight leg raise in chronic pelvic girdle pain subjects. *Manual Therapy*, 15(2), pp. 190–199.

Brophy, R., Backus, S., Pansy, B. et al., 2007. Lower extremity muscle activation and alignment during the soccer instep and side-foot kicks. *Journal Orthopaedic Sports Physical Therapy*, 37(5), pp. 260–268.

Cibulka, M. and Delitto, A., 1993. A comparison of two different methods to treat hip pain in runners. *Journal Orthopaedic Sports Physical Therapy*, 17(4), pp. 172–176.

Dutton, M., 2004. *Orthopaedic Examination, Evaluation and Intervention*. 2nd ed. New York: McGraw-Hill.

Feddock, C., 2007. The lost art of clinical skills. *American Journal Medicine*, 120(4), pp. 374–378.

Fryer, G., 2011. Muscle energy technique: an evidence-informed approach. *International Journal Osteopathic Medicine*, 14(1), pp. 3–9.

Furman, M. and Johnson, S., 2019. Induced lumbosacral radicular symptom referral patterns: a descriptive study. *Spine*, 19(1), pp. 163–170.

Gibbons, S., 2007. Assessment and rehabilitation of the stability function of psoas major. *Manuelletherapie*, 11, pp. 177–187.

Greenman, P., 1996. *Principles of Manual Medicine*. 5th ed. Philadelphia: Lippincott Williams and Wilkins.

Haneline, M., Cooperstein, R., Young, M. et al., 2008. Spinal motion palpation: a comparison of studies that assessed intersegmental end feel vs excursion. *Journal Manipulative Physiological Therapeutics*, 31(8), pp. 616–626.

Harris-Hayes, M., Sahrmann, S. and Van Dillen, L., 2009. Relationship between the hip and low back pain in athletes who participate in rotation-related sports. *Journal Sport Rehabilitation*, 18(1), pp. 60–75.

Hegedus, E., Goode, A., Campbell, S. et al., 2008. Physical examination tests of the shoulder: a systematic review with meta-analysis of individual tests. *British Journal Sports Medicine*, 42(2), pp. 80–92.

Hodges, P., Gurfinkel, V., Brumagne, S. et al., 2002. Coexistence of stability and mobility in postural control: evidence from postural compensation for respiration. *Experimental Brain Research*, 144(3), pp. 293–302.

Hodges, P., Moseley, G., Gabrielsson, A. et al., 2003. Experimental muscle pain changes feedforward postural responses of the trunk muscles. *Experimental Brain Research*, 151(2), pp. 262–271.

Hölmich, P., 2007. Long-standing groin pain in sportspeople falls into three primary patterns, a "clinical entity" approach: a prospective study of 207 patients. *British Journal Sports Medicine*, 41(4), pp. 247–252.

Hölmich, P., Hölmich, LR., Bjerg, AM., 2004. Clinical examination of athletes with groin pain: an intraobserver and interobserver reliability study. *British Journal Sports Medicine*, 38(4), pp. 446–451.

Hungerford, B., Gilleard, W., Moran, M. et al., 2007. Evaluation of the ability of physical therapists to palpate intrapelvic motion with the stork test on the support side. *Physical Therapy*, 87(7), pp. 879–887.

Inscoe, E., Witt, P., Gross, M. et al., 1995. Reliability in evaluating passive intervertebral motion of the lumbar spine. *Journal Manual Manipulative Therapy*, 3(4), pp. 135–143.

Jacob, H. and Kissling, R., 1995. The mobility of the sacroiliac joints in healthy volunteers between 20 and 50 years of age. *Clinical Biomechanics*, 10(7), pp. 352–361.

Jung, J. and Kim, N., 2018. Changes in training posture induce changes in the chest wall movement and respiratory muscle activation during respiratory muscle training. *Journal of Exercise Rehabilitation*, 14(5), pp. 771–777.

Lamontagne, M., Kennedy, M. and Beaulé, P., 2009. The effect of cam FAI on hip and pelvic motion during maximum squat. *Clinical Orthopaedics and Related Research*, 467(3), pp. 645–650.

Laslett, M., McDonald, B., Aprill, C. et al., 2006. Clinical predictors of screening lumbar zygapophyseal joint blocks: development of clinical prediction rules. *Spine*, 6(4), pp. 370–379.

Lee, D. 2011. *The Pelvic Girdle: An Integration of Clinical Expertise and Research*. 4th ed. Edinburgh: Churchill Livingstone/Elsevier.

Lequesne, M., Mathieu, P., Vuillemin-Bodaghi et al., 2008. Gluteal tendinopathy in refractory greater trochanter pain syndrome: diagnostic value of two clinical tests. *Arthritis & Rheumatism*, 59(2), pp. 241–246.

Lewit, K., 1999. *Manipulative Therapy in Rehabilitation of the Locomotor System*. 3rd ed. Oxford: Butterworth, pp. 26–29.

Loghmani, M. and Whitted, M., 2016. Soft tissue manipulation: a powerful form of mechanotherapy. *Journal Physiotherapy Physical Rehabilitation*, 1(4), p. 122.

Macintyre, J., Johson, C. and Schroeder, E., 2006. Groin pain in athletes. *Current Sports Medicine Reports*, 5(6), pp. 293–299.

Magee, D., 2014. *Orthopedic Physical Assessment*. 6th ed. St Louis: Elsevier/Saunders.

Main, CJ. and George, SZ., 2011. Psychologically informed practice for management of low back pain: future directions in practice and research. *Physical Therapy*, 91(5), pp. 820–824.

McCarthy, C. 2010. *Combined Movement Theory: Rational Mobilization and Manipulation of the Vertebral Column*. Edinburgh: Churchill Livingstone/Elsevier.

Mens, J., Vleeming, A., Snijders, C. et al., 2002. Reliability and validity of hip adduction strength to measure disease severity in posterior pelvic pain since pregnancy. *Spine*, 27(15), pp. 1674–1679.

Mens, J., Damen, L., Snijders, C. et al., 2006. The mechanical effect of a pelvic belt in patients with pregnancy-related pelvic pain. *Clinical Biomechanics*, 21(2), pp. 122–127.

Michael, J., Gyer, G. and Davis, R., 2017. *Osteopathic and Chiropractic Techniques for Manual Therapists*. London and Philadelphia: Singing Dragon.

Morelli, V. and Smith, V. 2001. Groin injuries in athletes. *American Family Physician*, 64(8), pp. 1405–1414.

Naito, H., Yoshihara, T., Kakigi, R. et al., 2012. Heat stress-induced changes in skeletal muscle: heat shock proteins and cell signaling transduction. *Journal Physical Fitness Sports Medicine*, 1(1), pp. 125–131.

Naqvi, U., and Sherman, A., 2021. *Muscle Strength Grading*. [online] PubMed. Available at: <https://pubmed.ncbi.nlm.nih.gov/28613779/> [accessed June 14, 2020].

O'Sullivan, P., 2000. Masterclass. Lumbar segmental 'instability': clinical presentation and specific stabilizing exercise management. *Manual Therapy*, 5(1), pp. 2–12.

Panjabi, M., 1992. The stabilizing system of the spine. Part I. Function, dysfunction, adaptation, and enhancement. *Journal Spinal Disorders*, 5(4), pp. 383–389.

Panzer, D., 1992. The reliability of lumbar motion palpation. *Journal Manipulative and Physiological Therapeutics*, 15(8), pp. 518–524.

Pincus, T., Holt, N., Vogel, S. et al., 2013. Cognitive and affective reassurance and patient outcomes in primary care: a systematic review. *Pain*, 11, pp. 2407–2416.

Ranawat, AS., Guadiana, MA., Slullitel, PA. et al. 2017. Foot progression angle walking test: a dynamic diagnostic assessment for femoroacetabular impingement and hip instability. *Orthopaedic Journal Sports Medicine*, 5(1), p. 2325967116679641.

Reiman, M., Mather, R. and Cook, C., 2015. Physical examination tests for hip dysfunction and injury. *British Journal Sports Medicine*, 49(6), pp. 357–361.

Reiman, M. and Thorborg, K., 2014. Clinical examination and physical assessment of hip joint-related pain in athletes. *International Journal Sports Physical Therapy*, 9(6), pp. 737–755.

Rubinstein, S. and van Tulder, M., 2008. A best-evidence review of diagnostic procedures for neck and low-back pain. *Best Practice & Research Clinical Rheumatology*, 22(3), pp. 471–482.

Sahrmann, S., 2002. *Diagnosis and Treatment of Movement Impairment Syndromes*. Philadelphia: Mosby, p. 63.

Schon, D., 1983. *Reflective Practitioner*. New York: Basic Books.

Serner, A., Weir, A., Tol, J. et al., 2016. Can standardised clinical examination of athletes with acute groin injuries predict the presence and location of MRI findings? *British Journal Sports Medicine*, 50(24), pp. 1541–1547.

Shacklock, M., 2014. *Clinical Neurodynamics: A New System of Musculoskeletal Treatment*. London: Elsevier.

Shan, G. and Westerhoff, P., 2005. Soccer. *Sports Biomechanics*, 4(1), pp. 59–72.

Stuber, K., Lerede, C., Kristmanson, K. et al., 2014. The diagnostic accuracy of the Kemp's test: a systematic review. *Journal Canadian Chiropractic Association*, 58(3), pp. 258–267.

Swärd Aminoff, A., Agnvall, C., Todd, C. et al., 2018. The effect of pelvic tilt and cam on hip range of motion in young elite skiers and nonathletes. *Open Access Journal Sports Medicine*, 9, pp. 147–156.

Tidstrand, J. and Horneij, E., 2009. Inter-rater reliability of three standardized functional tests in patients with low back pain. *BMC Musculoskeletal Disorders*, 10(1), p. 58.

Todd, C., Kovac, P., Swärd, A. et al., 2015. Comparison of radiological spino-pelvic sagittal parameters in skiers and non-athletes. *Journal Orthopaedic Surgery Research*, 10(1), p. 162.

Todd, C., Sward, A. and Agnvall, C., 2016. Clinical spino-pelvic parameters in skiers and non-athletes. *Journal Sports Medicine*, 3(3), p. 22.

van Dieën, J. and de Looze, M., 1999. Directionality of anticipatory activation of trunk muscles in a lifting task depends on load knowledge. *Experimental Brain Research*, 128(3), pp. 397–404.

van Dieën, JH., Selen, LP. and Cholewicki, J. 2003. Trunk muscle activation in low-back pain patients, an analysis of the literature. *Journal Electromyography Kinesiology*, 13(4), pp. 333–351.

Verrall, G., Slavotinek, J., Barnes, P. et al., 2005. Description of pain provocation tests used for the diagnosis of sports-related chronic groin pain: relationship of tests to defined clinical (pain and tenderness) and MRI (pubic bone marrow oedema) criteria. *Scandinavian Journal Medicine Science in Sports*, 15(1), pp. 36–42.

Vleeming, A., Stoeckart, R., Volkers, A. et al., 1990a. Relation between form and function in the sacroiliac joint. *Spine*, 15(2), pp. 130–132.

Vleeming, A., Volkers, A., Snijders, C. et al., 1990b. Relation between form and function in the sacroiliac joint. *Spine*, 15(2), pp. 133–136.

Vleeming, A., Mooney, V. and Stoeckart, R., 2007. *Movement, Stability & Lumbopelvic Pain: Integration of Research and Therapy*. 2nd ed. Edinburgh: Churchill Livingstone, p. 113.

Wainner, R., Whitman, J., Cleland, J. et al., 2007. Regional interdependence: a musculoskeletal examination model whose time has come. *Journal Orthopaedic Sports Physical Therapy*, 37(11), pp. 658–660.

Waldén, M., Hägglund, M. and Ekstrand, J., 2015. The epidemiology of groin injury in senior football: a systematic review of prospective studies. *British Journal Sports Medicine*, 49(12), pp. 792–797.

Walheim, G. and Selvik, G., 1984. Mobility of the pubic symphysis in vivo measurements with an electromechanic method and a roentgen stereophotogrammetric method. *Clinical Orthopaedics Related Research*, 191, pp. 129–135.

Weir, A., Brukner, P., Delahunt, E. et al., 2015. Doha agreement meeting on terminology and definitions in groin pain in athletes. *British Journal Sports Medicine*, 49(12), pp. 768–774.

Youdas, J., Mraz, S., Norstad, B. et al., 2007. Determining meaningful changes in pelvic-on-femoral position during the Trendelenburg test. *Journal Sport Rehabilitation*, 16(4), pp. 326–335.

Chapter 3 structure

Introduction   53

Applied anatomy relating to the thoracopelvic canister   60

Applied anatomy of the functional slings   68

Conclusion   82

Introduction

In this chapter I would like to propose the fundamentals of anatomical knowledge that may be applied in both clinical and sporting environments. As previously mentioned, adopting a pathoanatomical approach to identifying tissue dysfunction has been heavily criticized (Koes et al., 2010), and evidence suggests this approach proves successful, for diagnostic purposes, in only 10–15 percent of cases (Cheung et al., 2009). While I can accept this in principle, my personal experience of working in sport has highlighted the necessity of appreciating the clinical application of anatomy to help inform diagnostic skills. This chapter will provide a general overview of applied anatomy relating to the spino-pelvic-hip complex. If you are looking for a greater, in-depth appreciation of this subject, I recommend the anatomical textbooks included in the reference list at the end of the chapter.

Spinal column

The spinal column (Figure 3.1) has several curvatures in the sagittal plane. The cranial and caudal lordotic curves are separated by the thoracic kyphotic curve (Muyor et al., 2013; Roussouly and Nnadi, 2010). These curvatures must be capable of fulfilling two mechanical requirements: rigidity and plasticity (Kapandji, 1995). The spinal column extends from the base of the skull to the pelvis and consists of a series of vertebral bodies, which increase in size from the cervical to the lumbar region. The cervical region has seven vertebrae, whereas the thoracic region has twelve and the lumbar region five. The sacral region is fused and is composed of five vertebrae. The vertebral column has an anterior pillar and a posterior pillar; the anterior pillar is formed of intervertebral disks and the posterior pillar is comprised of paired facet joints and a vertebral arch, which separates the vertebral bodies (Palastanga, 1997).

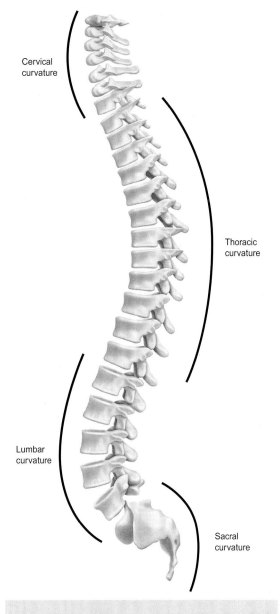

Cervical curvature

Thoracic curvature

Lumbar curvature

Sacral curvature

Figure 3.1
Vertebral column with spinal curvatures.

Vertebra–disk–vertebra, the vertebral motion segment (Figure 3.2) or functional spinal unit (FSU), has a superior and an adjacent inferior vertebra with an intervertebral disk, facet joints and ligamentous attachments. The intervertebral disk (IVD) houses the central nucleus pulposus, the circumferential annulus fibrosis and two hyaline cartilage endplates that connect to the superior and inferior vertebral bodies (Pezowicz et al., 2005; Boos et al., 2002). The different tensile properties of the IVD ensure it can withstand and transfer heavy spinal loads and accommodate spinal motion (Niosi and Oxland, 2004).

The range and type of movement possible between two vertebrae is largely determined by the shape and orientation of the facet joints (Palastanga, 1997). The vertebral column is capable of flexion, extension, lateral flexion and rotation; however, movement within the column varies between regions. For example, in the lumbar spine, the orientation of facet joints is more sagittal (flexion and extension), which limits spinal rotation compared to the thoracic region, where the orientation is more frontal (abduction and adduction), allowing for greater rotation.

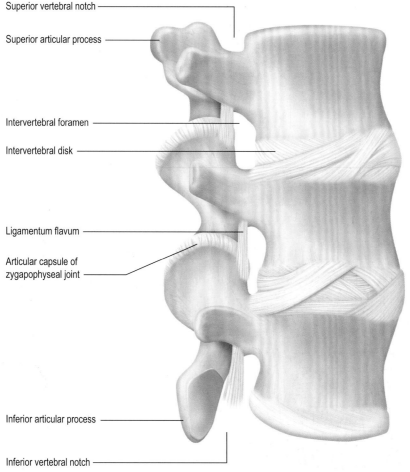

Superior vertebral notch

Superior articular process

Intervertebral foramen

Intervertebral disk

Ligamentum flavum

Articular capsule of zygapophyseal joint

Inferior articular process

Inferior vertebral notch

Figure 3.2
Vertebral motion segment.

The anterior and posterior pillars have different roles. The anterior pillar is static and the posterior pillar is dynamic; there appears to be a functional link between the two pillars, whereby they help absorb compression from passive and active stresses. The multiple structural components of each pillar, interlinked by the complex attachments of ligaments and muscles (Muyor et al., 2013), create the dynamic plasticity of the spinal column.

Spinal alignment is the integration of anatomical regions, which provide shape, position, form and function between the spine, pelvis and hips (Mac-Thiong et al., 2007; Berthonnaud et al., 2005). This integration helps humans to maintain an upright posture, forward gaze and bipedal locomotion, while minimizing energy expenditure (Roussouly and Nnadi, 2010; Berthonnaud et al., 2005; Descamps et al., 1999; Duval-Beaupère et al., 1992). To maintain sagittal spinal balance, the cervical lordosis, thoracic kyphosis and lumbar lordosis are intrinsically related. Analysis of lordosis and kyphosis reveals that the superior arc of the lumbar lordosis is equal to the inferior arc of the thoracic kyphosis. Each curve has the capacity to react to compensate for degenerative changes in the other, allowing humans to maintain a forward gaze (Figure 3.3). In addition, spinal alignment is not just a static entity, but the result of a dynamic evolution in response to mechanical loads.

Studies suggest that spinal curvatures assist with force distribution throughout the spinal column (Hardacker et al., 1997; Uetake et al., 1998). The curvatures are fundamentally related and can influence the form and function of the pelvis and hips (Roussouly and Pinheiro-Franco, 2011; Mac-Thiong et al., 2007; Berthonnaud et al., 2005). A good example is when loss of lumbar lordosis results in a posterior pelvic tilt, with subsequent shortening of the hamstring muscles. This can be compared to an increase in lumbar lordosis, which may lead to an anterior pelvic tilt and the subsequent shortening of the hip flexor and quadricep muscles, or an increase in thoracic kyphosis, which may result in an insufficient lumbar lordosis and increased anterior pelvic tilt (Legaye, 2011).

Pelvic girdle

The pelvic girdle is at the base of the trunk; it supports the abdomen and links the vertebral column to the lower limbs. Kapandji (1995) describes it as "A closed osteo-articular ring, made up of three bony parts and three joints." The two innominate bones are each composed of three bones: the ilium, ischium and pubis. Anteriorly, the symphysis pubis forms the articulation between the innominate bones, whereas posteriorly, the sacroiliac joints (SIJs) form the articulation with the vertebral column (Figures 3.4 and 3.5).

Stability is provided by the conformity of articular surfaces, joint capsules and the ligaments that bind the joints together, in combination with the muscles that act around them (Palastanga, 1997). This arrangement of joint shape and capsule, ligaments and muscles, providing stability, holds true for all joints in the body. When function is reviewed, the innominate bone should be considered as a lower-extremity bone, and the two SIJs as the junction of the vertebral axis and the lower extremities. Palastanga (1997) suggested that one key role of the pelvis during the gait cycle (walking) is the translation from side to side by a rotatory movement at the lumbosacral articulation.

Sacroiliac and pubic symphysis joints

The two sacroiliac joints (SIJs), as previously described in Chapter 2, are designed to provide stability through form and force closure and help counterbalance the load of the upper and lower extremities (Vleeming et al., 1990ab) (Figure 3.6). These joints are covered by two different kinds of cartilage: hyaline cartilage on the sacral surface and fibrocartilage on the iliac surface (Vleeming et al., 2012). Range of motion (ROM) in the SIJs is small, estimated to be between 0.4 and 4.3° of rotation, and 0.7 mm of translation (Jacob and Kissling, 1995). The pubic symphysis is a secondary cartilaginous joint located between the two pubic bones; similarly to the SIJ, a small ROM occurs in the pubic symphysis. It is estimated that 2 mm of vertical motion and 3° in the coronal axis are available (Walheim and Selvik, 1984).

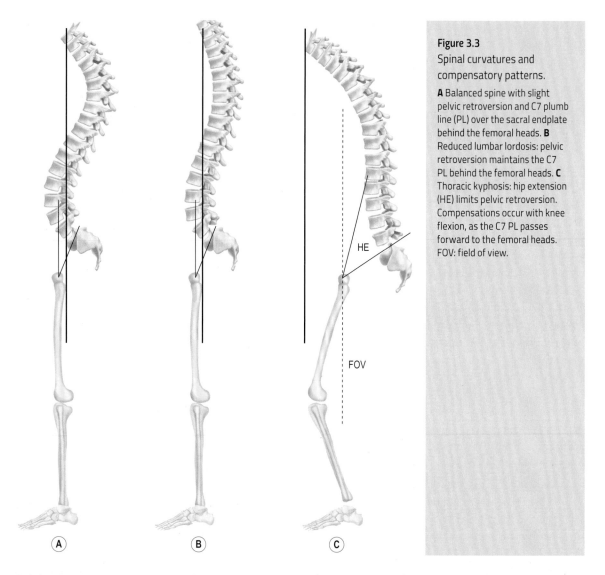

Figure 3.3
Spinal curvatures and compensatory patterns.

A Balanced spine with slight pelvic retroversion and C7 plumb line (PL) over the sacral endplate behind the femoral heads. **B** Reduced lumbar lordosis: pelvic retroversion maintains the C7 PL behind the femoral heads. **C** Thoracic kyphosis: hip extension (HE) limits pelvic retroversion. Compensations occur with knee flexion, as the C7 PL passes forward to the femoral heads. FOV: field of view.

Pelvic parameters

An understanding of the pelvic parameters is useful if the pelvic girdle is viewed as the functional link between the torso and the lower extremities (Figure 3.7). Pelvic parameters are a concept that is used to compare three different measurements by means of pelvic geometry:

- pelvic incidence (PI)
- pelvic tilt (PT)
- sacral slope (SS).

These parameters have been shown to play a significant role in maintaining balanced spinal alignment in the sagittal plane (Roussouly and Pinheiro-Franco, 2011; Jackson et al., 2000; Duval-Beaupère et al., 1992). The anatomical relationship between the spine and the pelvis assists in the modulation of an erect posture, through the pelvic girdle balancing lumbar lordosis with hip joint extension (Roussouly and Pinheiro-Franco, 2011).

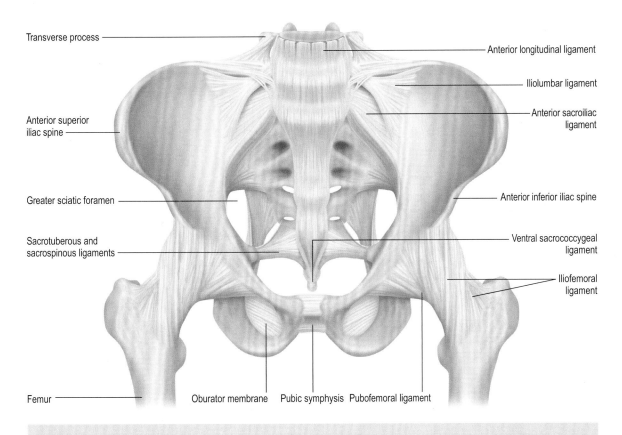

Transverse process

Anterior longitudinal ligament

Iliolumbar ligament

Anterior sacroiliac ligament

Anterior superior iliac spine

Greater sciatic foramen

Anterior inferior iliac spine

Sacrotuberous and sacrospinous ligaments

Ventral sacrococcygeal ligament

Iliofemoral ligament

Femur

Oburator membrane · Pubic symphysis · Pubofemoral ligament

Figure 3.4
Anterior view of the pelvic girdle.

Pelvic incidence (PI)

PI is a morphological parameter relating to the angle measured from a perpendicular line to the mid-point of the sacral plate, extending to the center of the femoral head. It is a fixed parameter that remains constant after an individual attains skeletal maturity. The angle of PI is described as an essential anatomical pelvic parameter and is used to classify the morphology and functional context of how the pelvis is behaving, especially with regard to pelvic compensation (Roussouly and Pinheiro-Franco, 2011; Jackson et al., 2000; Duval-Beaupère et al., 1992).

Studies show that in an asymptomatic low back pain (LBP) population, PI values range from 35° to 85° with

an approximate mean of 52° (Roussouly et al., 2005). Those with a low PI angle are shown to have a more vertical-shaped pelvis, a lower tolerance for producing posterior PT and reduced lumbar lordosis (Boulay et al., 2006; Guigui et al., 2003; Marty et al., 2002; Duval-Beaupère et al., 1998). Those with a high PI angle have been shown to have a more horizontal-shaped pelvis, a greater tolerance for posterior active PT (Roussouly et al., 2003) and increased lumbar lordosis (Boulay et al., 2006; Guigui et al., 2003; Marty et al., 2002; Duval-Beaupère et al., 1998). There is evidence that dynamic changes in PT have a clinical significance for hip joint mobility. For example, posterior PT will increase hip

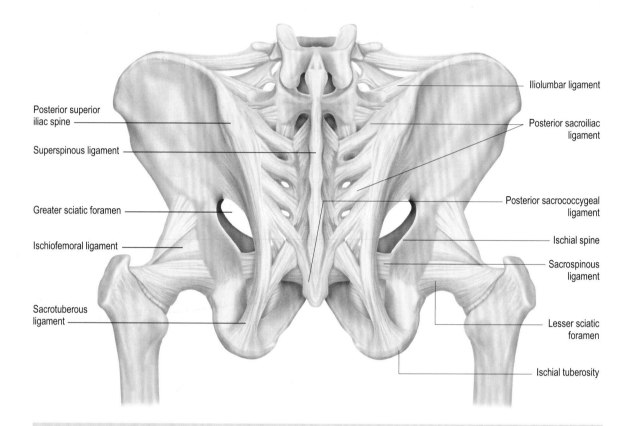

Figure 3.5
Posterior view of the pelvic girdle.

joint flexion and internal rotation, while anterior PT reduces hip joint flexion and internal rotation (Swärd Aminoff et al., 2018; Ross et al., 2014).

Pelvic tilt (PT)

The angle of PT is measured from a perpendicular line starting at the center of the femoral head and extending to the mid-point of the sacral plate. It is a positional (functional) parameter. The mean value of the PT angle is approximately 12° within a 5–30° range (Van Royen et al., 1998). In addition, as this is a compensatory angle, PT changes with posture, decreasing with anterior pelvic rotation and increasing with posterior pelvic rotation.

Sacral slope (SS)

SS is also a positional parameter; the angle is measured from the superior endplate of S1 and a horizontal axis (Boulay et al., 2006; Guigui et al., 2003). The mean value for the SS angle is approximately 40° in a 20–65° range (Labelle et al., 2004; Van Royen et al., 1998). Similarly to PT, the SS is a compensatory angle and adapts to posture. There is a geometrical relationship between the morphological PI angle and the functional parameters PT and SS, which results in the equation PI=PT+SS (Van Royen et al., 2000).

A coordinated dynamic muscular action is required for an individual to sit from standing. The action of

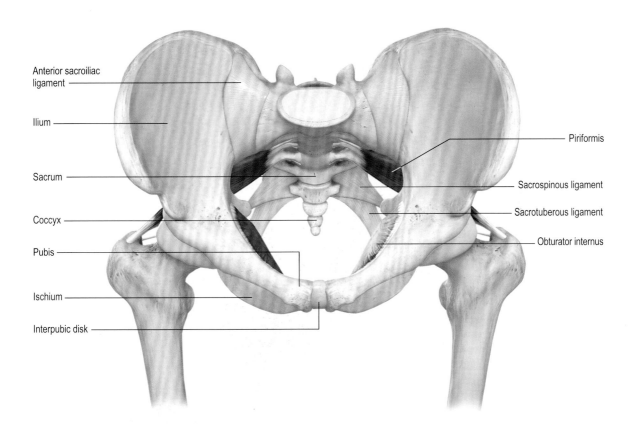

Figure 3.6
Sacroiliac joint and pubic symphysis.

Anterior sacroiliac ligament

Ilium

Sacrum

Coccyx

Pubis

Ischium

Interpubic disk

Piriformis

Sacrospinous ligament

Sacrotuberous ligament

Obturator internus

sitting involves hip flexion, knee flexion, ankle dorsiflexion and lumbar flexion. During this movement, the PI angle remains constant, while the PT angle increases and the SS angle decreases accordingly. This would mean that an individual's ability to perform active PT has huge ramifications for their ability to engage in normal functional movement. Similarly, any variability that reduces active PT may increase an individual's vulnerability to LBP, hip and groin-related pain.

Hip joint

The hip joint is a synovial ball and socket joint. The architecture of the hip joint allows for the round femoral head to articulate with the concave acetabulum of the pelvis (Figure 3.8). Movement in all three planes is possible at the hip joint: sagittal (flexion and extension) and frontal (abduction and adduction) are combined with transverse (internal and external rotation). These movements have a similar ROM to that available at the glenohumeral joint but due to the larger loads imposed on the hip joint there is a greater demand for stability. Micro-instability may occur from subtle anatomical abnormalities of the acetabular labrum, or from ligamentous laxity and weakening of the joint capsule and surrounding muscles (Shu and Safran, 2011; Boykin et al., 2011). The joint capsule is reinforced with strong ligaments to enhance stability

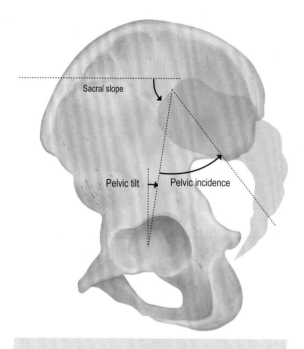

Figure 3.7
Geometrical evaluation of pelvic parameters.

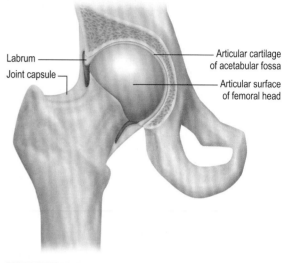

Figure 3.8
Architecture of the hip joint.

but also functions to influence the ROM within the joint. Anteriorly, the iliofemoral ligament limits extension; inferiorly, the pubofemoral ligament limits abduction; and posteriorly, the ischiofemoral ligaments limit internal rotation.

The joint capsule is further reinforced posteriorly by the annular ligament, which attaches to the greater trochanter of the femur and runs circumferentially around the neck of the femur, helping to resist distraction forces on the joint (Ito et al., 2009). Hip joint stability is enhanced by the labrum, which is a fibrocartilaginous structure located along the bony circumference of the acetabulum. Inferiorly, the anterior and posterior portions are connected by the transverse ligament but superiorly it runs continuously with the acetabular cartilage. The labrum increases the effective depth of the socket and the coverage of the femoral head, increasing both joint stability and congruity (Ferguson et al.,

2000). An intra-articular connection between the pelvis and femur occurs through the ligamentum teres. This arises from the transverse ligament and inferior aspect of the acetabulum and inserts into the fovea capitis on the head of the femur, functioning as an intrinsic hip joint stabilizer (Cerezal et al., 2010).

Applied anatomy relating to the thoracopelvic canister

From a holistic standpoint, it is essential to include the thoracic spine when evaluating the lumbar spine. While the thoracic spine may appear relatively stiff, it actually has more joint articulations than the lumbar spine. This knowledge suggests the lumbar spine should be interpreted as the more stable structure, while, by comparison, the thoracic spine may be interpreted as more mobile. Observing from the side makes it easy to visualize the thoracolumbar spine and ribcage, which sit on the pelvis like a canister. The muscles and fascia form the walls of the canister, while the top and bottom of the canister are composed of the fascial layers that form the thoracic diaphragm and pelvic floor, respectively (Figure 3.9). The thoracopelvic canister must be capable of maintaining two functional roles: mobility and stability.

- Mobility is required to perform the normal activities of daily life, in addition to the dynamic actions necessary in a sporting environment.

- Stability is required when performing functional tasks that need stiffness and rigidity. For example,

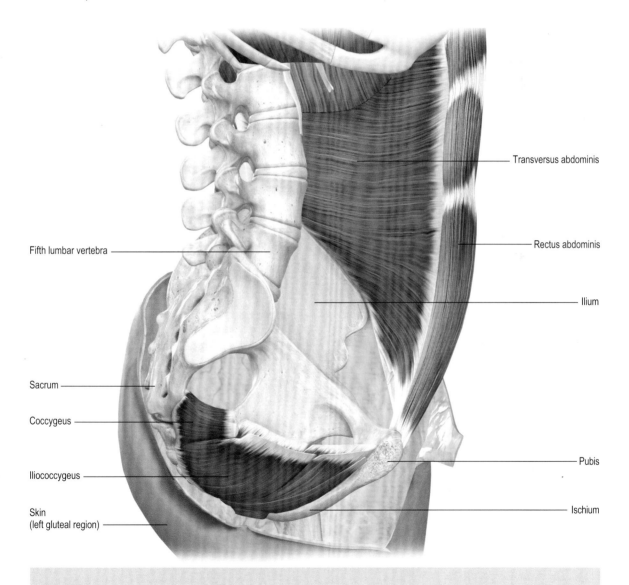

Figure 3.9
The thoracopelvic canister.

lifting heavy weights, such as in a deadlift, may require bracing of the thoracopelvic canister, with the resulting stability enabling the effective transfer of forces during the lifting action.

The muscles essential for maintaining the function of the thoracopelvic canister include (Figures 3.10–3.12):

- diaphragm
- psoas major and the smaller psoas minor (if present)
- quadratus lumborum
- transversus abdominis
- external and internal obliques
- pelvic floor.

Diaphragm

The diaphragm (see Figure 3.10) is the primary muscle of ventilation, separating the thorax from the abdomen into two distinct cavities (Osar and Bussard, 2016). Innervation is from the phrenic nerve and the intercostal nerves. Optimal or diaphragmatic breathing involves the synchronized motion of the diaphragm, upper and lower ribcage and abdomen (Kaminoff, 2006; Pryor and Prasad, 2002). As well as playing a primary role in breathing, the diaphragm also performs a postural role. If one of its functions is challenged, it may influence the capacity to perform the other (Hodges et al., 2007). For example, movement pattern dysfunctions have been shown to be more prevalent in patients with breathing pattern disorders (Bradley and Esformes, 2014; Roussel et al., 2007; O'Sullivan et al., 2002), which suggests that altered respiratory mechanics are associated with changes in movement.

Psoas major

Psoas major (see Figure 3.10) originates from the anterior lateral surfaces of the vertebral bodies and the transverse processes of vertebrae T12–L5 and the intervertebral disk L1–4. Superiorly, the fascia attaches to the crura of the diaphragm and is continuous with transversus abdominis (Myers, 2014; Gibbons, 2005ab). Posteriorly, the fascia from the diaphragm blends with quadratus lumborum and psoas (Myers, 2014; Bordoni and Zanier, 2013). The psoas major muscle plays a huge role in connecting the torso with the lower extremities.

Distally, psoas major integrates by fascial attachments to the pelvic floor, transversus abdominis and internal oblique, before descending inferiorly to insert into the lesser trochanter of the femur.

Innervation to the anterior fascicles is through a branch of the femoral nerve, and the posterior fascicles are innervated from the ventral rami of T12 to L1–5 with or without S1 (Myers, 2014). The fibers are unipennate, approximately 3–8 cm in length anteriorly and 3.5 cm posteriorly. When contracted, the length of the anterior fascicles shortens by 1–2.5 cm and the posterior fascicles shorten by 1–1.5 cm. Contrary to popular belief, psoas major is unable to produce sufficient force to be an effective hip flexor (Gibbons, 2007). This may challenge current views held by some clinicians, who view psoas major as predominantly a hip flexor. In my opinion, this is a misconception that has been poorly taught for many years and I challenge those clinicians not to let prior education get in the way of continued learning and development.

Psoas minor, if present, originates from the 11th and 12th thoracic vertebrae, adjoining ribs and intervertebral disks, and inserts into the superior ramus of the pelvis; it may be absent in approximately 40–50 percent of the population (Yoshio et al., 2002).

Iliacus

Although iliacus is not technically a muscle that forms part of the thoracopelvic canister, I am mentioning it at this point because of its integral relationship with psoas major. Anatomy textbooks often describe psoas and iliacus together as the iliopsoas muscle. I also used to teach this many years ago and this view can be explained by the similarity of their insertions. The iliacus muscle (see Figure 3.10) originates from the iliac fossa and descends inferiorly over the iliopubic eminence of the pelvis before it inserts into the lesser trochanter of the femur. Iliacus

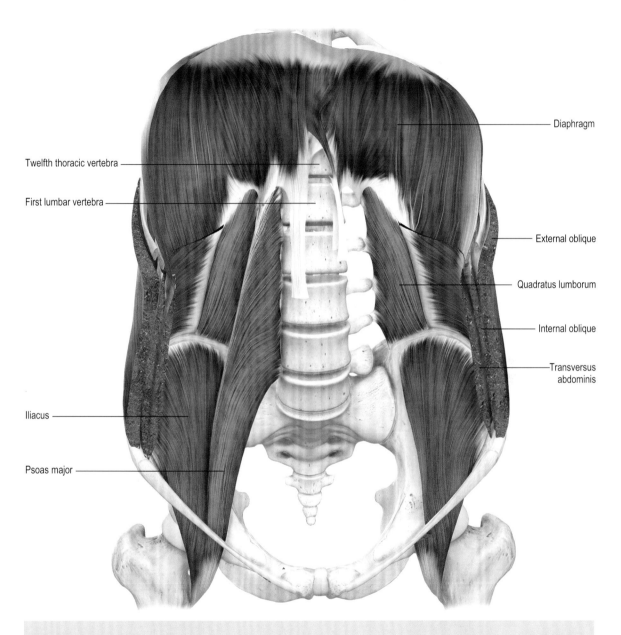

Diaphragm

Twelfth thoracic vertebra

First lumbar vertebra

External oblique

Quadratus lumborum

Internal oblique

Transversus abdominis

Iliacus

Psoas major

Figure 3.10
Thoracopelvic canister posterior muscles.

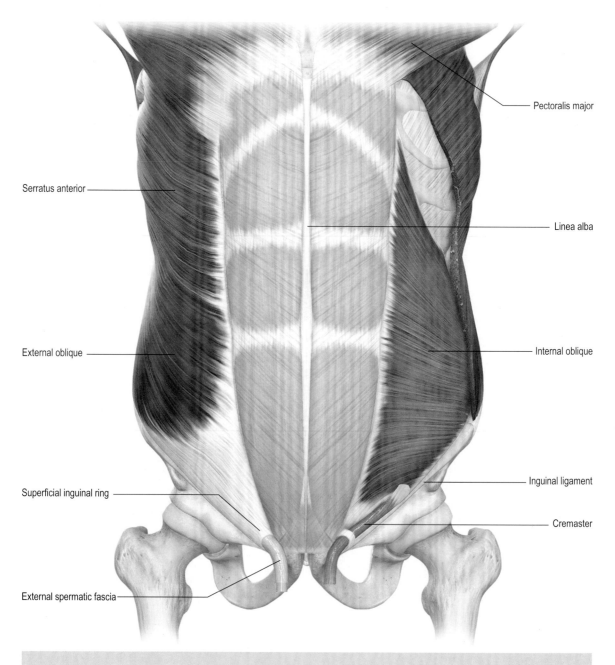

Pectoralis major

Serratus anterior

Linea alba

External oblique

Internal oblique

Inguinal ligament

Superficial inguinal ring

Cremaster

External spermatic fascia

Figure 3.11
Thoracopelvic canister anterior muscles.

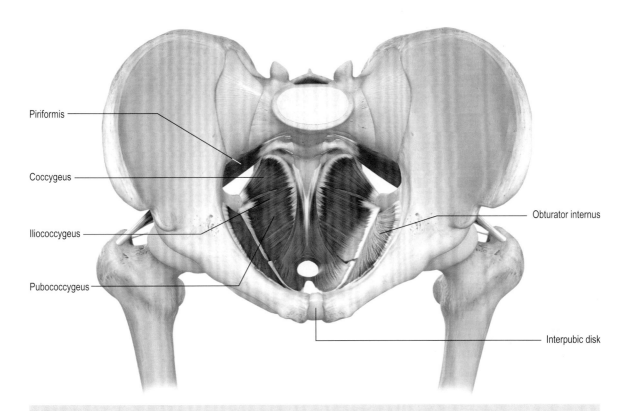

Piriformis

Coccygeus

Iliococcygeus

Pubococcygeus

Obturator internus

Interpubic disk

Figure 3.12
Muscles of the pelvic floor.

and the psoas each have their own individual insertions (McGill, 2007). Innervation of iliacus is from femoral nerve L2–4, and as this is different from the psoas muscle, it may indicate that they function independently from each other (Retchford et al., 2013).

Quadratus lumborum

Quadratus lumborum (QL) (see Figure 3.10) is a deep quadrilateral-shaped muscle that is positioned in the posterior abdominal wall. Originating from the ilio-lumbar ligament and the internal aspect of the posterior iliac crest, the fibers of QL run superiorly and insert into the medial half of the lower border of the 12th rib and

transverse process of the lumbar vertebrae. Innervation is from the T12 subcostal nerve, L1 iliohypogastric nerve and ilioinguinal nerve and from branches of the L2–3 ventral rami (Bordoni and Varacallo, 2020). The QL stabilizes the 12th rib and diaphragm during inspiration, ipsilateral contraction of the QL creates lateral flexion of the spine and bilateral contraction produces extension of the spine.

Transversus abdominis

Transversus abdominis (TA) (see Figure 3.9) is the deepest layer of the abdominal musculature. The fibers of this layer of muscle run horizontally and anteriorly. It originates from the deep surface of the lower six costal cartilages, lumbar fascia, the anterior two-thirds of the iliac crest and the lateral third of the inguinal ligament. The TA inserts into the xiphoid process, linea alba and symphysis pubis. The lowest fibers, similar to the internal oblique (discussed later), help to form the conjoint tendon, which is located at the pubic crest and pectineal line (Gray, 1989). Like the internal oblique, they are innervated by the lower six thoracic nerves, the iliohypogastric and ilioinguinal. The function of the TA is to stabilize the lumbar spine nerves in preparation for movement and to assist in breathing and compression to offset tensile forces (Lee, 2011).

Rectus abdominis

Rectus abdominis (RA) (see Figure 3.11) is located across the entire length of the anterior abdominal wall and its two halves are separated by the linea alba. Originating from the anterior aspect of the symphysis pubis and the pubic crest, it inserts into the costal cartilage of ribs and the xiphoid process. The aponeuroses of the external and internal obliques and TA enclose the RA muscle and collectively form the rectus sheath. Innervation is from the lower six thoracic nerves (Drake et al., 2015; Gray, 1989). The RA is an important postural muscle. When the pelvis is fixed, the RA performs lumbar flexion; when the ribcage is fixed, the contraction of the RA assists with posterior pelvic tilt. It also plays a role in forced expiration and increase of intra-abdominal pressure (Drake et al., 2015).

External oblique

The external oblique (EO) (see Figure 3.11) is the largest and most superficial layer of the abdominal muscles. It originates from the external surface and inferior borders of the lower right ribs. The fibers from the lower ribs run inferiorly, inserting into the anterior half of the iliac crest. The middle and upper fibers run inferiorly, inserting anteriorly into the xiphoid process, linea alba, pubic crest and pubic tubercle (Gray, 1989). They are innervated by the lower six thoracic nerves and the iliohypogastric and

ilioinguinal nerves (Mantle et al., 2004). Functioning together, they can assist with spinal flexion, or unilaterally, with lateral flexion and contralateral rotation (Drake et al., 2015).

Internal oblique

The internal oblique (IO) (see Figure 3.11) layer lies deeper than the EO, arising from the thoracolumbar fascia, the anterior two-thirds of the iliac crest and the lateral two-thirds of the inguinal ligament. The muscle fibers run superomedially, inserting into the inferior borders of the lower three ribs and their costal cartilages, the xiphoid process, the linea alba and the symphysis pubis. The lowest tendinous fibers blend with the transversus abdominis fibers to form the conjoint tendon. They are innervated by the lower six thoracic nerves, the iliohypogastric nerve and the ilioinguinal nerve (Mantle et al., 2004). Functioning unilaterally, contraction of the IO results in ipsilateral lateral flexion and rotation of the trunk. The IO also assists with compression of internal viscera and forced expiration.

Pelvic floor

The pelvic floor (Figure 3.12) is composed of a number of muscles that form a dome-shaped sheet separating the pelvic cavity from the perineal region (Bharucha, 2006). This broad muscular and fascial sling extends from the symphysis pubis to the coccyx, and from one lateral side wall to the other.

Levator ani

The two levator ani muscles are thin, broad structures that stretch across the pelvic floor. While the two muscles unite in the midline, they are separated by the prostate in males and the urethra and vagina in females. Levator ani comprises two distinct parts, pubococcygeus and iliococcygeus. Pubococcygeus arises from the dorsal surface of the pubis and fascia of obturator internus and inserts into the anococcygeal body and the sides of the coccyx. Iliococcygeus arises from the fascia over obturator internus and inserts into the anococcygeal body and sides of the coccyx (Ashton-Miller and DeLancey, 2007).

Coccygeus

This muscle lies posteriorly to levator ani. Flat and triangular in shape, coccygeus forms a sheet that stretches from the ischial spine and inserts into the lower two segments of the sacrum and the upper two segments of the coccyx and the supraspinous ligament (Ashton-Miller and DeLancey, 2007).

The main function of coccygeus and levator ani is to support the abdominal and pelvic viscera, and to help maintain continence, bowel and bladder movement, and sexual activity (Mantle et al., 2004).

Piriformis

Piriformis is a flat, pyramidal muscle that originates from the anterior aspect of S2,3 and S4, as well as the ventral capsule of the SIJ, the anterior aspect of the posterior superior iliac spine (PSIS) and sometimes the upper part of the sacrotuberous ligament. The muscle descends through the greater sciatic notch to insert into the superior margin of the greater trochanter of the femur (Oatis, 2009). Innervation is from the sacral plexus L5 and S1–2.

The function of piriformis is to perform external rotation when the hip is in extension, abduction when the hip is in flexion, and a slight lateral pelvic tilt; it also assists with posterior pelvic tilt (Oatis, 2009). Acting as an important stabilizer of the SIJ, piriformis is important in functional activities: for example, from a seated position abducting and externally rotating the hip to lift the leg out of a car prior to standing up, and during the loading phase of gait, maintaining balance and stabilizing the pelvis when the trunk is rotated (Palastanga, 1997).

Obturator internus

Obturator internus is a deep intrinsic muscle of the hip that forms part of the lateral wall of the pelvis. Originating from the inferior margin of the superior ramus and from the pelvic surface of the obturator membrane, it exits the pelvis through the lesser sciatic foramen and inserts onto the greater trochanter of the femur (Ramirez et al., 2018). Innervation is by the obturator internus nerve (L5–S2). The functions of obturator internus include external rotation of the hip and abduction of the hip; it also acts as a hip joint stabilizer (Byrne et al., 2017; Hodges et al., 2014).

Clinical implications

 Dysfunction in any of the muscles that form the thoracopelvic canister will provoke an increased compensatory mechanism. This, in turn, increases global muscle recruitment, leading to postural changes and compromised breathing patterns (Bradley and Esformes, 2014; Roussel et al., 2007; O'Sullivan et al., 2002). Eventually, this affects the entire kinetic chain and can result in increased stiffness of the thoracic spine and ribcage, with inhibition of the deep muscles that are responsible for respiration and stabilization (Umphred, 2007). The potential musculoskeletal consequences of progressive changes affecting the kinetic chain are as follows:

- Compensatory hypermobile patterns commonly observed in the thoracolumbar and lumbosacral junctions. These often result in non-functional movements and loss of segmental motor control. The lumbar extensor muscles produce a posterior shear force at L4–5 and an anterior shear force at L5–S1. Clinically, this may present as an extension "hinging" of the lower lumbar spine (Sahrmann, 2002).

- Reflexive stiffness leading to a loss of joint centration affecting the hip joints, and psoas inhibition with over-activity in the tensor fasciae latae (TFL) and rectus femoris muscles (Oscar, 2012).

- Compromised respiratory mechanics leading to over-recruitment of the accessory respiratory muscles of ventilation. If diaphragmatic breathing is compromised, every movement becomes altered and inefficient (Lewit, 1999).

There are many clinical implications for the psoas muscle: it plays a stability role in producing force on the lumbar spine, through axial compression (Bogduk, 2005), assists with posterior rotation across the SIJs and influences the stability of the pelvic girdle. When the lower extremity is fixed, psoas assists with spinal flexion and, eccentrically, helps to control spinal extension. In a functional exercise such as a deep squat, psoas helps to control spinal flexion (Comerford and Mottram, 2012). The psoas and multifidus muscles function collectively to create stability in the lumbar spine. Patients with LBP and sciatica have been shown to have a decreased cross-sectional area, with atrophy of psoas and multifidus (Barker et al., 2000b).

Across the hip joint, psoas acts a stabilizer, creating acetabular compression of the femoral head in the acetabulum (Richardson et al., 2004). This supports the movement of hip flexion, with psoas stabilizing the femoral head and eccentrically controlling hip extension. In respiration, psoas assists breathing mechanics by stabilizing the thoracolumbar spine to aid optimal diaphragm function (Osar and Bussard, 2016). Psoas and iliacus can be described as functional antagonists – two muscles that oppose each other but function together cooperatively (Osar and Bussard, 2016). Across the hip joint, psoas aligns and controls the femoral head in the acetabulum, while iliacus flexes the hip joint. Contraction of iliacus creates an anterior tilt of the pelvis, which subsequently increases the lumbar lordosis and spinal curvature. Compare this with the contraction of psoas, which tilts the pelvis posteriorly and helps compress the lumbar spine.

Evidence of the clinical implications of pelvic floor dysfunction suggests that muscle insufficiency may be a significant factor in involuntary urine loss, as experienced during an abrupt increase in intra-abdominal pressure, such as when coughing, sneezing, lifting or laughing (Nygaard et al., 2008; Sapsford, 2004). Developing muscle synergies within the pelvic floor is an important mechanism to promote continence, by resisting increased intra-abdominal pressure (Junginger et al., 2010). Coactivation of the pelvic floor, acting in synergy with muscles of the abdominal cavity, contributes to spinal stiffening and stability (Bussey et al., 2019; Pool-Goudzward et al., 2004; Sapsford, 2004; Sapsford and Hodges, 2001).

Applied anatomy of the functional slings

Within a theory of human movement science, spinal rotation has been proposed as being fundamental. Gracovetsky (2008) suggests that the efficient harmony within the muscle systems plays a significant part in human movement, with the limbs amplifying the movement originating in the muscles and joints of the spine. Gracovetsky's "spinal engine" theory is reinforced by showing that a quadruple amputee could walk on the bones at the base of the pelvis, by using the spinal engine as a way to propel themselves forward.

The anatomy slings play a huge role in an individual's ability to generate efficient dynamic activity (Osar and Bussard, 2016). Combining superficial muscle activity with that of the deep muscles is considered to be an integral component of this movement approach. The anatomy slings are comprised of numerous tissues, muscles, fascia, tendons and ligaments, which function collectively to provide stability and mobility. Muscle contraction generates force that is transmitted through other structures in the sling. The resultant force vector is what enables movement to occur distally, away from the origin of the initial muscle that contracted. Myofascial slings may often overlap and interconnect with other slings, which may determine the change in the force vectors required for appropriate dynamic movement. If the force vectors are balanced, then they provide optimal alignment of the skeletal system. Imbalances within the force vectors may result in altered tension within the myofascial slings, creating malalignment and increased vulnerability to injury, due to loss of stability during either static or dynamic tasks (Lee, 2011). To illustrate this, let's view the anterior and posterior oblique slings as having an agonist and antagonist relationship. When one sling contracts, the other sling may be controlling or stabilizing the movement that is being produced: for example, in maintaining optimal load transfer when running uphill or stepping up onto a box.

Anterior oblique sling

The anterior oblique sling (Figure 3.13) helps to control the stability of the pubic symphysis and controls rotation of the thoracic spine and pelvis. The muscles that assist with this are serratus anterior, the external obliques and the contralateral internal obliques and adductors. It has been observed that activity in the anterior oblique system increases during acceleration from walking to running (Basmajian, 1967). Multi-directional sports, such as tennis, soccer, rugby, hockey and basketball, place great demands on the anterior oblique sling because it contributes significantly to acceleration, deceleration and spinal and hip rotation, to facilitate changing direction (Brookbush, 2013). Clinically, it is not uncommon to find dysfunctions in this sling, as a result of soft tissue overload from accelerating and decelerating activities. For example, in my experience, patients and athletes presenting with adductor-related groin pain often also present clinically with over-activity on palpation of the EO, and inhibition and pain on clinical testing to the contralateral IO.

Adductors

The adductor muscles (Figure 3.14) are situated between the flexor and extensor muscles of the femur. They originate from the lower pelvic bone and attach to the lower femur and around the knee. They are comprised of pectineus, adductor brevis, adductor longus, adductor magnus and gracilis. Innervation is from the obturator nerve L2, L3, L4. While most anatomy texts define these muscles as hip joint adductors, they have a vast myofascial network of attachments, suggesting that they may have a much more functional role (Oscar, 2012). For example, the adductor complex may assist the lateral sling (TFL and gluteus medius and minimus)

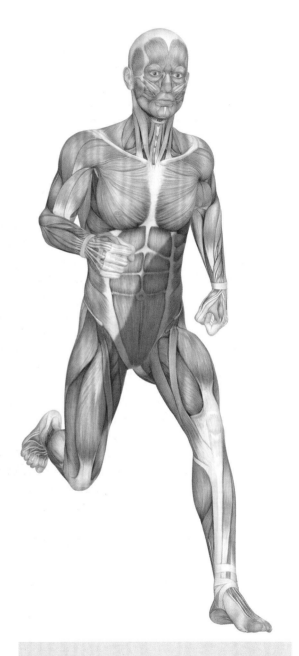

Figure 3.13
Anterior oblique sling.

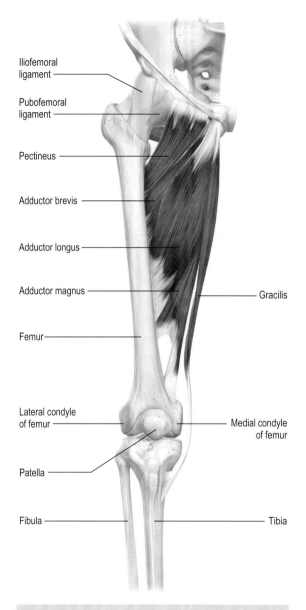

Figure 3.14
The adductors.

Labels on figure:
- Iliofemoral ligament
- Pubofemoral ligament
- Pectineus
- Adductor brevis
- Adductor longus
- Adductor magnus
- Femur
- Lateral condyle of femur
- Patella
- Fibula
- Gracilis
- Medial condyle of femur
- Tibia

with frontal plane pelvic stability during single-leg stance and, as previously mentioned, assist the anterior oblique sling to provide transverse plane stabilization during rotational movements. Furthermore, in the transverse plane, the adductor brevis, longus and magnus muscles may also contribute by eccentrically controlling internal rotation of the femur at the hip joint (Leighton, 2006).

A deeper anatomical understanding of the structures that cross the groin was suggested by Falvey et al. (2009). One approach that I often use to locate the soft tissue structures crossing this region is to take the example of a compass that I visually superimpose over the pubic bone, as illustrated in Figure 3.15.

The EO muscle connects with the contralateral adductor longus, via the superficial layer of the anterior pubic ligament located anteriorly to the pyramidalis muscle. The superficial inguinal ring forms the mediocaudal end of the inguinal canal and can be found superolaterally to the pubic tubercle. The mediocaudal fibers of the IO and transversus abdominis (conjoint tendon) run caudally, attaching to the inferior section of the rectus sheath and, with the EO, form the mediosuperior border of the inguinal ring.

There are three functional connections between the abdominal and adductor muscles:

- external oblique with the contralateral adductor longus
- pyramidalis with the ipsilateral adductor longus
- rectus abdominis with the ipsilateral gracilis.

Pyramidalis helps to provide tension in the abdominal aponeurosis, assisting the rectus abdominis muscle to transfer force to the oblique and transverse muscles (Schilders et al., 2017).

Clinical implications

Although these structures can be described separately, it is clear that these anatomically blended close fasciae associations assist each

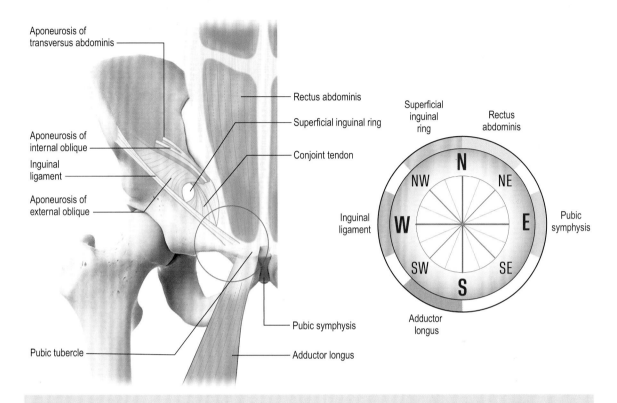

Figure 3.15
Structures that cross the groin.

other with functional movement. It is thought that the numerous myofascial connections control and transfer forces between the upper body and lower extremities during sports actions. In doing so, they influence and control pelvic movement (Robertson et al., 2009). If we consider the groin as the anterior junction of the spino-pelvic-hip complex, it would be expected that the complexity of this region's anatomy might often lead to clinical presentations that involve multiple entities. While it is logical to break down structures (adductor, inguinal, abdominal, psoas-related groin pain) and test them in relation to their anatomical capabilities, this very often produces a mixed bag of results and can be confusing. My clinical experience has led me to believe that

pain may not always be a good indicator of pathology (Orchard et al., 2000). For example, an obturator muscle strain is often associated with kicking sports. The mechanism of injury is normally overuse and the presentation is often initial pain in the groin, similar to the pain associated with an adductor muscle injury (Byrne et al., 2017; Khodaee et al., 2015). Strengthening obturator internus not only may to help prevent this but also may play a significant role in maintaining normal function of the pelvic floor (Tuttle et al., 2016).

Posterior oblique sling

The posterior oblique sling (Figure 3.16) helps to control the stability of the lumbosacral junction (LSJ) and

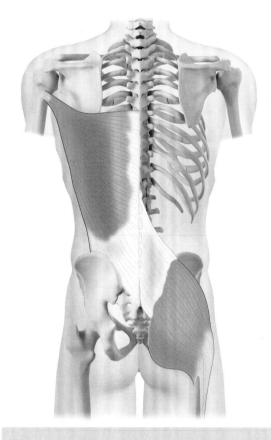

Figure 3.16
The posterior oblique sling.

stabilize the lumbar spine and SIJ (Lee, 2011). The proposition is that energy is stored in the GMx and latissimus dorsi as they lengthen during the gait cycle. Kinetic energy is then released when the muscles contract from their respective lengthening phase (Vleeming et al., 2007). It is believed that the gait cycle is more efficient as a result of this proposed mechanism, which reduces the unnecessary expenditure of energy from the surrounding muscles involved in locomotion (Chek, 2011; Vleeming et al., 2007).

Gluteus maximus

Gluteus maximus (GMx) (see Figure 3.16) is the most powerful muscle in the body. It is quadrilateral in shape and consists of two layers. The upper attachment is to the gluteal surface of the ilium, behind the posterior gluteal line, the posterior border of the ilium and the adjacent part of the iliac crest. It originates from the side of the coccyx, the posterior aspect of the sacrum and the upper part of the sacrotuberous ligaments. The upper fibers attach to the aponeurosis of the erector spinae, while the deep fibers originate from the fascia that covers gluteus medius (GMed). The fibers pass inferiorly and anteriorly to the upper end of the femur, attaching to the iliotibial tract and the gluteal tuberosity of the femur. GMx innervation is from the inferior gluteal nerve L5, S1,2. The skin covering the muscle is supplied by L2 and S3 (Palastanga, 1997).

Latissimus dorsi

Latissimus dorsi (see Figure 3.16), a broad, flat, triangular muscle of the back, has extensive attachments from the spinous processes of the 7th thoracic to 5th lumbar vertebrae, iliac crest, thoracolumbar fascia and the lower three to four ribs; it inserts into the bicipital groove of the humerus (Drake et al., 2014). Innervation is from the thoracodorsal nerve C6–C8. The primary actions of latissimus dorsi are adduction, extension and internal rotation of the glenohumeral joint, and it has a role in scapular function (Calais-German, 1993). Secondary actions are to assist longissimus thoracis and iliocostalis lumborum with

the SIJ, combined with contributing to control of rotation through the spine, pelvis, hips and lower extremity. The structures involved with this sling are latissimus dorsi, the thoracolumbar fascia and the contralateral gluteus maximus (GMx). During the propulsive gait phase, the GMx and the contralateral latissimus dorsi contract concentrically, from lengthened positions, resulting in extension of the arm, while at the same time propelling the opposite leg. When both these mechanisms operate together, they create a coupled contraction of the GMx and the contralateral latissimus dorsi (Chek, 2011). The subsequent tension in the thoracolumbar fascia helps to spinal extension, rectus abdominis with spinal flexion, QL and rectus abdominis with spinal lateral flexion, and rectus femoris with anterior and lateral pelvic tilt. Latissimus dorsi also participates in breathing mechanics, during deep inhalation and forced exhalation (Schünke et al., 2007).

Thoracolumbar fascia

The thoracolumbar fascia (TLF) is a broad, diamond-shaped area of connective tissue covering the lumbar, thoracic and sacral regions and enclosing the intrinsic muscles of the erector spinae (Figure 3.17). The TLF

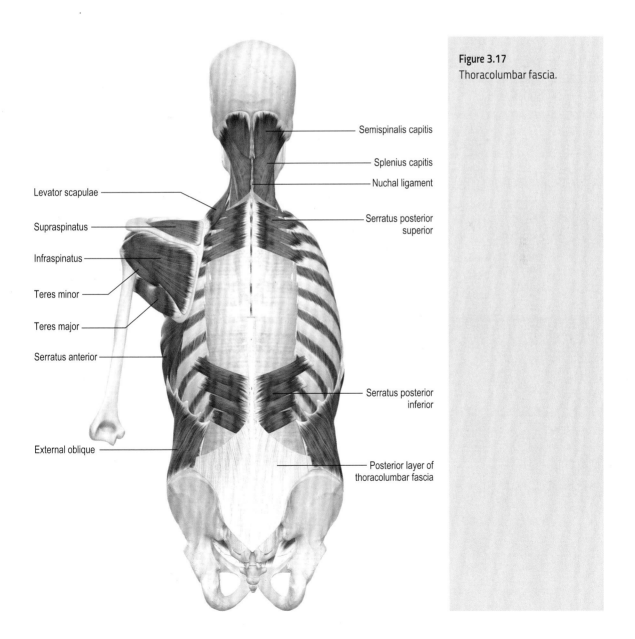

Figure 3.17
Thoracolumbar fascia.

Semispinalis capitis

Splenius capitis

Nuchal ligament

Serratus posterior superior

Levator scapulae

Supraspinatus

Infraspinatus

Teres minor

Teres major

Serratus anterior

Serratus posterior inferior

External oblique

Posterior layer of thoracolumbar fascia

comprises several layers. In the thoracic region it forms a thin covering for the extensor muscles of the vertebral column, attaching medially to the thoracic vertebrae and laterally to the ribs. In the lumbar region it is attached to the vertebral bodies but has a strong aponeurosis that is connected laterally to the muscles of the abdominal wall. Medially, it separates into three layers: the anterior and middle layers which surround the QL and the middle and posterior layers which form a sheath to envelop the erector spinae and multifidus. Inferiorly, it attaches to the iliolumbar ligament, the iliac crest and the SIJ; due to its extensive attachments to the vertebral bodies, the TLF also attaches to the supraspinous and interspinous ligaments, the joint capsule and the facet joints (Barker et al., 2004a).

Clinical implications

The TLF performs two distinct roles: stabilization and load transfer (Vleeming et al., 2012; 1995). Stabilization occurs through the increased fascial tension that develops when the vertebral column is flexed (Gracovetsky, 1986). When the spine is placed in full range of flexion, the TLF increases in length by about 30 percent (Gracovetsky et al., 1981). The expansion in length is accompanied by a stiffening in width, and this creates a deformation of the tissue, with reduced muscle activation required when it recovers into an extended position (Gracovetsky et al., 1981). Load transfer occurs in functional movement by coordinated contralateral motions of the upper and lower extremities, such as those seen in the posterior oblique sling, during activities such as running and sprinting (Vleeming et al., 1995).

Clinically, it is fairly common to find dysfunction occurring in this sling: for example, that arising from GMx weakness or inefficiency, leading to over-activity in the hamstring muscles as they attempt to stabilize the pelvis. Another common clinical presentation is a patient with LBP or SIJ pain caused by lack of shoulder ROM from over-activity in latissimus dorsi, which has affected the neuromuscular efficiency of the contralateral GMx. Primarily an extensor of the hip joint, the GMx is also capable of rotating the thigh laterally during extension. The lower fibers can adduct the thigh, while the upper fibers may help in abduction. The deeper and lower fibers of the GMx can help to draw the femoral head posteriorly within the acetabulum. Functionally, the GMx can also be seen as a synergist to psoas, performing hip joint centration (Gibbons, 2007; 2005ab). The GMx forms part of the posterior oblique sling through its attachment to the contralateral latissimus dorsi muscle, assisting with load transfer between the spine, the shoulder complex and the lower extremity.

Posterior longitudinal sling

Functionally, the posterior longitudinal sling (Figure 3.18) contributes to allowing sagittal plane movement, while helping to influence local stability (Comerford and Mottram, 2012). The sling consists of the erector spinae, multifidus, thoracolumbar fascia, sacrotuberous ligament and biceps femoris muscle. Stability of the SIJ is promoted by a chain reaction triggered by musculature contraction within this sling. The superficial erector spinae aponeurosis descends from the thoracic spine and attaches to the sacrum and ilium. Contraction of the superficial erector spinae creates lumbar extension and promotes stability across the SIJ. The superficial multifidus muscles assist in spinal extension, and the deep multifidus muscles increase segmental spinal stability. The erector spinae and multifidus are enclosed within a "fascial envelope" derived from the thoracolumbar fascia. When these muscles contract, they increase tension in the thoracic canister and help spinal stability. Contraction of the biceps femoris muscle produces tension in the sacrotuberous ligament, which stabilizes the SIJ (Vleeming et al., 2007).

Erector spinae

The erector spinae mass (Figure 3.19) comprises the iliocostalis, longissimus and spinalis muscles, which are divided into two groups: superficial and deep. The superficial group consists of the lateral iliocostalis and the

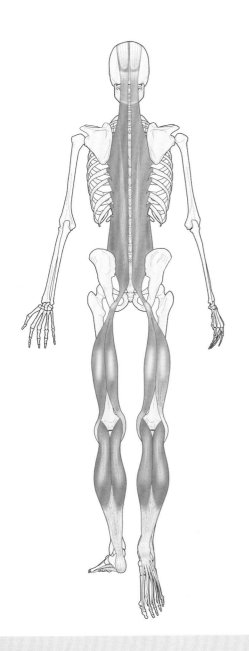

Figure 3.18
Posterior longitudinal sling.

medial longissimus muscles. They originate from the pelvis and run superiorly to insert into the thoracolumbar fascia and the ribs. Although these muscles do not attach directly to the lumbar spine, they are capable of producing between 40 and 80 percent of its extension movement as a direct result of their optimal lever arm (Bogduk et al., 1992). Contraction of the superficial erector spinae muscles will also produce anterior pelvic tilt.

The deep erector spinae group originates from the ilium and the deep surface of the thoracolumbar fascia, inserting into the transverse processes of the lower lumbar vertebrae. Contraction of the deep erector spinae group produces a compression and posterior shear force on the lower lumbar spine, and more importantly, helps to prevent an anterior shear force. Activity in these muscles assists with counterbalance of the anterior shear force from the deep abdominal wall muscles, specifically psoas.

Multifidus

Multifidus (Figure 3.20) is the deepest and most medial of the spinal muscles that assist with producing spinal stiffness and stability. There are two groups within the muscle: superficial and deep (Mosley et al., 2002). In the superficial group, the fibers originate from the spinous processes and extend inferiorly, across three vertebral segments. The fibers in the deep group originate from the posterior aspect of the spine and insert two segmental levels below. The multifidus fibers that originate from the lower lumbar segments insert into the pelvis, sacrum and SIJ, at the base of the spine. Innervation is from the dorsal rami of the associated spinal nerve. The deep fibers of multifidus maintain segmental and postural control, and demonstrate anticipatory movement, similarly to what is observed in the TA (Richardson et al., 2004). The superficial fibers create an extension movement to the lumbar spine.

Biceps femoris

Biceps femoris (see Figure 3.18), along with semimembranosus and semitendinosus, forms the posterior

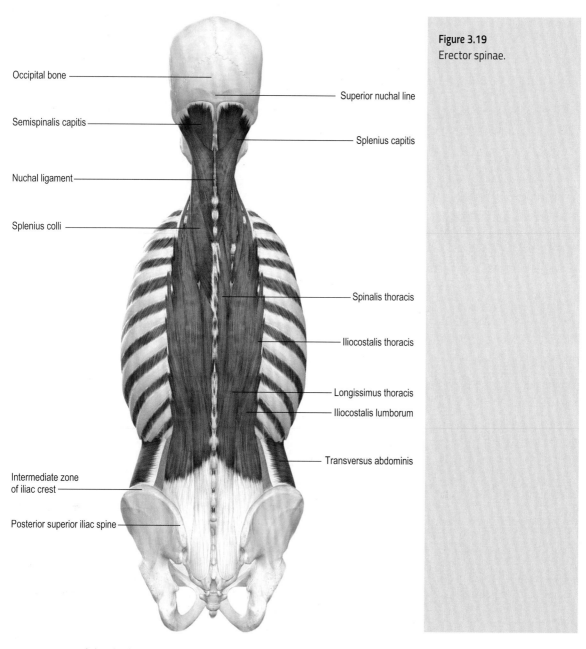

Occipital bone

Superior nuchal line

Semispinalis capitis

Splenius capitis

Nuchal ligament

Splenius colli

Spinalis thoracis

Iliocostalis thoracis

Longissimus thoracis

Iliocostalis lumborum

Transversus abdominis

Intermediate zone
of iliac crest

Posterior superior iliac spine

Figure 3.19
Erector spinae.

compartment of the thigh; they are collectively referred to as the hamstrings (Netter, 2014). More specifically, biceps femoris originates from two "heads." The "long head" arises from the ischial tuberosity, sharing a common origin with semitendinosus, and the "short head"

from the linea aspera and the lateral supracondylar line of the femur. The muscle travels inferiorly to insert into the lateral fibular head (Netter, 2014). Innervation of the "short head" is from the common peroneal component of the sciatic nerve, and the "long head" is innervated by

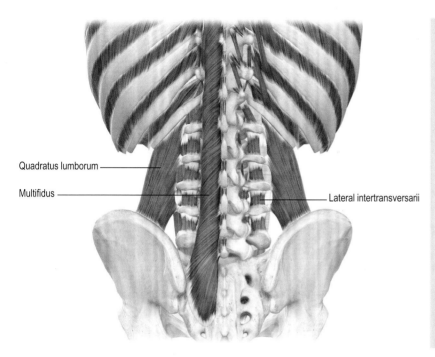

Quadratus lumborum ———————

Multifidus ————————

———————— Lateral intertransversarii

Figure 3.20
Multifidus.

the tibial component of the sciatic nerve (L5–S2) (Netter, 2014). Fascial attachments connect biceps femoris with the sacrotuberous ligament, and these muscles, together with the contralateral erector spinae and thoracolumbar fascia, form the posterior longitudinal sling.

The "long head" functions to flex the knee, extend the hip, and externally rotate the lower leg when the knee joint is flexed; it assists with external rotation when the hip is in extension. The "short head" externally rotates the lower leg when the knee is flexed (Netter, 2014; Palastanga, 1997). The "long head" provides posterior stability to the pelvis, and both heads contribute to rotational stability of the knee (Mofidi, 2019).

Clinical implications

The posterior longitudinal sling contains strong postural muscles that should be capable of activating throughout daily activity, contributing to movement and stability. The contribution to postural stability provided by this

sling is adjusted in accordance with the task or activity performed. Greater levels of stability are required to perform a deadlift exercise, compared to bending forward to tie your shoelaces. Clinically, on forward flexion testing of the lumbar spine, the erector spinae muscles should help to control increased translation motion in the lower lumbar segments. In an upright posture, the lumbar extensor muscles produce a posterior shear force at L1–4 and an anterior shear force at L5. Manual therapy treatment, or exercises that would provoke or increase compressive forces and extension-related symptoms in the lower lumbar spine, are contraindicated, as they may lead to an increase in translational motion and instability (McGill, 1998; Bogduk et al., 1992).

It is not unusual to find dysfunction within the posterior longitudinal sling that affects the stability role of the lumbar spine and SIJ, contributing to pain and movement restriction. Common examples are as follows:

- The cross-sectional area of the lumbar multifidus and psoas muscles has been shown to be different due to atrophy in patients with unilateral LBP (Woodham et al., 2014; Barker et al., 2004b).

- An inhibition, or weakness and tenderness on palpation, of biceps femoris is commonly seen in athletes as a result of training overload.

- Biceps femoris, through its attachment to the sacrotuberous ligament, contributes to deceleration; if biceps femoris becomes shortened, it will limit the degree of active pelvic tilt (Mofidi, 2019).

- A creep deformation of the erector spinae and thoracolumbar fascia may occur as a result of end-range loading: for example, when an athlete (or other patient) sits in sustained spinal flexion on a long-haul flight.

Lateral sling

The function of the lateral sling (Figure 3.21) is to provide frontal plane stability and to assist with dynamic movement and stability around the pelvis and hip joint. The QL works in synergy with the contralateral TFL, GMed, GMin and adductors, forming a lateral sling that maintains frontal plane stability of the pelvis (Wallden, 2014; Lee, 2011). During functional movement, the correct positioning of the pelvic girdle is to remain neutral in all three planes – coronal, sagittal and transverse – for example, in single-leg stance activities. The neutral position ensures that the forces placed through this region are evenly distributed, avoiding unnecessary strain occurring in any particular structure. A commonly observed clinical presentation is control failure of the lateral sling on single-leg stance. This failure results in a hip drop, or positive Trendelenburg sign. The impact of this dysfunction will be examined in Chapter 5.

Gluteus medius

Gluteus medius (GMed) (Figure 3.22) is naturally fanshaped and fills the space between the iliac crest and the greater trochanter of the femur. The muscle plays a significant role in walking, running and weight-bearing on one limb (Kapandji, 1995). The upper attachment is to the gluteal, or lateral, surface of the ilium, between the posterior and anterior gluteal lines. Covered by a strong layer of fascia from the deep surface, the GMed has a firm attachment to this fascia and often shares the posterior aspect of the fascia with the GMx. The posterior and middle fibers of the muscle pass inferiorly and anteriorly, and the anterior fibers pass inferiorly and posteriorly. The fibers come together to attach to the superolateral side of the greater trochanter of the femur. GMed innervation is from the superior gluteal nerve L4–5, S1. The skin covering the muscle is mainly supplied from L1–2 (Palastanga, 1997).

Gluteus minimus

Although gluteus minimus (GMin) is the smallest of the gluteal muscles, it takes the largest attachment from the gluteal surface of the ilium. The upper attachment arises from the gluteal surface of the ilium, in front of the anterior and above the inferior gluteal lines. Its fibers pass inferiorly, posteriorly and slightly laterally to form a tendon, which attaches to a small depression on the anterosuperior aspect of the greater trochanter of the femur. GMin innervation is from the superior gluteal nerve L4–5, S1. The skin covering the muscle is mainly supplied by L1 (Palastanga, 1997).

When the pelvis is fixed, the GMed will contract to pull the greater trochanter of the femur upwards into abduction. If the insertion of the muscle is fixed, it will pull the wing of the ilium down, producing a downward tilting of the pelvis to the same side and raising the pelvis on the opposite side. GMed anterior fibers, acting from a fixed pelvis, will produce a medial rotation of the femur. The posterior fibers are capable of assisting the GMx in lateral rotation (Kapandji, 1995).

If the upper part of the pelvis is fixed, contraction of the GMin will cause the femur to abduct. Medial rotation can also occur, due to the femoral attachment situated laterally to the fulcrum of the hip joint. An element of lateral rotation may take place with contraction of the most posterior fibers of GMin in assisting GMx (Kapandji, 1995).

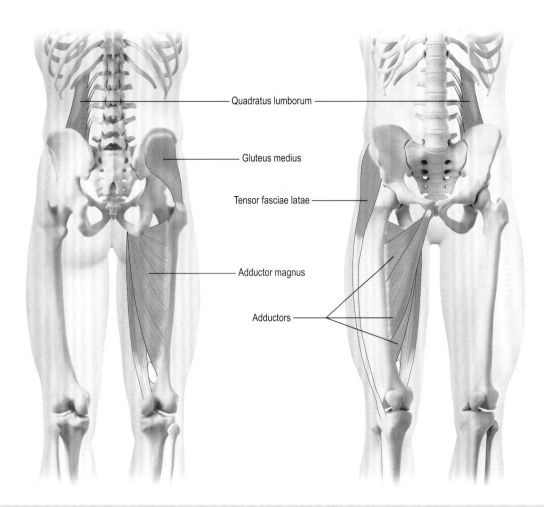

Figure 3.21
Lateral sling.

Tensor fasciae latae

The tensor fascia latae muscle (TFL) (Figure 3.23) is located anterolateral to the hip joint and the superficial fibers of the GMed. Originating from the anterior superior iliac spine (ASIS) and anterior aspect of the iliac crest, together with the GMx, it blends with the iliotibial tract and inserts into the lateral tibial condyle (Moore et al., 2014; Drake et al., 2014). The TFL is innervated by the superior gluteal nerve, which originates from the segments of L4–5 (Miller et al., 2009). The TFL has many functions. Together with the GMx and the iliotibial band, it assists centration of the head of the femur in the acetabulum and contributes to knee joint stability. As a prime mover, in hip joint medial rotation, it acts as an accessory muscle of hip flexion and abduction, and as part of the iliotibial tract it contributes to external rotation of the

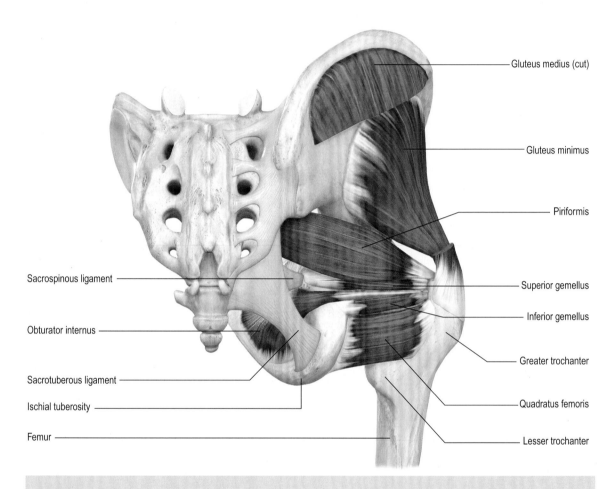

Figure 3.22
Deep gluteal muscles.

leg. In gait, it assists the lateral stability mechanism of the pelvis, linking the pelvis, femur and tibia during weight-bearing movements (Oscar, 2012; Palastanga, 1997).

Clinical implications

 Many athletes and patients present with lack of lateral control of the pelvic girdle, which may present, for example, as lateral transla-tion or anterior rotation of the ilium on the femur in single-leg stance. If the lateral stability mechanism

is considered as three different muscle layers, the superfi-cial layer consists of the upper fibers of the GMx and TFL, the intermediate layer consists of the GMed and piriformis, and the deep layer consists of the GMin (Grimaldi et al., 2009). Whereas prolonged inactivity has been shown to lead to atrophy of the deep stabilizing muscles (Grimaldi et al., 2009), no atrophy was observed in muscles of the super-ficial layer. There is evidence of a similar pattern of selec-tive atrophy in patients with degenerative changes in the hip joint (Grimaldi et al., 2009). Clinically, I often identify

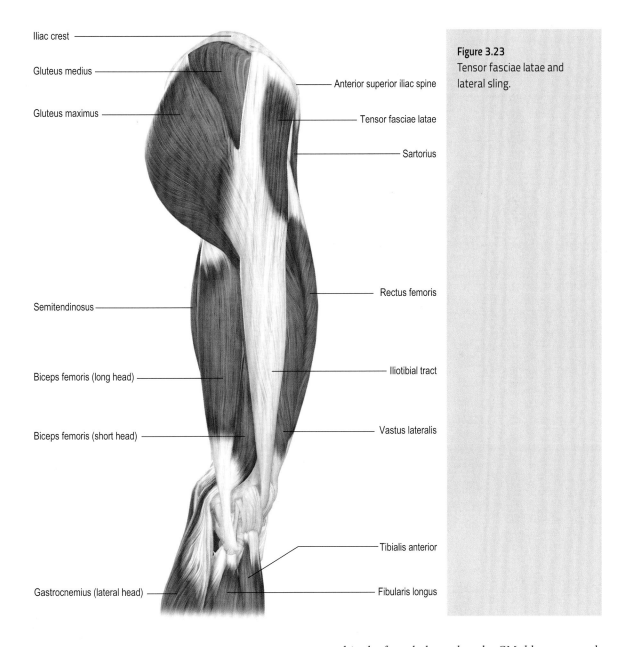

Iliac crest

Gluteus medius

Gluteus maximus

Anterior superior iliac spine

Tensor fasciae latae

Sartorius

Rectus femoris

Semitendinosus

Iliotibial tract

Biceps femoris (long head)

Biceps femoris (short head)

Vastus lateralis

Tibialis anterior

Gastrocnemius (lateral head)

Fibularis longus

Figure 3.23
Tensor fasciae latae and lateral sling.

inhibition of the deep and intermediate layers, resulting in GMed inhibition and over-activation of the TFL muscle. It is not uncommon to find tender points (TnPs) and trigger points (TrPs) within this superficial layer. The TFL often becomes over-active and dominant in the sagittal plane when weakness or inhibition of the psoas is apparent,

and in the frontal plane when the GMed becomes weak or inhibited. The TFL's ability to act as a strong hip joint internal rotator may lead to increased femoral anteversion, often observed in single-leg stance. This will increase the lateral pull on the knee, which in turn may cause patella tracking issues and lead to over-pronation of the foot.

Conclusion

This chapter has provided an anatomical overview of the spino-pelvic-hip complex. I have made a conscious decision to simplify some aspects, to demonstrate how application of anatomical knowledge in the sporting and clinical environments is a fundamental component of my work. My rationale is straightforward: there are many anatomical textbooks available that offer more detailed descriptions and explanations, and it is my fervent hope that this chapter will whet your appetite for further knowledge. In the next chapter, I will discuss pain, pathology and dysfunction in the spino-pelvic-hip complex, so please read on!

References

Ashton-Miller, JA. and DeLancey, JOL., 2007. Functional anatomy of the female pelvic floor. *Annals New York Academy of Sciences*, 1101(1), pp. 266–296.

Barker, K., Shamley, D. and Jackson, D., 2000. Changes in the cross-sectional area of multifidus and psoas patients with unilateral back pain: the relationship to pain and disability. *Clinical Journal Sports Medicine*, 10(4), pp. 239–244.

Barker, PJ., Briggs, CA. and Bogeski, G., 2004a. Tensile transmission across the lumbar fasciae in unembalmed cadavers: effects of the various muscle attachments. *Spine*, 29, pp. 129–138.

Barker, K., Shamley, D. and Jackson, D., 2004b. Changes in the cross-sectional area of multifidus and psoas in patients with unilateral back pain. *Spine*, 29(22), pp. E515–E519.

Basmajian, JV., 1967. *Muscles Alive: Their Functions Revealed by Electromyography*. 2nd ed. Baltimore: Williams & Wilkins.

Berthonnaud, E., Dimner, J. and Roussouly, P. et al., 2005. Analysis of the sagittal balance of the spine and pelvis using shape and orientation parameters. *Journal Spine Disorders*, 18(1), pp. 40–47.

Bharucha, AE., 2006. Pelvic floor: anatomy and function. *Neurogastroenterology and Motility*, 18(7), pp. 507–519.

Bogduk, N., 2005. *Clinical Anatomy of the Lumbar Spine and Sacrum*. 4th ed. Elsevier: New York.

Bogduk, N., Macintosh, J. and Peracy, M., 1992. A universal model of the lumbar back muscles in an upright position. *Spine*, 17(8), pp. 897–913.

Boos, N., Weissbach, S., Rohrbach, H. et al., 2002. Classification of age-related changes in lumbar intervertebral discs: Volvo Award in basic science. *Spine*, 27(23), pp. 2631–2644.

Bordoni, B. and Varacallo, M., 2020. *Anatomy, Abdomen and Pelvis, Quadratus Lumborum*. [Updated 2018 Dec 19]. In: StatPearls [Internet]. Treasure Island, FL: StatPearls Publishing; Jan–. Available at: <https://www.ncbi.nlm.nih.gov/books/NBK535407/> [accessed February 11, 2022].

Bordoni, B. and Zanier, E., 2013. Anatomic connections of the diaphragm: influence of respiration on the body system. *Journal Multidisciplinary Healthcare*, 3(6), pp. 281–291.

Boulay, C., Tardieu, C., Hecquet, J. et al., 2006. Sagittal alignment of spine and pelvis regulated by pelvic incidence: standard values and prediction of lordosis. *European Spine Journal*, 15(4), pp. 415–422.

Boykin, R., Anz, A., Bushnell, B. et al., 2011. Hip instability. *Journal American Academy Orthopaedic Surgery*, 19(6), pp. 340–349.

Bradley, H. and Esformes, J., 2014. Breathing pattern disorders and functional movement. *International Journal Sports Physical Therapy*, 9(1), pp. 28–39.

Brookbush, B., 2013. *Intrinsic Stabilization Subsystem*. Available at: <http://brentbrookbush.com/intrinsic-stabilization-subsystem> [accessed February 11, 2022].

Bussey, ND., Aldabe, D., Riberio, DC. et al., 2019. Is pelvic floor dysfunction associated with development of transient low back pain during prolonged standing? A protocol. *Clinical Medicine Insights: Women's Health.* DOI:10.1177/1179562X19849603.

Byrne, C., Alkhayat, A., O'Neil, P. et al., 2017. Obturator internus muscle strains. *Radiology Case Reports*, 12(1), pp. 130–132.

Calais-German, B. 1993. *Anatomy of Movement*. Seattle: Eastland Press.

Cerezal, L., Kassarjian, A. and Canga, A., 2010. Anatomy, biomechanics, imaging, and management of ligamentum teres injuries. *RadioGraphics*, 30, pp. 1637–1651.

Chek, P., 2011. *Core Stability: The Outer Unit*. International Association of Athletics Federations/New Studies in Athletics (IAAF/NSA) 1-2.00.

Cheung, KM., Karppinen, J., Chan, D. et al., 2009. Prevalence and pattern of lumbar magnetic resonance imaging changes in a population study of one thousand forty-three individuals. *Spine*, (5), pp. 24–35.

Comerford, M. and Mottram, S., 2012. The management of uncontrolled movement. In: *Kinetic Control*. Melbourne: Elsevier Australia.

Descamps, H., Commare, M., Marty, C. et al., 1999. Modifications des angles pelviens, dont l'incidence pelvienne, au cours de la croissance humaine. *Biometrie Humaine et Anthropologie*, 17, pp. 59–63.

Drake, R., Vogl, A. and Mitchell, A., 2014. *Gray's Anatomy for Students*. 3rd ed. Philadelphia: Churchill Livingstone/Elsevier.

Duval-Beaupère, G., Schmidt, C. and Cosson, P., 1992. A barycentre-metric study of sagittal shape and pelvis: the conditions required for an economic standing position. *ANN Biomedical Engineering*, 20, pp. 451–462.

Duval-Beaupère, G., Legaye, J., Hecquet, J. et al., 1998. Pelvic incidence: a fundamental parameter for three-dimensional regulation of spinal sagittal curves. *European Spine Journal*, 7, pp. 99–103.

Falvey, EC., Franklyn-Miller, A. and McCrory, PR., 2009. The groin triangle: a patho-anatomical approach to the diagnosis of chronic groin pain in athletes. *British Journal Sports Medicine*, 43(3), pp. 213–220. DOI:10.1136/bjsm.2007.042259.12.

Ferguson, S., Bryant, J., Ganz, R. et al., 2000. The influence of the acetabular labrum on hip joint cartilage consolidation: a poroelastic finite element model. *Journal Biomechanics*, 33(8), pp. 953–960.

Gibbons, S., 2005a. *Integrating the psoas major and deep sacral gluteus maximus muscles into the lumbar cylinder model.* Proceedings of 'The Spine': World Congress on Manual Therapy, October 7–9, Rome, Italy.

Gibbons, S., 2005b. *Assessment and Rehabilitation of the Stability Function of the Psoas Major and the Deep Sacral Gluteus Maximus Muscles.* Ludlow: Kinetic Control.

Gibbons, S., 2007. Assessment and rehabilitation of the stability function of the psoas major. *Manuelle Therapie*, 11, pp. 177–187.

Gracovetsky, S., 1986. Determination of safe load. *British Journal Industrial Medicine*, 43 (2), pp. 120–133.

Gracovetsky, S., 2008. *The Spinal Engine.* Montreal, Canada. Available at: <gracovetsky@videotron.ca> [accessed February 11, 2022].

Gracovetsky, S., Farfan, HF. and Lamy, C., 1981. The mechanism of the lumbar spine. *Spine*, 6, pp. 249–262.

Gray, H., 1989. *Gray's Anatomy.* 37th ed. Edinburgh: Churchill Livingstone.

Grimaldi, A., Richardson, C., Stantonb, W. et al., 2009. The association between degenerative hip joint pathology and the size of the gluteus medius, minimus and piriformis muscles. *Manual Therapy*, 14(6), pp. 605–610.

Guigui, P., Levassor, N., Rillardon, L. et al., 2003. Physiological value of pelvic and spinal parameters of sagittal balance: analysis of 250 healthy volunteers. *Revue de Chirurgie Orthopédique et Réparatrice de l'Appareil Moteur*, 89, pp. 496–506.

Hardacker, J., Shuford, R., Capicotto, R. et al., 1997. Radiographic standing cervical segmental alignment in adult volunteers without neck problems. *Spine*, 22, pp. 1472–1480.

Hodges, P., Sapsford, R. and Pengel, L., 2007. Postural and respiratory functions of the pelvic floor muscles. *Neurourology Urodynamics*, 26: pp. 362–371.

Hodges, PW., McLean, L. and Hodder, J., 2014. Insight into the function of the obturator internus muscle in humans: observations with development and validation of an electromyography recording technique. *Journal Electromyography and Kinesiology*, 24(4), pp. 489–496.

Ito, H., Song, Y., Lindsey, D. et al., 2009. The proximal hip joint capsule and the zona orbicularis contribute to hip joint stability in distraction. *Journal Orthopaedic Research*, 27(8), pp. 989–995.

Jackson, R., Kanemura, T., Kawakami, N. et al., 2000. Lumbopelvic lordosis and pelvic imbalance on repeated standing lateral radiographs of adult volunteers and untreated patients with constant low back pain. *Spine*, 25(5), pp. 575–586.

Jacob, H. and Kissling, R., 1995. The mobility of the sacroiliac joints in healthy volunteers between 20 and 50 years of age. *Clinical Biomechanics*, 10(7), pp. 352–361.

Junginger, B., Baessler, K., Sapsford, R. et al., 2010. Effect of abdominal and pelvic floor tasks on muscle activity, abdominal pressure and bladder neck. *International Urogynecology Journal*, 21, pp. 69–71.

Kaminoff, L., 2006. What yoga therapists should know about the anatomy of breathing. *Internal Journal Yoga Therapy*, 16, pp. 67–77.

Kapandji, I., 1995. *The Physiology of the Joints. The Trunk and Vertebral Column.* Vol. 2. Edinburgh: Churchill Livingstone.

Khodaee, M., Jones, D. and Spitter, J., 2015. Obturator internus and obturator externus strain in a high school quarterback. *Asian Journal Sports Medicine*, 6(3), p. e23481.

Koes, BW., van Tulder, M., Lin, CW., et al., 2010. An updated overview of clinical guidelines for the management of non-specific low back pain in primary care. *European Spine Journal*, (19), pp. 2075–2094.

Labelle, H., Roussouly, P., Berthonnaud, E. et al., 2004. Spondylolisthesis, pelvic incidence and spine pelvic balance: a correlation study. *Spine (Phila Pa 1976)*, 29(18), pp. 2049–2054.

Lee, D. 2011. *The Pelvic Girdle.* 4th ed. Edinburgh: Churchill Livingstone/Elsevier.

Legaye, J., 2011. *Analysis of the Dynamic Sagittal Balance of the Lumbo-Pelvi-Femoral Complex.* Biomechanics in Applications, Dr Vaclav Klika (ed.), InTech. Available at: <https://www.intechopen.com/chapters/19659>.

Leighton RD., 2006. A functional model to describe the action of the adductor muscles at the hip in the transverse plane. *Physiotherapy Theory and Practice*, 22(5), pp. 251–262.

Lewit, K., 1999. *Manipulative Therapy in Rehabilitation of the Locomotor System.* 3rd ed. Oxford: Butterworth, pp. 26–29.

Mac-Thiong, J., Labelle, H., Bertonnaud, E. et al., 2007. Sagittal spinopelvic balance in normal children and adolescents. *European Spine Journal*, 16, pp. 227–234.

Mantle, J., Haslam, J. and Barton, S., 2004. *Physiotherapy in Obstetrics and Gynecology*. 2nd ed. Edinburgh: Butterworth Heinemann.

Marty, C., Boisaubert, B., Descamps, H. et al., 2002. The sagittal anatomy of the sacrum among young adults, infants, and spondylolisthesis patients. *European Spine Journal*, 11, pp. 119–125.

McGill, S., 1998. Low back exercises: evidence for improving exercise regimens. *Physical Therapy*, 78, p. 784.

McGill, S., 2007. *Low Back Disorders: Evidence-based Prevention and Rehabilitation*. 2nd ed. Champaign, IL: Human Kinetics.

Miller, A., Heckert, KD. and Davis, BA., 2009. The 3-Minute Musculoskeletal & Peripheral Nerve Exam. New York: Demos Medical Publishing, pp. 116–117.

Mofidi, A., 2019. Bilateral snapping biceps femoris tendon: a case report and review of the literature. *European Journal Orthopaedic Surgery & Traumatology*, 29(5), pp. 1081–1087.

Moore, KL., Dalley, AF. and Agur, AM., 2014. *Clinically Oriented Anatomy*. 7th ed. Baltimore: Lippincott Williams & Wilkins.

Moseley, GL., Hodges, PW. and Gandevia, SC., 2002. Deep and superficial fibers of the lumbar multifidus muscle are differentially active during voluntary arm movements. *Spine*, 27(2), pp. E29–36.

Muyor, J., Sánchez-Sánchez, E., Sanz-Rivas, D. et al., 2013. Sagittal spinal morphology in highly trained adolescent tennis players. *Journal of Sports Science and Medicine*, 12, pp. 588–593.

Myers, T., 2014. *Anatomy Trains*. Edinburgh: Churchill Livingstone/Elsevier.

Netter, FH., 2014. *Atlas of Human Anatomy*. Philadelphia: Elsevier.

Niosi, CA. and Oxland, TR., 2004. Degenerative mechanics of the lumbar spine. *Spine Journal* (6 Suppl), pp. 202S–208S.

Nygaard, I., Barber, MD. and Burgio, KL., 2008. Prevalence of symptomatic pelvic floor disorders in US women. *Journal American Medical Association*, 300, pp. 1311–1316.

Oatis, CA., 2009. *Kinesiology: The Mechanics and Pathomechanics of Human Movement*. 2nd ed. Baltimore: Lippincott Williams & Wilkins.

Orchard, J., Read, JW., Verrall, GM. et al., 2000. Pathophysiology of chronic groin pain in the athlete. *International Sports Medicine Journal*, 1(1), pp. 1–16.

Osar, E. and Bussard, M., 2016. *Functional Anatomy of the Pilates Core*. Chichester: Lotus.

Oscar, E., 2012. *Corrective Exercise Solutions to Common Hip and Shoulder Dysfunction*. Chichester: Lotus.

O'Sullivan, PB., Beatles, DJ., Bentham, JA. et al., 2002. Altered motor control strategies in subjects with sacroiliac joint pain during active straight leg raise test. *Spine*, 27(1), pp. E1–E8.

Palastanga, N., 1997. *Anatomy of Human Movement*. Vol. 5. 2nd ed. Oxford: Butterworth Heinemann.

Pezowicz, CA., Robertson, PA. and Broom, ND., 2005. Intralamellar relationships within the collagenous architecture of the annulus fibrosus imaged in its fully hydrated state. *Journal Anatomy*, 207(4), pp. 299–312.

Pool-Goudzwaard, A., van Dijkstra, GH., van Gurp, M. et al., 2004. Contribution of the pelvic floor muscles to stiffness of the pelvic ring. *Clinical Biomechanics*, 19, pp. 564–571.

Pryor, JA. and Prasad, SA., 2002. *Physiotherapy for Respiratory and Cardiac Problems*. Edinburgh: Churchill Livingstone.

Ramirez, PT., Frumovitz, M. and Abu-Rustum, NR., 2018. *Principles of Gynecologic Oncology Surgery E-Book*, Elsevier Health Sciences, pp. 3–49.

Retchford, T., Crossley, K., Grimaldi, A. et al., 2013. Can local muscles augment stability in the hip? A narrative literature review. *Journal Musculoskeletal Neuronal Interaction*, 13(1), pp. 1–12.

Richardson, C., Hides, J., Wilson, S. et al., 2004. Lumbo-pelvic joint protection against antigravity forces: motor control and segmental stiffness assessed with magnetic resonance imaging. *Journal Gravitational Physiology*, 11(2), pp. 119–122.

Robertson, B., Barker, P., Fahrer, M. et al., 2009. The anatomy of the pubic region revisited: implications for the pathogenesis and clinical management of chronic groin pain in athletes. *Sports Medicine*, 39(3), pp. 225–234. DOI:10.2165/00007256-200939030-00004.

Ross, JR., Nepple, MJ., Philippon, MJ. et al., 2014. Effect of changes in pelvic tilt on range of motion to impingement and radiographic parameters of acetabular morphologic characteristics. *American Journal Sports Medicine*, 42(10), pp. 2402–2409.

Roussel, NA., Nips, J. and Truijen, S., 2007. Cliometrics properties of the Trendelenburg test, active straight raise test and breathing pattern during active straight leg raising. *Journal Manipulative Physiology and Therapy*, 30(4), pp. 270–278.

Roussouly, P. and Nnadi, C., 2010. Sagittal plane deformity: an overview of interpretation and management. *European Spine Journal*, 19(11), pp. 1824–1836.

Roussouly, P. and Pinheiro-Franco, J., 2011. Biomechanical analysis of the spino-pelvic organization and adaptation in pathology. *European Spine Journal*, 20 Suppl (5), pp. 609–618.

Roussouly, P., Berthonnaud, E. and Dimnet, J., 2003. Geometrical and mechanical analysis of lumbar lordosis in an asymptomatic population: proposed classification. *Revue de Chirurgie Orthopédique et Réparatrice de l'Appareil Moteur*, 89, pp. 632–639.

Roussouly, P., Gollogly, S., Bertonnaud, E. et al., 2005. Classification of the normal variation in the sagittal alignment of the human lumbar spine and pelvis in the standing position. *Spine*, 30(3), pp. 346–353.

Sahrmann, S., 2002. *Diagnosis and Treatment of Movement Impairment Syndromes*. Philadelphia: Mosby, p. 63.

Sapsford, R., 2004. Rehabilitation of pelvic floor muscles utilizing trunk stabilization. *Manual Therapy*, 9, pp. 3–12.

Sapsford, RR. and Hodges, PW., 2001. Contraction of the pelvic floor muscles during abdominal maneuvers. *Archives Physical Medicine and Rehabilitation*, 82, pp. 1081–1088.

Schilders, E., Bharam, S., Golan, E. et al., 2017. The pyramidalis–anterior pubic ligament–adductor longus complex (PLAC) and its role with adductor injuries: a new anatomical concept. *Knee Surgery Sports Traumatology Arthroscopy*, 25(12), pp. 3969–3977. DOI:10.1007/s00167-017-4688-2.

Schünke, M., Schulte, E. and Schumacher, U., 2007. *Prometheus: Lernatlas der Anatomis*. Stuttgart and New York: Georg Thieme.

Shu, B., and Safran, M., 2011. Hip instability: anatomic and clinical considerations of traumatic and atraumatic instability. *Clinical Sports Medicine*, 30, pp. 349–367.

Swärd Aminoff, A., Agnvall, C., Todd, C. et al., 2018. The effect of pelvic tilt and cam on hip range of motion in young elite skiers and non athletes. *Open Access Journal Sports Medicine*, 6(9), pp. 147–156.

Tuttle, LJ., DeLozier, ER., Harter, KA. et al., 2016. The role of the obturator internus muscle in pelvic floor function. *Journal Womens Health Physical Therapy*, 40 (1), pp. 15–19.

Uetake, T., Ohtsuki, F., Tanaka, H. et al., 1998. The vertebral curvature of sportsmen. *Journal of Sports Sciences*, 16, pp. 621–628.

Umphred, H. 2007. *Neurological Rehabilitation*. 5th ed. St Louis: Mosby/Elsevier.

Van Royen, B., Toussaint, H., Kingma, I. et al., 1998. Accuracy of the sagittal vertical axis in a standing lateral radiograph as a measurement of balance in spinal deformities. *European Spine Journal*, 7(5), pp. 408–412.

Van Royen, B., De Gast, A. and Smith, T., 2000. Deformity planning for sagittal plane corrective osteotomies of the spine in ankylosing spondylitis. *European Spine Journal*, 9(6), pp. 492–498.

Vleeming, A., Stoeckart, R., Volkers, A. et al., 1990a. Relation between form and function in the sacroiliac joint. *Spine*, 15(2), pp. 130–132.

Vleeming, A., Volkers, A., Snijders, C. et al., 1990b. Relation between form and function in the sacroiliac joint. *Spine*, 15(2), pp. 133–136.

Vleeming, A., Pool-Goudzwaard, AL., Stoeckart, R. et al., 1995. The posterior layer of the thoracolumbar fascia: its function in load transfer from spine to legs. *LRSpine (Phila Pa 1976)*, 20(7), pp. 753–758.

Vleeming, A., Mooney, V. and Stoeckart, R. 2007. *Movement, Stability & Lumbopelvic Pain: Integration of Research and Therapy*. Edinburgh: Churchill Livingstone.

Vleeming, A., Schuenke, MD., Masi, AT. et al., 2012. The sacroiliac joint: an overview of its anatomy, function and potential clinical implications. *Journal of Anatomy*, 221(6), pp. 537–567.

Walheim, G. and Selvik, G., 1984. Mobility of the pubic symphysis in vivo measurements with an electromechanic method and a Roentgen stereophotogrammetric method. *Clinical Orthopaedics and Related Research*, 191, pp. 129–135.

Wallden, M., 2014. The middle-crossed syndrome: new insights into core function. *Journal Bodywork and Movement Therapies*, 18(4), pp. 616–620.

Woodham, M., Woodham, A., Skeate, J. et al., 2014. Long-term lumbar multifidus muscle atrophy changes with magnetic resonance imaging: a case series. *Journal Radiology Case Reports*, 8(5), pp. 27–34.

Yoshio, M., Murakami, G., Sato, T. et al., 2002. The function of the psoas major muscle: passive kinetics and morphological studies using donated cadavers. *Journal Orthopaedic Science*, 7(2), pp. 199–207.

Chapter 4 structure

Low back pain	87
Specific LBP	92
Non-specific LBP	96
Sensitization in chronic LBP	98
Active healthcare in the management of chronic LBP	99
Factors that influence LBP	100
Hip pain in young athletes	104
Management of extra-/intra-articular hip and groin-related pain	107
Pelvic girdle physiology and dysfunction	111
Conclusion	114

Low back pain

While this chapter sets out to provide an overview of pain, pathology and dysfunction, I am not going to provide an in-depth explanation for every low back pain (LBP) condition that may affect athletes. There are many published texts on this subject that are widely available for further exploration, and these are listed in the references at the end of this chapter. From a learning perspective, understanding LBP may be broken down into an appreciation of the stages of healing, the differences between specific and non-specific LBP, and the bio-psychosocial model of this condition. I would like to add a reminder that clinicians should not become obsessed with a particular model for classifying LBP but should include within their clinical reasoning the multiple dimensions of LBP, to help inform them during the evaluation, treatment and management of the distinct and overlapping entities that may present.

LBP is a leading worldwide cause of disability and one of the most common non-communicable diseases (Owen et al., 2019). Currently, it affects 70–85 percent of the adult population. There are many classification models for LBP but few have been validated by evidence from clinical trials (Foster et al., 2009). Approximately 15 percent of patients presenting with LBP demonstrate clinical findings consistent with a specific pathoanatomical LBP diagnosis (Nijs et al., 2015). This suggests that up to 85 percent of patients with LBP may not have a specific pathoanatomically derived marker to support a precise description or diagnosis (Tschudi-Madsen et al., 2011; Dankaerts et al., 2009; Airaksinen et al., 2006). Perhaps in the attempt to label LBP with a specific pathology, the issue has been catastrophized by over-medicalization, subjecting patients to a needless battery of tests and investigations in an effort to find the source of pain (O'Sullivan et al., 2018).

Unfortunately, clinical tests and investigations reveal a high frequency of false positives and incidental findings, such as an intervertebral disk bulge, osteoarthritis (OA) or a lumbar anomaly. These findings only serve to label a patient as having a "bad back." They reinforce behavioral patterns, increase anxiety and loss of confidence, and can introduce (or exacerbate) a fear of movement and avoidance of activity (O'Sullivan, 2000). In addition, these findings are often reported in the aging population and may also be observed in patients that are pain-free, so are poorly correlated with pain or disability (Brinjikji et al., 2015; Steffens et al., 2014). In my experience, over-medicalization of LBP can have an impact on patient recovery. While clinical investigations may be required, pathologizing pain can often lead to patients and athletes being subjected to unnecessary levels of stress and anxiety.

Acute LBP

Reactive phase

Reactive or acute spinal pain is normally a single episode that resolves within 6 weeks (Liebenson, 2006). Normally, the reactive phase lasts from 24 hours to 1 week and is associated with a loss in range of movement (ROM) due to associated muscle spasm, swelling and pain from damage to nociceptive tissues. It is common at this stage for individuals to report that they are fearful of moving, as they do not want to aggravate their back any further. Symptoms can vary from pain that is very localized to the lumbar spine to that emanating from the buttock region. Initially, it can be asymmetrical but, in time, can develop a symmetrical distribution across the lower back and buttock region. Pain may initially be sharp on specific movements but resolve into a constant, dull ache with rest. Symptoms are sometimes described as burning, tingling and numbness, which often refer into the lower extremities. The working environment may be seen to aggravate symptoms; static loading, such as that involved in sitting for prolonged periods, driving or office work, may become troublesome. Similarly, jobs

Chapter 4

Table 4.1 Examples of low back pain differential diagnosis		
Specific pathoanatomical LBP	**Non-mechanical LBP**	**Visceral-related LBP**
• Sprain or strain • Herniated disk • Degenerative disk and facet joints • Spondylolysis/spondylolisthesis • Spinal stenosis • Traumatic fracture • Osteoporotic fracture	• Primary and secondary tumors • Myelopathy • Osteomyelitis • Seronegative spondyloarthropathies: ankylosing spondylitis, psoriatic arthritis • Scheuermann's disease	• Chronic pelvic inflammatory disease • Aortic aneurysm • Gastrointestinal involvement • Pancreatitis • Cholecystitis • Penetrating ulcer

that entail dynamic loading and place high loads on the spine, such as manual activity, may also be observed (reported) to increase symptoms. Sleep disturbance is frequently described and, in my opinion, can often prolong LBP recovery. Table 4.1 highlights examples that the practitioner should be alert to in the differential diagnosis of mechanical, non-mechanical and visceral-related LBP.

Having the opportunity to make a thorough evaluation is extremely important at this stage, as it assists with triaging the 1–2 percent of patients who fall into the category of having a serious underlying medical condition (Henschke et al., 2009). During the evaluation and taking of a case history, red flag questions should be asked by the clinician to assess whether there is a serious underlying spinal condition, such as cauda equina syndrome, tumor or fracture. The clinician must advise the patient to seek immediate and urgent medical attention if there are any signs or symptoms that indicate something may be seriously wrong:

• unremitting night pain
• sudden weight loss or loss of appetite
• fever
• malaise
• bladder or bowel incontinence
• history of saddle anesthesia.

Below is a case study highlighting the importance of being alert to potential red flags and non-musculoskeletal pathologies in clinical practice.

Case study: Patient B

 Patient B is a 22-year-old male triathlete, presenting with a dull, constant pain, specifically over his sacral region. The onset was 6 months previously, when he had visited his family doctor (GP) and was subsequently referred to a back clinic at the local hospital. There was no particular incident related to the onset of his symptoms and he reported that his training load had not really changed much in the past year. On questioning, he reported that the pain was worse in the morning and at night; he felt better with exercise but his symptoms did not change with rest. A symptom review highlighted that he had less energy and that one of his eyes had started to become blurred and painful. He was not aware of any familial history of inflammatory arthritis. On clinical testing, he was tender to palpation over the sacral region, although there were no signs of swelling or heat. Lumbar spinal ROM was reduced in all ranges but the most compromised was flexion. Neurological testing highlighted nothing abnormal.

My suspicions were raised due to the vague nature and history of his symptoms, and the fact that he was still reporting pain, despite having previously participated in a back clinic rehabilitation program at the local hospital. I referred Patient B back to his family doctor (GP) for a blood test, to rule out elevated inflammatory markers. The patient did, in fact, have raised levels of inflammatory markers and subsequently tested positive for the *HLA-B27* gene. He was diagnosed with ankylosing spondylitis (AS) and acute iritis, and was placed on a course of non-steroidal anti-inflammatory drugs (NSAIDs) to control his LBP and to help manage his iritis; he was encouraged to continue exercising. AS is an inflammatory spinal pathology that affects breathing mechanics, posture and spinal mobility. My clinical intervention, once the diagnosis had been made, was to provide manual therapy and exercise rehabilitation to educATE Patient B with posture, breathing mechanics and maintenance of mobility.

I have highlighted this case early in this chapter, as a reminder that not every presentation that we as clinicians are exposed to is musculoskeletal. Moreover, it should never be assumed that although an individual has been through the medical healthcare system, all investigations have been adequately completed. It is entirely possible that Patient B may not have presented to the other healthcare practitioners he had encountered previously with signs and symptoms related to an inflammatory pathology, and consequently did not at that stage raise any concerns that would indicate a requirement for further investigation.

What concerns most patients and athletes alike, during the reactive stage, is that their LBP may appear to get slightly better and then become worse for no apparent reason. A very general rule of thumb, which I often use, is to establish how the patient's symptoms are first thing in the morning, compared to the end of the day. For example, if a patient wakes up feeling really stiff but starts to feel better with movement, then I try to provide reassurance that this is typical of inflammation in an articular or joint-related structure. During sleep, inactivity has increased localized swelling and movement helps to disperse this. However, if the patient tells me that they wake up feeling much better every morning but their symptoms start to increase as the day progresses, I try to reassure them that this is more indicative of a muscle issue and explain that the reason why symptoms become worse as the day progresses is probably muscular fatigue. Of course, it is possible to have both articular and muscular issues occurring at the same time; and if this is the case, it is a matter, clinically, of prioritizing what to do initially so as to have the biggest impact on reducing their pain. Far and away the most important thing is to reassure patients that they will get better. I often use this analogy: "LBP is like a common cold; you will get over it."

Manual therapy techniques can have a huge pain-modulating effect, reducing muscle spasm, improving joint mobility and enhancing fluid dynamics, all of which may have a major impact on pain reduction. Advice on positions that modify symptoms, such as sitting, driving, work station ergonomics and sleep position – and in athletes, modifying training load – can help to calm the tissues down. Use of taping, belts and back supports may also provide some short-term relief. I often use these in a prophylactic capacity for some athletes, especially those that have a history of LBP, when they are traveling long distances by plane or coach. It works on the principle that preventative taping is better than the reaction to a static position on a long flight or coach journey. Pain relief medication and NSAIDs can play an important part during the reactive phase and have also been shown to be beneficial in reducing pain, swelling, severity and length of symptoms.

Regeneration phase

The regeneration or subacute phase starts as soon as the inflammatory stage becomes quiescent, which is generally from 5 days, and continues for approximately 3 weeks.

This is the repair stage, when symptoms start to subside and pain levels reduce. Normally during this stage, patients report having to take less medication, with functional activities, such as getting out of a chair, driving a car and walking for a longer duration, becoming easier. The goal in the regeneration phase is to encourage tissue healing, and both manual therapy and exercise have been shown to be extremely beneficial during this stage. Generally speaking, I think there should be less emphasis on *manipulATE* and a greater emphasis on *educATE*, with exercise progression from mobility and stretching to low-threshold strengthening and functional movements. Often, during this stage, it is common for patients to have a reaction or an acute flare-up of their symptoms. This is normally because they have been pain-free and progressed too quickly to a higher-threshold exercise which, at this stage, their tissues cannot cope with. I have found this type of reactive flare-up usually settles relatively quickly. This is an important point; *educATE* and encourage patients and athletes to remain active at a previously tolerated level of rehabilitation.

Remodeling phase

After 3 weeks, the remodeling phase starts; this is the stage at which the healing tissues become reasonably mature. During this period, progressive exercise rehabilitation makes a major contribution to helping restore elasticity and flexibility to the muscles and joints. As the tissue compliance to load is increased, the normal adaptation to exercise is stiffness, and so manual therapy techniques to maintain ROM and improve circulation and oxygenation to the tissues are extremely useful. I explain to patients that stiffness is a normal physiological response to exercise, and that the purpose of the manual therapy is to assist recovery of the previously damaged tissue, enabling them to continue progressively loading. Unfortunately, patients often associate stiffness with pain and it is quite common for them to report that their symptoms have returned. At this stage, I like to remind them of how far, or how regularly, they are now walking, running, riding and using the gym, compared to when they first reported their acute incident.

 It is crucial to *educATE* by reassuring patients and dispelling beliefs because the extra activities they are undertaking have a huge impact on tissue load and compliance. I want to make sure they understand that it is absolutely normal to feel stiff.

Chronic pain

Chronic LBP relates to an episode lasting for 12 weeks or longer, and is identified as being localized, below the costal margin and above the inferior gluteal folds, with or without leg pain (Owen et al., 2019; Hoy et al., 2010; Koes et al., 2010; van Tulder et al., 2006). Historically, most healthcare professionals have relied on biomedical and biomechanical models to manage chronic pain (Fryer, 2017). While they are still widely used, the issue with these particular models is that they do not take into account an individual's level of distress or previous experiences with pain (Smith et al., 2019). Reassurance, education and empowerment have been shown to result in positive outcomes, reducing anxiety, stress, fear and activity avoidance. Over 20 years ago, O'Sullivan (2000) proposed classifying chronic LBP patients as having movement and control impairments. In recent years this approach has evolved to embrace the bio-psychosocial aspect of LBP, placing a greater emphasis on *educATE* and patient-centered care (O'Sullivan et al., 2018).

Additionally, it has been suggested that using appropriate language can have a direct impact on the attitudes and beliefs of chronic LBP patients (Thomas and Collyer, 2017). Words and phrases such as "slipped disk" or "pelvis out of alignment" may heighten stress and anxiety or reinforce misbeliefs and fallacies. While I agree that the correct terminology should be used and common sense should always be applied, I would advise clinicians to be cautious. Using terms such as "non-specific LBP" or telling patients that their radiological investigation was "normal" and that there is "nothing wrong with them" or they "should just get on with it" is likely to end in patient dissatisfaction (Borkan et al., 1998). Dissatisfied patients will cancel appointments or fail to return for any follow-up treatment and this may significantly impact the confidence of a newly qualified clinician and affect the outcome of integrating the "five 'ATEs" framework.

Case study: Patient C

Consider the case of Patient C, who has complained of 3–4 days of LBP and has asked the question: "Do you think it's my disk?" I am always amazed at a patient's look of anxiety when they ask this, as if the term "disk" is a guarantee of long-term back pain, surgery and an extended recovery process. The answer I would give to Patient C is "No, it isn't." I would communicate this by going through a logical process of elimination and by reassuring them that their symptoms are not related to their "disk" because:

- they do not have radicular pain or neural sensitivity

- they demonstrate full power and reflexes on neurological testing

- they demonstrate adequate ROM in the spine

- and in the last week, they have had a significant increase in training volume, on a harder playing surface, which has more than likely increased axial spinal loading and could have resulted in low back symptoms.

While a response like this may go a long way towards quickly recovering this situation, manual therapy and rehabilitation exercises may also be used in preparation for training and for recovery. An important point to drive home is that these comments need to be effectively communicated to the medical team, ensuring there is one consistent message. This avoids any confusion between the athlete and the medical staff, the athlete and the coaching staff, and the medical staff and the coaching staff.

Sporting environments can be highly pressurized and stressful. It is common for a manager, coach or athlete to push the medical team for a definitive answer to their problem, by requesting or demanding an investigation. Is it that they doubt the medics' ability to perform effective clinical testing and to hypothesize using a clear, clinical reasoning process? More than likely not. What the coach is likely doing is formulating a return to play (RTP) plan for that athlete: that is, establishing "when will they be available for me?" Patients with chronic LBP may be strongly influenced by the medical profession, perhaps much more than by their families and friends (Darlow, 2016), but do all athletes behave in a similar manner, especially in the current climate when so many ex-athletes become coaches or managers? Not only do they have friends and family offering advice, but also agents, other athletes and other medical professionals they may have had previous contact with. These will all be on hand to lend advice and opinions. I have even come across cases where other healthcare professionals offer advice on how they can help with the athlete's particular condition, despite the fact that neither the athlete nor I have ever had any previous contact with them. Quite simply, everyone is an expert!

Managing these situations can be extremely difficult; actually, I think it becomes more of an art. This could be a reason why those who practice only evidence-based medicine seem to have a limited shelf life in high-performance sport. I am not dismissing evidence-based medicine, but rather suggesting that there is a requirement to combine evidence-based medicine within a performance framework: that is, while evidence-based medicine is not to be challenged as such, how it is carried out in the elite environment may require modifications in the approaches of the practitioner and the whole team. Perhaps it comes back to the use of effective communication skills. While reassurance and education are crucial, the practitioner's clinical skills, experiences and clinical reasoning processes are equally important, and this should not be forgotten. Is it good enough to tell an elite athlete that their LBP will get better with time and that in the interim they should try to continue to train? Sometimes, in medicine, the hardest thing to do is nothing, and this can be especially true in a sporting environment. With all these points in mind, if an investigation is planned, then it is normally for a specific reason, which might be to reduce the possibility of potential red flags, assist with making a pathoanatomical diagnosis that correlates with clinical testing, and help with planning an appropriate recovery and rehabilitation period, taking into account any future competitions.

Specific LBP

When a precise pain-provoking tissue can be diagnosed, specific LBP may be divided into two categories: nociceptive and neuropathic. Nociceptive LBP relates to pain-provoking tissues that may be muscular, myofascial, ligamentous, capsular or articular in nature but excludes non-neural tissue damage (Schilder et al., 2014; Smart et al., 2010; Tsao et al., 2010; Merskey, 1994). The site and location may be important: midline LBP increases the probability of intervertebral disk lesions, while para-midline LBP increases the probability of facet joint or sacroiliac joint (SIJ) pain (Nijs, 2015).

Neuropathic LBP is a specific subset of LBP, affecting 20–30 percent of patients (Freynhagen and Baron, 2009). It relates to a history or specific incident affecting the nervous system, either central or peripheral. Pain distribution is neuroanatomically logical: that is, it is segmentally related. For example, the femoral nerve may refer to the anterior thigh and knee joint. Pain is often described as burning, shooting or pricking.

Below are some examples of the pathoanatomical structures related to specific LBP and the types of clinical examination recommended in the current literature. Refer to Chapter 5 for more details on performing these tests.

1. In patients with lumbar disk herniation, the slump test has been shown to have 84 percent sensitivity, compared to the straight leg raise (SLR) test, which has considerably less at 52 percent. However, the SLR was shown to be slightly more specific at 89 percent, compared to the slump test at 83 percent (Majlesi et al., 2008).

2. Lumbar facet joint syndrome pain was ruled out with a negative lumbar extension and rotation ROM test with 100 percent sensitivity, following a local facet joint injection block (Laslett et al., 2006).

3. SIJ pain was ruled out with three or more clinical SIJ tests with 94 percent sensitivity and 78 percent specificity, following a local anesthetic injection into the SIJ (Laslett et al., 2005).

LBP in athletes

The prevalence of LBP appears to differ, depending on the type of sporting activity and the duration of sporting participation (Hangai et al., 2010). The incidence of LBP is well documented in many sports and is shown to be correlated with increased spinal loading in up to 89 percent of elite athletes (Table 4.2). While LBP has been shown to have a higher prevalence in athletes participating in high-performance sports, it should be noted that it is also reported among non-athletes: that is, the general

Table 4.2 Incidence of LBP in various sports

Sporting discipline	Incidence of LBP (%)
Gymnastics	67
Water-ski jumping	45
Soccer	53
Weight-lifting	71
Wrestling	77
Orienteering	55
Ice hockey	89
Diving	89
Tennis	50
Alpine and cross-country skiing	67

population. Sports in which there is a high incidence of reported LBP in athletes, suggesting a potential increase in risk of LBP, are summarized in the table.

Athlete technique

Poor athlete training techniques, whether they are gym-based or track and field-based, have the potential to increase the risk of LBP and spinal injury. An example may be an athlete that has a poor understanding or lack of education and is required to perform an intricate movement or specific drill. This may lead to compensatory movement patterns, dysfunction and increased loading on specific contact points of the functional spinal units (FSUs), previously described in Chapter 3.

Spinal loading

A greater frequency of spinal radiological abnormality, such as intervertebral disk degeneration, has been previously shown among athletes in sports that place a heavy demand on the spine. Examples include wrestling, diving, gymnastics, soccer, ice hockey, orienteering, skiing and tennis (Witwit et al., 2018; Thoreson et al., 2015; Baranto et al., 2010; 2006; Sward et al., 1990). While it is difficult to correlate radiological findings with an individual's pain, a greater prevalence of LBP has been reported in young athletes who participate in sports that place a heavy demand on the spine (Witwit et al., 2020; Baranto et al., 2009; 2005; Sward et al., 1991).

Posture

Posture has become a contentious subject, especially on social media over the past few years. Previously, it was suggested that LBP had a strong correlation with poor posture. Of course, the human population is subject to the rigors of gravity and the way we position our vertebral segments, under gravitational load, will have an impact on our musculoskeletal system. Perhaps a better way to explain posture may be to say that poor posture can influence habitual movement patterns, which may lead to muscular imbalance and influence how movement is regulated. Such imbalances can lead to dysfunction

and occur in athletes: for example, after intense spikes in training load, during normal periodization of training and in competitions. While I believe there is no such thing as perfect posture, when an athlete stands with their weight distributed evenly through their feet, they are promoting an optimal length–tension relationship of the agonist and antagonist muscles. Such a relationship assists with maintaining joint centration and provides optimum efficiency for transferring load and force during functional movement.

Spinal curvatures

A lot of research has been dedicated to this subject since the turn of the century. When I think back to my doctoral degree, we were able to highlight, with clinical and radiological studies, that the standing sagittal spino-pelvic alignments of athletes are different to those of non-athletes (Todd et al., 2015; 2016). Sports-specific training or the accumulation of a high training load at a young age can affect skeletal curvatures and has been correlated with spinal pathologies. For example, radiological studies have shown that a larger sacro-horizontal angle, which increases the lumbar lordotic curvature in young athletes, is correlated with spinal pathologies such as spondylolysis and spondylolisthesis (Sward et al., 1991).

Pelvic parameters

The pelvic girdle is essential for the maintenance of spinal sagittal balance. The relationship between the trunk and the lower extremities helps to modulate an erect posture. As previously discussed in Chapter 3, individuals with a narrow pelvic incidence (PI) angle are shown to have a flatter back and as a result do not have a very efficient spine for performing high-performance sports (Todd et al., 2015; Roussouly et al., 2003). Recently, work has been carried out to investigate the possibility that the pelvic parameters may indicate a potential risk factor for an athlete's susceptibility to hip pain. While I can accept this possibility, there is a distinct lack of evidence to support it at the moment.

Age

People who strive to become top-level athletes are exposed from a young age to high levels of intense training and consequently experience heavy loads on their spine. The downside is the repetitive nature of strenuous physical exercise and the increased vulnerability to overuse repetitive injuries. In a young athlete who is skeletally immature, repetitive movements after the adolescent growth spurt may lead to an array of potential pathologies, ranging from intervertebral degenerative disk disease and other abnormalities which affect the vertebral endplates and the vertebral ring apophyses. There are some sports, such as gymnastics and competitive diving, that subject the adolescent spine to a greater risk of injury due to the extreme range of movement or the high level of axial spinal loading (Witwit et al., 2020; Baranto et al., 2009; 2005; Sward et al., 1991).

Repetitive micro- or acute macro-trauma

LBP in athletes is normally caused by acute macro-trauma or repetitive micro-trauma/over-use injuries, or a combination of both (Baranto et al., 2010; 2009; Sward et al., 1991). Acute trauma injury patterns are different between adults and children. Young athletes may suffer avulsion injuries to the vertebral endplate, whereas adults suffer vertebral fracture or rupture of the intervertebral disk (Baranto et al., 2005). Repetitive micro-trauma may increase accessory motion on the contact points of the FSUs. This results in loss of segmental stability and control, challenging the compliance of the soft tissues as they are subjected to increased strain and leading to a creep deformation. Over time, this may lead to degenerative spinal changes (Sahrmann, 2002).

Experimental studies in animal models have shown that the growth zone is the weakest portion in a young spine, and this is also found in spinal units created to examine disk degeneration experimentally (Baranto et al., 2005). Clinical studies in young athletes have highlighted that the weakest parts of the skeletally immature spine are the growth zone and the endplates (Baranto et al., 2005; Sward et al., 1991). It can be hypothesized that frequent exposure to high-level loading in a young, skeletally immature spine may create repetitive micro-trauma to the FSUs, which could lead to a greater incidence of LBP in young athletes.

LBP in young athletes is often vague in presentation, and less distinct compared to their adult counterparts. Differential diagnosis may include diskogenic back pain, traumatic or atypical Scheuermann's kyphosis, spondylolysis and spondylolisthesis (Sassmannshausen and Smith, 2002; Waicus and Smith, 2002). Clinicians should be alert to the possibility of these pathologies and ensure that the correct diagnostic investigations and appropriate management plans are instigated. Once a diagnosis has been ascertained, symptom modification techniques (SMTs) may help to inform an effective clinical reasoning process. An understanding of the global impact of human movement on local tissue pathology, including the regional interdependence model, has huge ramifications for assisting with the management of acute or chronic related pathologies.

Case study: Patient D

Consider the case of this young soccer player, who was previously diagnosed with spondylolysis. After allowing some time for the symptoms to resolve and following a computed tomography (CT) scan review, the player returned to training. During this period of RTP, I used an approach to help improve the stability of the lower lumbar spine, while improving dynamic mobility in the thoracic spine, thoracolumbar region and hip joints.

 Dynamic mobility of the thoracic spine, thoracolumbar region and hip joints was achieved using manual therapy techniques to address restrictions in soft tissue and joint mobility (see Chapter 6). This was integrated into motor control exercises such as heel to pelvis in four-point kneeling for lumbar stabilization and thoracic dissociation, and reverse lunge for lumbar stabilization and hip dissociation (see Chapter 7).

Stability of the lumbar spine was introduced pre-training to *activATE* the deep spinal stability mechanism (Gibbons, 2005; McGill, 2004). This included exercises such as a modified short-lever side-lying plank and psoas suction, combined with inner-range hip flexion motor control techniques (see Chapter 7).

 This is another example of applying the *manipulATE* and *activATE* components of the "five 'ATEs'" to manage pathology in the spino-pelvic-hip complex successfully in high-performance sport. Functional movement combined with a regional interdependence model, alongside monitoring of health status for any flare-up in symptoms, meant that Patient D remained asymptomatic, was able to be available for training and made a successful RTP.

Movement and control dysfunctions

Movement and control dysfunctions of the lumbar spine were first proposed by O'Sullivan (2000) as a way of helping to plan recovery strategies for patients with LBP. Movement dysfunction (Figure 4.1) relates to a specific structure such as "tight" hamstrings that may limit the ability of an individual to perform (in this example)

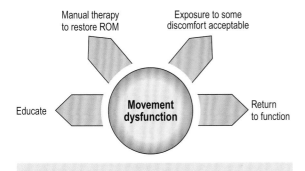

Figure 4.1
Management of LBP movement dysfunction.

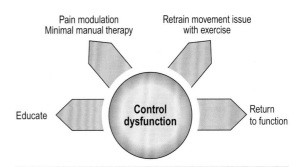

Figure 4.2
Management of LBP control dysfunction.

lumbar flexion. Control dysfunction (Figure 4.2) is when an individual has the ability to demonstrate lumbar flexion, but when asked to perform this task repeatedly may start to experience symptoms and report pain. This is due to a loss of segmental motor control of the deep stabilizing muscles of the spine and is often characterized by patients reporting pain as they return from flexion to an upright standing position.

While it appears straightforward to define chronic movement and control impairments of the lumbar spine as completely separate entities, clinical experience highlights the fact that many patients will present with a combination of both issues. For example, extension movement may be restricted in the thoracic spine, while capacity to limit extension may be lost in the lower lumbar segments. Classically, this would present with "extension hinging" or "extension-related" LBP. It is important to make the distinction. This is not a result of loss of mobility in the lower lumbar facet joints, such as an acute facet joint capsular strain. On the contrary, in this case, pain during extension is a result of increased accessory motion in the lower lumbar segments due to hypomobility in the thoracic spine, and "extension hinging" and an acute facet joint capsular strain would have to be managed very differently. Their management will be discussed in Chapter 6 and Chapter 7.

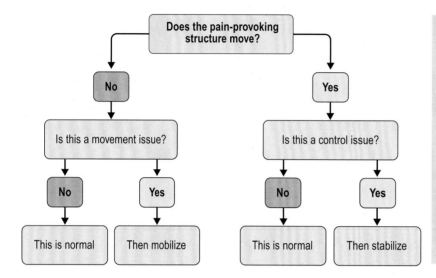

Figure 4.3
Flow chart highlighting LBP management.

Clinicians may be confused and commonly make the mistake of trying to manage control impairments as movement issues, administering copious manual therapy techniques in an attempt to resolve the issue, often unsuccessfully. The same can be said for clinicians attempting to manage movement impairments as control issues, prescribing a regime of exercises that simply ramp up pain levels as patients are wrongly encouraged to move into a pain-provoking ROM. The skill of the clinician is to know when to mobilize and when to stabilize (Figure 4.3), and it is my intention for this to become clearer as you progress through this book.

The fundamental theme behind managing both movement and control impairments is to *"educATE."* In Chapters 1 and 2, I referred to SMTs or "mini treatments" as a means to validate this. Manual therapy to restore ROM in movement impairments (see Figure 4.1) may be indicated, and some exposure to discomfort is acceptable. This differs from control impairments (see Figure 4.2), where minimal manual therapy is required, as the emphasis here lies specifically with retraining the movement impairment issue. Remember, a combination of both problems is usually found in most cases, so the art is to know which structures to mobilize and which to stabilize.

It is a challenge to remain alert for potential red flag pathologies, while at the same time appreciating the continuum of pathoanatomical changes that may occur to the spino-pelvic-hip complex as a result of high-performance sport. This challenge can lead to the practitioner having a deeper understanding of how dysfunctional movement presents in an elite individual. The practitioner will develop management strategies that reflect these experiences and develop a differential appreciation of dysfunctional presentations within this population.

Non-specific LBP

If only 15 percent of specific LBP cases in the general population demonstrate pathoanatomical features, it follows that a precise pathoanatomical diagnosis cannot be given to approximately 85 percent of the population (Tschudi-Madsen et al., 2011; Dankaerts et al., 2009; Airaksinen et al., 2006). Non-specific LBP can be extremely complex and challenging for clinicians, as there may be no structural change, no inflammatory response and no specific disease attributed as a cause (O'Sullivan, 2000). It may therefore be proposed that functional issues, such as loss of stability and/or movement control in the spine, may be persistent contributors to non-specific LBP. A reduction in the cross-sectional area of the deep spinal muscles, with increased deposits of intramuscular fat and reports of increased levels of fatiguability, have all been reported in association with non-specific LBP, which suggests that changes in muscle tissue may accompany this condition. Altered postural control of the hip and pelvis has, in particular, been shown to occur in individuals with non-specific LBP (Koch and Hansel, 2019), examples being an inability to maintain load transfer during single-leg (SL) stance or reduced active pelvic tilt due to loss of inner-range hip flexion control, which further supports a proposal of altered lumbopelvic movement regulation in non-specific LBP.

With this in mind, is it reasonable to assume that non-specific LBP could be managed as a functional issue? Perhaps it is not as straightforward as this. Chronic pain is accompanied by alterations within the central nervous system (CNS), such as increased responsiveness to stimuli perceived to be painful or threatening, leading some researchers to suggest that chronic pain contributes to dysfunction at the level of the CNS. Sometimes patients may report an amplification of symptoms that have no direct correspondence or anatomical relationship with the region of nociceptive damage, and the distribution of pain may be diffuse or, alternatively, not segmentally related to the source of pain (Nijs et al., 2014; 2010). Patients exhibiting these issues require treatment that targets the CNS (brain) rather than the low back. This approach to treating non-specific LBP is referred to as "top-down," to distinguish it from a "bottom-up" approach, which focuses on addressing nociceptive (pain) aspects of the presentation in the periphery (Nijs et al., 2015).

Bio-psychosocial non-specific LBP

Managing patients with chronic LBP may involve addressing many aspects that relate to their physical or biological traits (Ng et al., 2015; Steffens et al., 2015), cognitive and emotional or psychological characteristics (Darlow et al., 2016; Hannibal and Bishop, 2014), and cultural, societal or social factors (Hoogendoorn et al., 2000): hence the common use of the term "bio-psychosocial

model" (O'Sullivan et al., 2018) to describe this multidimensional approach. Practitioners should be able to recognize any potential traits in patients presenting with LBP, such as pain-related fear, negative emotional states, kinesiophobia and depression (Stubbs et al., 2016).

Pain may not be simply the result of injury or pathology but may be the response to "an unpleasant sensory and emotional experience, associated with actual or potential tissue damage" (Merskey and Bogduk, 1994). As a consequence, pain can be seen as a combination of a physical, noxious sensation and an emotional experience, which is heavily influenced by nociception and the individual's perception, beliefs or attitude towards pain. Emotional and cognitive factors may result in fear of movement or avoidance of activity, which will eventually progress to deconditioning and tissue sensitization (Nijs et al., 2015).

The longer pain persists, the less relationship it may have with the tissue that was initially damaged. Given the evidence that mental health issues, such as depression and anxiety, are closely associated with LBP, and the rising costs for managing LBP, perhaps a more active approach should be encouraged to manage these conditions (Gerrits et al., 2015). Similarly, cognitive functional therapy (CFT) (Figure 4.4) has evolved from behavioral psychology and neuroscience as an integrated approach for clinicians to manage non-specific LBP (O'Sullivan et al., 2018). While it is not within the scope of this book to discuss CFT in detail, this mode of therapy could, in general, be viewed as the point where understanding pain, lifestyle changes and exposure with control all converge and encourage the clinician to take the patient on an individualized journey, as summarized in Figure 4.4.

Understanding pain

Understanding pain is a complex process that attempts to make sense of the patient's story, their previous experiences and the narrative of their symptoms. Clinicians may outline why previously held negative beliefs, contextual factors and unhelpful emotional and behavioral

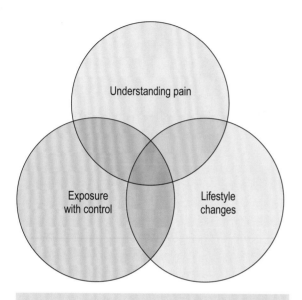

Figure 4.4
Cognitive functional therapy intervention.

responses may influence pain and disability and discuss how to dispel them, using a non-judgmental approach (O'Sullivan et al., 2018). Reinforcing the structural integrity of the spine and explaining the meaning of radiological imaging can be beneficial to patients at this stage (McCullough et al., 2012). For example, it can help a patient to overcome fears of having a "broken" or "abnormal" spine, especially if they have built up negative thoughts around their back pain, perhaps from comments made by other clinicians during previous examinations.

Exposure with control

This process attempts to encourage behavioral change through experiential learning: specifically, by controlled activity exposure to painful, fear-inducing, functional tasks that may have been avoided previously. This allows the patient to return gradually to activities they previously enjoyed, through a graded exposure to exercise, without any escalation in pain (Caneiro et al., 2017).

Lifestyle changes

An individualized exercise program is designed for the patient, based on their preferences, and can be specifically linked to pre-determined goals. It is important for this type of exercise program to consider variables such as financial cost, availability and the possibility of social engagement (O'Keefe et al., 2017). Some patients will indulge in over-activity, while other more sedentary patients will be under-active. In both cases, an activity diary may be beneficial to manage patients effectively.

Sensitization in chronic LBP

Chronic pain sensitivity may involve peripheral and/or central elements. Peripheral and central sensitization occur in a similar manner. The fundamental difference between them is that peripheral sensitization (often called primary hyperalgesia) occurs as a result of sensitization to the peripheral nerve endings, whereas central sensitization (secondary hyperalgesia) is caused by changes in the spinal cord and brain (Vardeh and Naranjo, 2017).

Peripheral sensitization

When peripheral tissue damage or inflammation occurs, nociceptors up-regulate their activity, leading to an increased neurogenic inflammatory response mediated by neuropeptides (Pezet and McMahon, 2006). The endogenous chemicals released from the site of injury can activate and sensitize peripheral nerve endings, resulting in peripheral sensitization. This in turn leads to the injured tissue becoming hypersensitive to heat and touch, and this effect is termed "primary hyperalgesia." Primary hyperalgesia equates to peripheral sensitization, while secondary hyperalgesia (a pain state that is not reactive to heat) suggests central sensitization (Bolay and Moskowitz, 2002). Clinically, this is an important point because if a patient presents with chronic pain and their symptoms can be modulated by heat, then it would suggest a diagnosis of peripheral sensitization. Alternatively, if their pain symptoms are not modulated by heat, it suggests central sensitization.

Central sensitization

Central sensitization, or secondary hyperalgesia, is an amplification of neural signaling within the CNS that elicits pain hypersensitivity, normally as a direct result of a noxious experience or from repetitive noxious stimuli (Nijs et al., 2015). Essentially, the patient becomes more sensitive and experiences greater levels of pain with less tissue provocation. This encompasses dysfunctions within the CNS and contributes to greater responsiveness to stimuli such as mechanical pressure, chemical substances, light, sound, cold, heat, stress and electrical activity (Woolf, 2011; Nijs et al., 2010; Meyer et al., 1995). Central sensitization may result in altered sensory processing in the brain, increased activity in the nociceptive pathways and reduced function of the descending, anti-nociceptive pathways. Often, the pain that patients report is disproportionate to the mechanism, nature and extent of their injury (Nijs et al., 2015). In recent times, it has been suggested that the immune system plays a role in the development of chronic pain states, and although this is not fully understood, it is thought that it may be associated with central sensitization (Nicotra et al., 2012; Guo and Schluesener, 2007; DeLeo et al., 2004).

Clinical examination of LBP patients exhibiting central sensitization often reports what can only be interpreted as neuroanatomically illogical pain, with increased levels of sensitivity at segmental levels, unrelated to the primary source of nociception (Nijs et al., 2014; 2010). Examples of this may be bilateral symmetrical pain patterns, widespread pain and hyperalgesia that appears neuroanatomically illogical. For example, an individual suffering with LBP may report an increase in pain when they are hugged. The spinal cord may become sensitized 6–10 segments above or below the site that may have been exposed to either macro-trauma or repetitive micro-trauma (Brooks et al., 2012). Perhaps this may help explain why there is often what appears to be an illogical neuroanatomical distribution of pain.

The best evidence for how to treat chronic pain sensitivity supports the benefit of improving general health, as opposed to fixing specific "issues in the tissues." Encouraging an active lifestyle has been shown to have a positive outcome, and exercise training is an effective treatment for non-specific chronic LBP; however, the best mode of training is still unknown (Owen et al., 2019). Exercise-induced hypoalgesia is considered to be a response that involves many different mechanisms that contribute to pain analgesia (Naugle et al., 2012). Exercise can trigger the endogenous opioid system due to changes in blood pressure and heart rate. It is well recognized that the function of the immune system is enhanced through regular exercise. If illnesses such as diabetes and heart disease have been shown to reduce with general exercise, then why not non-specific chronic LBP?

 Below is an example of a clinical solution to assist with the management of non-specific chronic LBP:

- reassurance that there are no signs of any particular disease and patient education to dispel any negative disbeliefs

- emphasis on functional issues that contribute to LBP, such as lack of fitness, in the absence of any findings from clinical investigation

- emphasis on training movement, not muscle, and cognitive advice directed at making lifestyle changes that will have the greatest impact

- reassurance given to the patient that the sooner function improves, the quicker the symptoms reduce.

Active healthcare in the management of chronic LBP

Over the last few years, it has become increasingly common to acknowledge that there is no "quick fix" for LBP. In fact, I often explain to patients that they will get *themselves* better and I will merely *facilitate* and *guide* them through the process. Perhaps, from a clinician's perspective, managing LBP is in part an acknowledgment of our role in educating the patient, and therefore means empowering patients with the correct tools to self-manage and to help themselves.

Athletes and patients alike demonstrate changes in behavioral patterns if they are labeled with a "bad back." If a sporting activity becomes painful for athletes as a result of LBP, they may demonstrate a reduction in levels of performance. In this case, limitations may be due to both psychological and physical factors. Increased levels of stress, muscle guarding and pain are common, and often athletes and patients will need reassurance, advice and guidance to dispel mistaken beliefs, help develop coping mechanisms and increase levels of self-confidence, for a quick and successful return to previous athlete activity (Main and Watson, 1999). It makes complete sense to create an active healthcare management plan that endorses the bio-psychosocial model of LBP and includes Pilates, stabilization/motor control, and aerobic and resistance training, all of which have been shown to be the most effective strategies for managing non-specific LBP (Owen et al., 2019).

However, active healthcare also endorses the biomechanical model of human movement. Advising athletes to avoid prolonged periods of bed rest and inactivity, while encouraging safe and effective exercise activity – modified, if necessary – is extremely important. Similarly, athletes should be educated to understand that LBP can be a result of inactivity or over-activity, and may affect particular regions of the body. Sahrmann (2002) suggested that creep deprivation may occur from prolonged lengthening of a muscle, specifically in poor sitting positions. This may occur as a result of the relative flexibility between adjacent joints. For example, an athlete with reduced hip flexion ROM would be forced to adopt a sitting position which could increase segmental translation in their lower lumbar spine, similar to a young athlete who returns home after training and sits for a prolonged period on a low sofa, while playing games on a PlayStation®. Such a reduction in hip mobility and increase in lumbar spine mobility would create a creep deprivation of the lower lumbar segments and subsequent LBP.

 Low-threshold motor control activation exercises appear to be useful for pain modulation in LBP. Encouraging neuromuscular activation to help control specific segments of the spine (to improve dynamic alignment within regions of the spine) may assist with enhancing stiffness within those segments that may have become inhibited due to pain.

 I try to *educATE* patients that stiffness can be negatively viewed, often misinterpreted and associated with having to "release tight tissues." However, improving spinal stiffness can be extremely beneficial for helping reduce segmental translation and increased accessory spinal motion. Agonist and antagonist muscle activation becomes disturbed in the presence of LBP, as do the endurance and coordination of the spinal flexors and extensors (Richardson et al., 2002; Cholewicki et al., 2000; 1997). Encouraging the athlete or patient to resume activities may not only reduce pain symptoms, but also influence tissue healing positively.

Factors that influence LBP

Three major factors have been identified as the medical reasons that have precipitated the LBP epidemic in modern society (Waddell, 1987):

- over-emphasis on a pathoanatomical diagnosis
- poor advice, such as prolonged bed rest
- over-use of surgery.

Over-emphasis on a pathoanatomical diagnosis

Modern healthcare clinicians often use radiological investigations unnecessarily, although it is true that these are used to rule out any potential red flags. The rate of incidental findings and false-positive investigations is alarming, with patients receiving unnecessary treatment after being mislabeled with a particular condition. The problem arises when there is a negative result from imaging and the patient is told that their symptoms are non-specific. This may drive the patient's impression that their symptoms are "all in their head." Currently, in the UK, the National Institute for Health and Care Excellence (NICE) guidelines suggest that individuals with LBP, with or without sciatica, should be told that they may not need imaging.

Prolonged bed rest

When a specific LBP pathoanatomical structure cannot be diagnosed, bed rest and medication are sometimes the only advice and treatment offered. Prescribing bed rest for LBP may have contributed to a huge financial burden on the welfare state in time lost and absenteeism from work. In the UK, current LBP and sciatica guidelines state that patients should be given "encouragement to continue with normal activities, which includes going back to work."

Over-use of surgery

Surgery is recommended only for patients who have not responded to their treatment and exercise rehabilitation plans. Even if a conservative approach to managing the condition has not worked for a patient, it does not necessarily mean they are suitable candidates for surgery. While surgery clearly has a place in managing LBP, it should be a last resort after all other avenues have been explored.

I started this chapter by making a statement that clinicians should not become obsessed with the classifications of LBP. In clinical practice, I have mostly found that patients and athletes present with a mixed combination of the many aspects attributed to both biomedical and bio-psychosocial LBP. It is necessary, as a clinician, to keep an open mind when formulating a successful management plan. Table 4.3 highlights the "five 'ATEs", the patient/athlete management strategy I currently use for managing chronic LBP. A significant emphasis is placed on the patient understanding how to manage their symptoms quickly and effectively, and how to return to normal activity as rapidly and as safely

Table 4.3 The "five 'ATEs" patient/athlete management strategy

"ATE"	Components
EvaluATE	<ul><li>Case history and clinical evaluation to reduce likelihood of red flags</li><li>Establishing whether this is an acute or chronic issue</li><li>Pathoanatomical features</li><li>Functional performance</li><li>Bio-psychosocial aspects of patient presentation</li><li>Referral for further investigations if necessary</li><li>Symptom modification techniques to reduce biomechanical strain</li><li>Clinical and functional re-evaluation</li></ul>
EducATE	<ul><li>Reassurance of patient</li><li>Dispelling beliefs and previous misconceptions</li><li>Empowerment and self-confidence through understanding</li><li>Clinical and functional re-evaluation</li></ul>
ManipulATE	<ul><li>If appropriate, use of manual therapy</li><li>Pain modulation with soft tissue or joint manipulation</li><li>Clinical and functional re-evaluation</li></ul>
ActivATE	<ul><li>Return to activities of daily living (ADLs)</li><li>Symptom modification techniques to reduce biomechanical strain</li><li>Clinical and functional re-evaluation</li></ul>
IntegrATE	<ul><li>Return to functional activity and sports-specific exercise</li><li>Clinical and functional re-evaluation</li></ul>

as possible. This will be discussed further in subsequent chapters. The "five 'ATEs" management strategy involves regularly re-evaluating the patient or athlete. Clinically, I find this to be an extremely powerful tool. Pain modification, empowerment, improving self-confidence and overcoming fear and anxiety can all act as markers against which patient progress can be assessed in order to assist patients to progress and they enable clinicians to plan specific strategies for managing a successful resolution.

There follows an example of a modified case report that I presented at a conference in London in 2016. The case reflects many aspects of my approach to addressing movement and control deficits around the spino-pelvic-hip complex. RTP considerations and conservative approaches adopted in the management of LBP in elite soccer appear to lack structured clinical guidelines, with limited levels of published evidence available. Standardized criteria for the conservative management of spinal pathologies in athletes against which athlete RTP could be benchmarked have not been established (Iwamoto et al., 2010). The majority of decisions on RTP appear, therefore, to be based on expert opinion and clinical experience (Huang et al., 2016). The purpose of this case report was to present the management of a soccer player presenting with chronic low back, hip and groin pain, highlighting a successful RTP after a conservative management strategy was adopted.

Case study: Patient E

Patient E, a 23-year-old male soccer player, had a presenting complaint of long-term LBP and groin pain. Sprinting aggravated his symptoms, as did striking a ball and sitting for prolonged periods. His previous medical history highlighted an L4–5 spondylolysis on magnetic resonance imaging (MRI); he had previously undergone right hip arthroscopy for cam-type femoroacetabular impingement (FAI) revision, combined with labral reconstruction and subsequent right-sided psoas tenotomy. Quantitative measurements were recorded, which included the use of (1) a visual analogue scale (VAS) and (2) a 66fit® pressure biofeedback unit (PBU).

Standing active spinal and pelvic examination revealed pain at end-of-range lumbar flexion and extension. Hypermobility was noted on active flexion at the L4–5,

L5–S1 segments, and on active extension "hinging" was noted at the L4–5 segment. He tested positive for loss of force transfer through the pelvis and lower extremity with SL stance on the right. Passive evaluation highlighted segmental facet joint restrictions at T12–L1 and T7–9, and increased spinal hypermobility was noted on palpation over right-sided lower lumbar segments and SIJ.

Hip examination highlighted pain and restriction in motion on active hip flexion in standing and sitting, and he tested positive for impingement with hip joint flexion, adduction and internal rotation (FADIR). Active straight leg raise (ASLR) was labored but improved with pelvic force closure (reinforced external compression of pelvis). VAS was 6/10. PBU squeeze test on first consultation was straight leg (SL) 150 mmHg and bent knee (BK) 60° 120 mmHg.

My working hypothesis was that this was a presentation involving a triad of multi-faceted, related issues: suboptimal spino-pelvic motor control combined with movement restrictions higher up the kinetic chain. A reduction in hip flexor motor control and intolerance to load, as a result of the previous surgery, may have compounded the breakdown of spinal and pelvic compensatory mechanisms, leading to a loss of axial spinal stability and anterior hip joint and SIJ stability. This was noticeable on ASLR, alongside signs of a positive hip impingement in spite of surgery for hip joint cam revision.

Management of this patient involved four treatment sessions over a 5-week period, covering patient education, correction of spinal dysfunctions at T12–L1, T7–9, and soft tissue mobilization to address over-active muscles such as tensor fasciae latae (TFL), rectus femoris and deep external rotators.

Activation techniques were included to improve inhibited muscles, progressing through a program to increase muscle

capacity (exercise tolerance) and improve spinal conditioning, which encompassed segmental motor control and regional dissociation, combined with concentric/eccentric anterior and posterior trunk muscular endurance training. Initially, the player used an SIJ belt for 2 weeks to help reinforce pelvic closure and took part in daily water-based recovery sessions. He was able to resume modified training at 10 days, and played 45 minutes after 3 weeks and 90 minutes at 5 weeks with no reaction.

He was followed up over the course of a year:

- Follow-up at 1 week revealed the VAS score was reduced to 4/10, with pain-free spinal ROM and negative (symptomatically) on load/unload. Therefore, the Sorensen test (see Chapter 5) was used to review trunk muscle capacity (170 seconds) (this was because Patient E had a significant reduction in LBP after the initial consultation); the PBU squeeze test SL was 150 mmHg and BK 60° 120 mmHg.

- Follow-up at 3 weeks revealed VAS 1/10, pain-free spinal ROM, negative on load/unload, Sorensen test 220 seconds, PBU squeeze test SL 240 mmHg and BK 60° 280+ mmHg.

- Follow-up at 5 weeks revealed VAS 0/10, Sorensen test 240+ seconds, PBU squeeze test SL 280 mmHg and BK 60° 300+ mmHg.

- By follow-up at 1 year, the participant had played over 40 games and remained injury-free.

In treating this particular patient, SMT helped inform my clinical reasoning. For example, reduction of lower segmental spinal "hinging" during spinal extension was achieved by restoring function to the thoracic spine through manual therapy. Re-education of movement control helped the player to restore hip joint centration and use his functional antagonists (gluteals and psoas) appropriately, which assisted with improving lumbar flexion control. As evaluation

showed, pelvic reinforcement (external compression) helped to reduce symptoms during the ASLR test; prescribing an SIJ belt was beneficial in the short term, as it helped with transferring load and force through the pelvis and enabled this player to train in a modified way (Figure 4.5).

This case reports on the conservative approach to return to play, in a soccer player with chronic low back and groin pain. Although criteria for RTP after LBP in soccer players are limited, the general consensus is that players should be symptom-free and without neurological deficits, have full ROM and have developed appropriate (adequate for performance) muscle capacity tolerance to load and strength (Huang et al., 2016). Moreover, some studies have shown that the timescale for RTP with conservative management is similar to that after surgical intervention (Mortazavi et al., 2015). However, a more rapid RTP has been demonstrated for the conservative management of specific spinal pathologies (Iwamoto et al., 2010). It has been suggested that in the conservative management of a soccer player with chronic low back, hip and groin pain, the spino-pelvic-hip complex should be viewed as a functional, integrated unit and treated as such (Mortazavi et al., 2015).

This case demonstrates how control and movement dysfunction issues can occur together. In the case of this player, I reasoned that his spino-pelvic complex was over-compensating, as shown in the altered movement strategies revealed during testing and assessment, which could have resulted from an incomplete rehabilitation plan following his previous hip surgery. It was hypothesized that the lower lumbar segments may have developed increased translation motion due to the impact of inappropriate hip joint flexion, perhaps even for many years prior to his hip surgery, alongside the previous diagnosis of a spondylolysis. The psoas tenotomy may have had an impact on both hip joint centration and spinal stability. Pelvic reinforcement improved

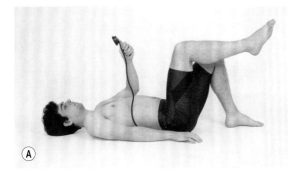

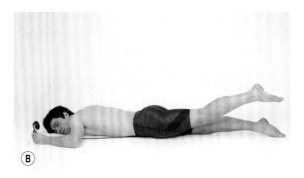

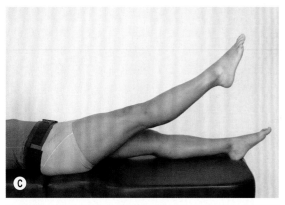

Figure 4.5
Evaluation and management of Patient E.
A Use of pressure biofeedback unit (PBU) in supine.
B Use of PBU in prone. **C** Use of a sacroiliac joint stability belt.

ASLR, highlighting the need for restoring neuromuscular motor control and tissue capacity across the pelvic girdle, to transfer force and load optimally.

Hip pain in young athletes

Hip joint and groin injuries in young athletes appear to be diagnosed with increasing levels of frequency (Griffin et al., 2016). Evidence suggests that understanding and diagnosing these injuries has been challenging. This may

be due in part to the complexity of the anatomical structures that cross the pelvic girdle and the upper thigh. Athletic hip pain may encompass either intra- or extra-articular pathologies, or a combination of both, and can often refer from the lumbar spine or SIJs. These symptoms may stem from progressive, repetitive microtrauma or be the result of a specific incident.

Assessment of risk factors suggests that a reduction in neuromuscular coordination and proprioceptive awareness may be related to these types of injuries. This may occur in response to a linear growth spurt during puberty, initially affecting the bones of the lower limbs, which lengthen at a different rate to the surrounding soft tissues (Hawkins and Metheny, 2001). The consequence is a loss of ROM and flexibility of the soft tissue across the hip joint, primarily affecting the hip flexors and hamstrings. Loss of ROM predisposes a young athlete to potential soft tissue injury, increasing their vulnerability to sprains, strains and avulsion fractures. They may also be more susceptible to growth-related injuries throughout this period, as compression and shear forces, which affect the open physes and cartilage growth plates of long bones, may result in premature closure, apophyseal avulsion and cartilage injuries (Kovacevic et al., 2011).

Serious pathology in a young athlete presenting with hip or groin-related pain should be investigated thoroughly to rule out any major concerns or potential red flags. Examples include a history of prostate cancer in males and in the reproductive organs in females, cancer-related metastases, an unexplained history of trauma, such as avascular necrosis fractures to the femoral neck and pelvic girdle, fever, weight loss, dysuria and night pain. At present, evidence supporting the diagnostic accuracy in predicting red flags appears to be limited and inconsistent in a clinical context (Downie et al., 2013). In light of this evidence, if assessment raises the suspicion of red flags, further investigation is always warranted.

The spino-pelvic complex should also be screened to rule this out as the source of referred pain reported in the hip and groin region. Chapter 2 included a description of tests with high sensitivity and specificity, which may be used to screen for lumbar intervertebral disk herniation, facet joint syndrome and SIJ pain. These will be discussed in greater detail in subsequent chapters.

Extra-articular hip pain

Extra-articular overload injuries around the hip joint include pathologies such as tendinopathy, bursitis, hernia and muscle strain (Griffin et al., 2016). High-load activities, such as kicking and sprinting, may render an athlete vulnerable to avulsion fractures, with the anterior superior and inferior iliac spines being the most common sites (Schuett et al., 2015). In recent years, a classification model has been developed to help clinicians examine certain clinical entities, with the aim of developing a common language (Weir et al., 2015; Hölmich, 2007; Hölmich et al., 2004). The Doha Agreement (Weir et al., 2015) and the Warwick Agreement (Griffin et al., 2016) are both useful clinical models that classify athletes according to particular clinical pathologies (Figure 4.6). Tenderness and pain on palpation, stretch and resistance testing may all be a recognizable symptom related to the anatomical structure being tested: for example, the adductor-iliopsoas-pubic and inguinal regions. The outcomes of multiple clinical tests can often be tricky for the clinician to navigate. For example, adductor-related groin pain has been shown to have a high accuracy on clinical testing for predicting and identifying injuries in this region (Serner et al., 2016). However, on clinical testing, it is much more difficult to distinguish between the iliopsoas and rectus femoris muscles of the hip flexor group (Serner et al., 2016). The absence of pain on palpation has been shown to have the most significant value for ruling out injuries to both the adductors and the

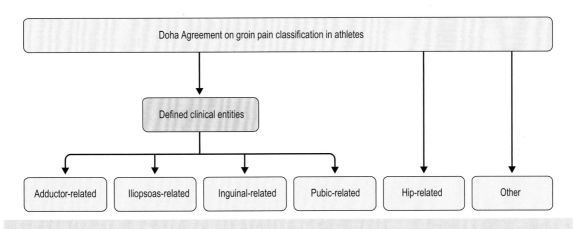

Figure 4.6
Classification by clinical pathology.

iliopsoas, with a reported accuracy of greater than 90 percent (Serner et al., 2016).

Hip-related pubic pain

Hip-related pubic pain (Figure 4.7) should be considered as a source of groin pain in both young and mature athletes. The pubic symphysis is the last anatomical structure to become skeletally mature and this may explain why adolescent athletes with hip-related groin pain are more susceptible to pubic apophysitis (Sansone et al., 2014). Although it is well documented in the literature that hip-related groin pain is more common in mature athletes, starting in their early twenties (Kivlan et al., 2017; Clohisy et al., 2009), in older athletes hip-related groin pain may be an indicator of premature OA, with symptoms referred from the hip into the pubic region (Clohisy et al., 2009).

Hip joint-related pain

Hip-related intra-articular overload injuries have also been shown to be common in young male athletes (Carsen et al., 2014; Brian et al., 2010; Siebenrock et al., 2013). Clinical tests are shown to be more beneficial in ruling out intra-articular hip pathology (negative test result), compared with "ruling in" the need for further investigation (positive test result) (Reiman et al., 2015). FAI has been defined as a motion-related clinical hip disorder with a triad of symptoms, clinical signs and imaging findings (Griffin et al., 2016). The primary symptoms are motion- or position-related pain in the hip or groin region, with potential clicking, catching, locking, stiffness, restricted hip ROM or the hip "giving way." Intra-articular hip joint symptoms may also be associated with an underlying pediatric issue, such as hip joint dysplasia, complex bony deformities or labral and cartilage lesions (Griffin et al., 2016). There are two types of FAI – "cam" (osteophytes in the zone of the femoral head–neck junction) and "pincer" (osteophytes at the acetabular edges) – and a combination of both cam and pincer may be present (Anderson et al., 2012; Byrd, 2010; Brunner et al., 2009; Martin and Philippon, 2007; Siebenrock et al., 2004; Ito et al., 2004; Ganz et al., 2003; Goodman et al., 1997). Hip joint cam-type FAI (Figure 4.8) has been shown to be common in young athletes (Carsen et al., 2014), resulting in suboptimal hip function (Harris-Hayes et al., 2009) with effects on spino-pelvic motion (Lamontagne et al., 2008). Cam-type FAI impingement is characterized by a non-spherical femoral head or by an insufficient offset between the femoral head and neck (Sink et al., 2008). Such abnormal joint morphology, combined with repetitive loading from the proximal femoral head abutting against the acetabulum (Anderson et al., 2012; Byrd, 2010; Brunner et al., 2009; Martin and Philippon, 2007;

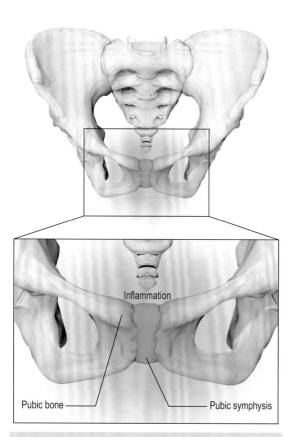

Inflammation

Pubic bone

Pubic symphysis

Figure 4.7
Hip-related pubic pain.

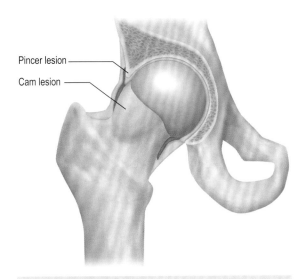

Pincer lesion

Cam lesion

Figure 4.8
Hip joint femoroacetabular impingement.

Siebenrock et al., 2004; Ito et al., 2004; Ganz et al., 2003; Goodman et al., 1997), may cause increased stress and damage to the articular cartilage during repetitive hip flexion and internal rotation (Kienle et al., 2012; Beall et al., 2005).

A greater prevalence of cam-type FAI impingement has been shown to occur in elite athletes, with prevalence ranging from 60 to 89 percent in sports such as basketball, ice hockey, soccer and American football (Siebenrock et al., 2011; Kapron et al., 2011). In athletes, the most common complaint relating to FAI is groin pain exacerbated by intense activity, including repetitive hip flexion movements. Moreover, symptoms may be vague and diffuse, with pain often being referred medially towards the pubic symphysis, laterally towards the greater trochanter or dorsally towards the gluteal muscles. The C sign is often used by individuals to describe the location of their pain, by placing their hand in a C shape around the hip (Frank et al., 2013). Clinically, the most common finding with FAI

examination relates to reduced ROM, specifically flexion and rotation (Audenaert et al., 2012; Kapron et al., 2012; Clohisy et al., 2009).

FAI diagnosis is based on clinical history, physical examination and investigations using plain radiographs, CT or MRI (Beall et al., 2005). The reliability of clinical tests for FAI, such as flexion, abduction, external rotation (FABER) and flexion, adduction, internal rotation (FADIR) (see Chapter 5), varies. Although both tests are shown to be sensitive, they lack specificity (Kapron et al., 2012; Maslowski et al., 2010; Clohisy et al., 2009). The FABER test also shows good reliability but the FADIR test appears to be more widely reported in studies regarding FAI (Ratzlaff et al., 2013; Kapron et al., 2012; Maslowski et al., 2010; Prather et al., 2010; Cibere et al., 2008; Martin and Sekiya, 2008). Jónasson et al. (2016), in a clinical and radiological study, found that athletes had a higher Tönnis grade (presence of hip joint OA), more pain on FADIR test and a significantly lower ROM in internal and external rotation.

Recent research has shown that the cam-type deformity may be linked to a mechanical etiology, emerging from the physeal (growth plate-related) scar of the proximal femoral physis (Siebenrock et al., 2004). It has been suggested that this may have developed during adolescence, as a response to vigorous sporting activity (Jónasson et al., 2015; Tak et al., 2015; Agricola et al., 2014). Similar growth disturbances and chronic physeal damage have also been reported to occur in other regions, such as the spine, in adolescent elite athletes, which further underlines how loading during development may impact on long-term athletic musculoskeletal health (Baranto et al., 2006; Lundin et al., 2001; Epstein and Epstein, 1991; Sward et al., 1990).

Management of extra-/intra-articular hip and groin-related pain

Most athletes can continue to train with hip and groin-related pain for many months, until they are eventually forced to withdraw from exercise due to pain. Unfortunately, continuing to train with pain can lead to the development of non-functional movement patterns and compensation strategies, which may further contribute to decreased function (dysfunction) and performance (Edwards et al., 2017; Franklyn-Miller et al., 2017). To date, it appears that there are similar time-frames for RTP in athletes with groin pain who elect to have a surgical intervention, compared to those who are managed conservatively (King et al., 2015). This emphasizes the need to include movement impairment and functional testing alongside more traditional clinical tests, especially if planning a conservative management approach. I have often found this conservative management strategy to be extremely successful in resolving symptoms in patients who continue to report hip and groin pain after surgery.

Range of motion testing

If side-to-side differences in mobility of greater than 5° are highlighted during hip ROM testing (Figure 4.9), it suggests the patient or athlete may benefit from specific, highly targeted strategies to manage their

symptoms (Griffin et al., 2016). However, it is important to realize that ROM restrictions may not only be affected by bony morphology in the joint, but also reflect the underlying chondral (joint surface) status and could be indicative of protective muscle guarding (Thorborg et al., 2018). As previously mentioned in relation to the adolescent hip, increased soft tissue tension may perhaps limit mobility as a result of a recent growth spurt, leading to the development of joint and myofascial stiffness.

Strength and capacity testing

Muscle strength deficits are a consistently reported finding in athletes presenting with hip and groin pain. This has previously been shown in pain related to the adductors, pubis and hip, as reported in FAI (Kloskowska et al., 2016), and it is also seen to occur after athletes have undergone surgery for FAI (Todd et al., 2020). Objective strength measurements, in all planes of motion, can be taken using hand-held dynamometry (Figure 4.10). Clinically, changes or differences in

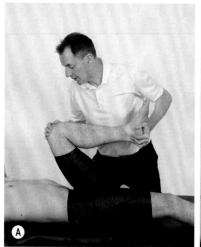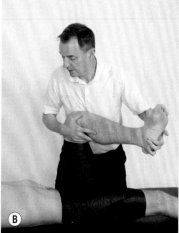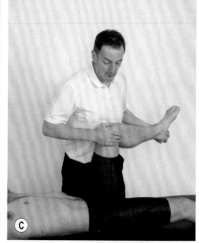

Figure 4.9
Hip joint ROM testing.
A Flexion. **B** External rotation. **C** Internal rotation.

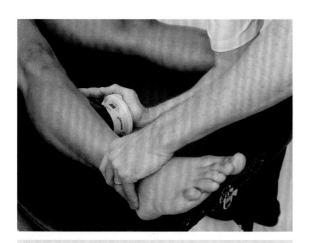

Figure 4.10
Adductor strength testing with hand-held dynamometer.

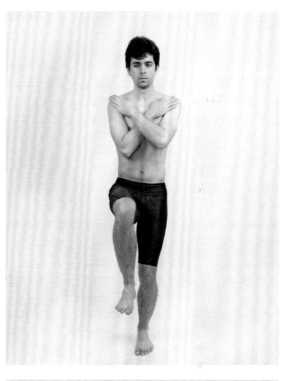

Figure 4.11
Functional evaluation single-leg stance test with small knee bend.

muscle strength ratios between limbs can be measured reliably by this method, and deficits of greater than 20 percent in adductors and abductors have been reported in athletes with adductor and pubic-related groin pain (Thorborg et al., 2014). I have also found a 20 percent deficit in muscle strength between limbs for hip flexor strength to be clinically significant and therefore, in my practice, I am especially attentive to asymmetry in muscle strength presentations in my patients. These individuals, in my experience, respond to techniques that *activATE* as opposed to *manipulATE*. Clinically, this highlights the significance of understanding control and movement impairments that can affect the hip, similar to that previously described for LBP earlier in this chapter.

Functional evaluation

In a clinical setting, testing for functional strength deficits (Figure 4.11), may be challenging, as not everyone has access to 3-D motion camera analysis. The use of SL stance, small knee bend (SKB) and the star excursion balance test for athletes has been supported in a systematic review by Diamond et al. (2015) and I

have highlighted this in Chapter 5, which contains an in-depth explanation and range of functional tests for assessing movement dysfunction.

Clinical implications

Hip and groin-related pain may have many causes that often present simultaneously: that is, coexisting alongside another pathology. A patient can present with either one or both, a combination of soft tissue and articular movement restrictions, alongside neuromuscular control deficits. Patients may often have developed a pattern of substitution strategies for coping and managing for themselves during movement and for pain avoidance (Casartelli et al., 2011). For example, FAI may be present alongside a proximal muscle issue. Hölmich et al. (2014) previously demonstrated that patients presenting with adductor-related groin pain achieved good results with an exercise program, in spite of the coexistence of a bony morphology related to FAI and hip dysplasia. This suggests that morphology may not be the sole driver of symptoms and, moreover, that symptoms that may be linked to a morphological finding can be addressed with an active exercise approach.

Hip flexor weakness and reduced hip joint ROM have also been shown to occur pre- and post-FAI surgery (Todd et al., 2020; Diamond et al., 2015; Casartelli et al., 2011). The iliopsoas tendon, due to its close anatomical proximity to the anterior capsule and labrum, may actually cause or mimic hip impingement and result in FAI symptoms (Blankenbaker and Tuite, 2008). A reduction in hip flexor muscle strength has also been shown in patients with acetabular labral pathology (Mendis et al., 2014). Decreased levels of strength might have implications for physical function, contributing to altered movement patterns in gait and during functional tasks. No difference was shown in the cross-sectional area of hip flexor muscle, demonstrated on MRI, between symptomatic hips and asymptomatic hips. This suggests that deficits in strength may be related to alteration of neuromuscular control, rather than muscle atrophy, and offers further support for the proposition that exercise targeting neuromuscular control and synergies, alongside strength training, may be beneficial.

In the presence of pain, neuromuscular control may be altered because of reduced afferent input from damaged joint tissues, and modulated motor control output via spinal reflex pathways, which may be affected by damage to joint receptors (Rice and McNair, 2010; Stokes and Young, 1984; Spencer et al., 1984). There is evidence of positive outcomes for exercise to address this; for example, hip flexor strength training, using resistance bands, has been shown to have a positive effect (17 percent improvement in hip flexor strength)

in an asymptomatic population after 6 weeks' training (Thorborg et al., 2015).

Case study: Patient F

 Player F, a 22-year-old male soccer player (stature 190 cm and body mass 82 kg), presented with an 18-month history of hip and groin pain. Twelve months previously, he had undergone bilateral arthroscopy surgery for cam-type FAI. He was complaining of constant groin pain that was preventing him from training. He had previously undergone an adductor-loading program at his club but in spite of this he still reported groin pain.

Examination revealed loss of ROM, specifically active and passive hip flexion and internal rotation. Strength measurements were recorded using a handheld dynamometer and highlighted significant weakness and pain on hip flexion and hip abduction testing. Functional testing demonstrated an inability to perform an SL stance with SKB, without collapsing into a knee joint valgus position.

 SMTs were used to restore hip flexion and internal rotation. Manual therapy techniques to restore the flexibility of TFL and adductor muscles helped to improve hip flexion and internal rotation ROM.

 Motor control techniques to restore deep hip flexors (psoas) and inner-range hip abduction (posterior fibers of gluteus medius) helped to improve ROM and control through the range. The clinical reasoning for these techniques was to address both movement and control issues around the hip joint.

 Treatment was given over 5 weeks, during five consultations, resulting in pain reduction (VAS 8/10 to 0/10). Improvement in hip joint strength in all ranges was shown, specifically right hip flexion (0.29–0.43 Nm/kg, 48 percent) and right hip abduction (0.35–0.46 Nm/kg, 31 percent).

In conclusion, SMT used in this case report supports the rationale for restoring hip joint neuromuscular control in the presence of anterior hip pain, post arthroscopic surgery for FAI.

Pelvic girdle physiology and dysfunction

The pelvic girdle makes anatomical and functional contributions to human movement and obstetrics (Rosenberg and DeSilva, 2017). Viewed functionally, it is a mobile platform facilitating the balance of lumbar lordosis with hip joint extension to maintain the human standing upright posture (Todd et al., 2016). Any impairment of pelvic movement may reduce an athlete's performance and induce a higher risk of recurrence and chronicity of injury (Walden et al., 2015). Pelvic morphology may influence the biomechanics of hip motion. Similarly, the pelvic girdle has been shown to affect spinal postures and curvatures in young athletes (Todd et al., 2016). There is scant documentation of the relationship between pelvic and hip ROM and groin pain in athletes. If we refer to the terms "form closure" and "force closure" (see Chapters 1 and 2), perhaps we can start to appreciate the functional role of the pelvis as a dynamic platform during human movement.

Form closure refers to the stability derived from the articular surfaces fitting tightly together. Hence this term is likened to the keystone concept in a Roman arch: according to this analogy, the articular surfaces of the sacrum and ilia can be visualized as being compressed together at the end of range of sacral nutation, and the transmission of load and force would occur through the articular surfaces. Force closure, as previously discussed, refers to the compression provided by active CNS-regulated muscular contributions to the passive system. Vleeming et al. (2007) proposed that, as the sacrum is wider cranially than caudally, and wider anteriorly than posteriorly, perhaps such a configuration helps to wedge the sacrum into the ilia. While this model appears reasonable, it is open to questioning. The performance of tasks in weight-bearing, which require load transfer of forces through the pelvic girdle, encourages intra-pelvic motion: that is, the sacrum moves anteriorly and inferiorly. During the gait cycle or tasks that require transverse or frontal plane motion in the trunk or lower extremities, an intra-pelvic torsion left or right will occur (Lee and Lee, 2011). Although this is only a small degree of movement, it may be clinically relevant in identifying a potential cause of pain.

If we accept the principle of the keystone concept – that is, that a small degree of intra-pelvic motion may occur between the joint surfaces – then it is plausible that degenerative changes may occur around these joints from friction occurring at the joint surfaces as they compress and stabilize the pelvic girdle. Ligamentous suspension has also been proposed as another concept to explain factors contributing to pelvic stability. Investigation of the SIJ ligaments in four-legged animals has shown that these ligaments assist in supporting the weight of the caudal vertebral column. Perhaps it could be argued that the human skeleton has been constructed similarly to that of other animals and that ligamentous suspension may actually be a more efficient stabilizing mechanism for the pelvic girdle, compared with the model of weight transfer (Haussler, 2012).

Injury to the ligaments that support the pelvis can result in increased ligamentous laxity, and this may lead to increased shear and compressive forces through the articular surfaces, causing degenerative changes. Therefore, force closure from the extra-articular structures may prove essential to holding the suspended sacrum tightly, compressing the SIJ against the ilia. Gluteus maximus (GMx) and the contralateral latissimus dorsi have both been shown to create force closure across the pelvic girdle (Snijders et al., 1993). Unfortunately, this has led many clinicians and fitness enthusiasts to assume that GMx exercises are essential for SIJ dysfunction, and the general population, including athletes, have become obsessed with gluteal exercises and the ability to "switch them on." So, what is the answer? Before you take this proposal on board without question, I would ask you to cast your mind back to Chapters 1 and 2 and the concept of movement function and dysfunction, and to think about the prospect of accepting that neuromuscular fatigue from excessive load, and maladaptive compensation patterns from previous injury, may be significant causal factors.

Clinical implications of increased or reduced force closure

 In my experience, most musculoskeletal pelvic girdle dysfunctions result either from increased force closure, such as an SIJ or pubic symphysis restriction, or from decreased force closure, stemming from a motor control deficit or weakness in the extra-articular structures. It is extremely important to bear in mind that an athlete or other patient may frequently present with asymmetrical imbalances: one side may test positive for increased force closure, while the other side tests positive for decreased forced closure. This is often the reason why some patients report pain when you clinically test the asymptomatic joint.

Active pelvic tilt is considered to be an integral component, acting as a central segment assisting in proximal-to-distal sequencing of high-speed body movements (Shan and Westerhoff, 2005). In sprinting, the pelvis tilts posteriorly during the early stance phase, then reverses quickly to anterior tilt. In kicking a ball, spinal flexion and posterior pelvic tilt appear to be coupled movements, which occur prior to ball impact (Naito et al., 2012). Any deficit in the ability of the pelvis to move may have a negative effect on energy transfer and result in compensatory movement strategies at the adjacent segments, with increased load being taken through the muscles associated with these segments. Soccer players with a history of groin injury demonstrate decreased

pelvic tilt during a kicking task. Similarly, the kinematics of the hip and pelvis during sport-specific tasks, such as an SL drop landing and a change of direction task, are different in athletes with a groin injury from those in athletes without (Severin et al., 2017; Janse van Rensburg et al., 2017; Franklyn-Miller et al., 2017). This suggests that restoring active pelvic tilt should always be considered an essential part of rehabilitation for injured athletes, as it allows optimal mechanical energy transfer during sports actions (Naito et al., 2012).

Clinical evaluation may be improved by using SMT to test for increased or decreased force closure across the pelvic girdle. The ASLR (Figure 4.12) is a clinically validated test for evaluating load transfer across the pelvic girdle, from the trunk to the lower extremity, in patients with peripartum pelvic pain (Mens et al., 1999; 2001; 2002). It has subsequently been proposed that varying the hand positions, when applying compression around the pelvic girdle during the ASLR, enables the clinician to gather more information pertaining to the structure and tissues involved, to help inform a clinical reasoning process (Lee, 2011).

Optimal function of the spino-pelvic-hip complex should result in the leg being raised without effort from the supine position, with no movement occurring in the pelvis relative to the thoracic region and/or lower extremity. Introducing pelvic compression has been shown to reduce the effort necessary to perform the leg raise, and to assist with force closure and improve pelvic reinforcement. Conversely, if pelvic compression results in the patient experiencing more difficulty in performing the ASLR test, then perhaps pelvic reinforcement needs to be reduced. Refer to Chapter 5, where this test is discussed in greater detail. This is a quick, yet effective SMT that can be applied clinically. I have used this approach many times in high-performance sport with athletes who have returned to the changing room at half-time in a game, reporting they had experienced groin or hip pain during the first half of a match.

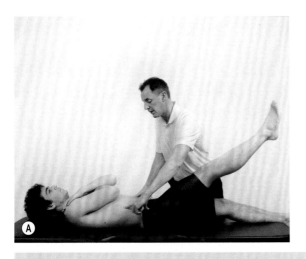
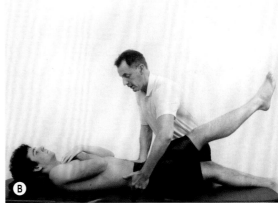

Figure 4.12
Active Straight Leg Raise (ASLR).
A The ASLR used to evaluate load transfer across the pelvis. **B** ASLR testing using external compression for pelvic reinforcement.

Case study: Patient G

Patient G is a 28-year-old female triathlete and endurance athlete, who had been struggling with an ongoing history of groin pain. Over a period of 5 years, she had undergone multiple investigations, and while she had been able to modify her training, she had unfortunately not been able to return to the competition levels she had once enjoyed.

Evaluation highlighted that Patient G had reduced active and passive adductor ROM. Although she tested strong in neutral, using handheld dynamometry, she reported central, pubic-related groin pain when she activated her adductors to contract. Testing showed that outer-range strength was virtually non-existent, weak and painful.

SMT, using manual pelvic reinforcement, helped to modify the pubic-related groin symptoms and enabled her to generate more power on her adductor squeeze (Mens et al., 1999). Manual therapy techniques were used to restore length to the adductor muscles, and when re-evaluated, the strength measurements in her outer range had also improved.

Management involved soft tissue manipulation to restore length to the adductor muscles, combined with education through a progressive strengthening program for the adductors, initially to improve motor control. This progressed from low-threshold to higher-threshold exercises to develop tissue capacity (Figure 4.13).

Initially, an SIJ stability belt was used to assist force closure across the pelvic girdle, but as Patient G began to function more optimally, the need to wear the SIJ belt reduced. Over the next 6 months, Patient G went from struggling to walk pain-free to being able to continue with her training. Initially, running was performed on a gravity-reducing treadmill to reduce load, and then

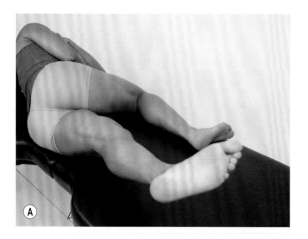

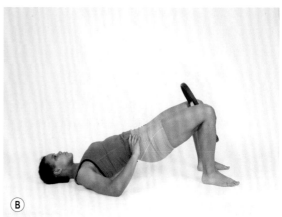

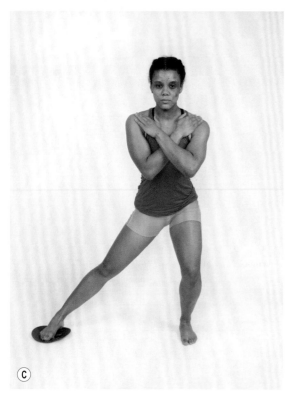

Figure 4.13
Progression of adductor exercises.
A Side-lying inner-range isometric holds. **B** Supine squeeze with Pilates ring. **C** Single-leg slider.

gradually transferred to road running while monitoring symptoms. The patient successfully ran a marathon at 4 months in an Ironman race in Frankfurt. Later the same year, she completed a 52 km ultra-run, followed by a 100 km 5-day competition.

In conclusion, SMT alongside manual therapy and motor control techniques was used to manage Patient G's pubic-related groin pain effectively and efficiently, while she progressively loaded her tissues to develop muscle capacity and compliance, resulting in a successful return to her sporting activity.

Conclusion

To summarize, it was the intention of this chapter to provide an overview of the more common musculo-skeletal presentations related to the spino-pelvic-hip complex. I cannot emphasize enough the importance of using our clinical skills, knowledge and understanding of pain, pathology and dysfunction in helping to determine a correct diagnosis for the many presentations associated with this region. In my opinion, clinicians should remain open-minded and embrace all aspects relating to the biomedical, biomechanical and bio-psychosocial models of pain, as this will help them to apply my "five 'ATEs" in a successful management strategy.

The following chapters are dedicated to specific aspects of this process and will serve to enhance your knowledge and clinical reasoning skills further.

References

Agricola, R., Heijboer, MP., Ginai, AZ. et al., 2014. A cam deformity is gradually acquired during skeletal maturation in adolescent and young male soccer players: a prospective study with minimum 2-year follow-up. *American Journal Sports Medicine*, 42(4), pp. 798–806.

Airaksinen, O., Brox, JI., Cedraschi, C. et al., 2006. Chapter 4 European guidelines for the management of chronic nonspecific low back pain. *European Spine Journal*, 15, pp. S192–S300.

Anderson, SE., Siebenrock, KA., Tannast, M., 2012. Femoroacetabular impingement. *European Journal Radiology*, 81(12), pp. 3740–3744.

Audenaert, E., Peeters, I., Vigneron, L. et al., 2012. Hip morphological characteristics and range of internal rotation in femoroacetabular impingement. *American Journal Sports Medicine*, 40(6), pp. 1329–1336.

Baranto, A., Ekstrom, L., Holm, S. et al., 2005. Vertebral fractures and separations of endplates after traumatic loading of adolescent porcine spines with experimentally-induced disc degeneration. *Clinical Biomechanics (Bristol, Avon)*, 20(10), pp. 1046–1054.

Baranto, A., Hellstrom, M., Nyman, R. et al., 2006. Back pain and degenerative abnormalities in the spine of young elite divers: a 5-year follow-up magnetic resonance imaging study. *Knee Surgery Sports Traumatology Arthroscopy*, 14(9), pp. 907–914.

Baranto, A., Hellstrom, M., Cederlund, CG. et al., 2009. Back pain and MRI changes in the thoracolumbar spine of top athletes in four different sports: a 15-year follow-up study. *Knee Surgery Sports Traumatology Arthroscopy*, 17(9), pp. 1125–1134.

Baranto, A., Hellstrom M. and Sward L., 2010. Acute injury of an intervertebral disc in an elite tennis player: a case report. *Spine (Phila Pa 1976)*, 35, pp. E223–E227.

Beall, D., Sweet, C., Martin, H. et al., 2005. Imaging findings of femoroacetabular impingement syndrome. *Skeletal Radiology*, 34(11), pp. 691–701.

Blankenbaker, DG. and Tuite, MJ., 2008. Iliopsoas musculotendinous unit. *Seminars Musculoskeletal Radiology*, 12, pp. 13–27. DOI:10.1055/s-2008-1067934.

Bolay, H., and Moskowitz, M., 2002. Mechanisms of pain modulation in chronic syndromes. *Journal of Neurology*, 59, pp. S2–S7.

Borkan, J., Koes, B., Reis, R. et al., 1998. A report from the second international forum for primary care research on LBP: re-examining properties. *Spine*, 23, pp. 1992–1996.

Brian, P., Bernard, S. and Flemming, D., 2010. Femoroacetabular impingement: screening and definitive imaging. *Seminars in Roentgenology*, 45(4), pp. 228–237.

Brinjikji, W., Luetmer, P., Comstock, B. et al., 2015. Systematic literature review of imaging features of spinal degeneration in asymptomatic populations. *American Journal Neuroradiology*, 36, pp. 818–816.

Brooks, JC., Kong, Y., Lee, MC. et al., 2012. Stimulus site and modality dependence of functional activity within the human spinal cord. *Journal Neuroscience*, 32(18), pp. 6231–6239.

Brunner, A., Horisberger, M. and Herzog, R., 2009. Sports and reaction activity of patients with femoroacetabular impingement before and after arthroscopic osteoplasty. *American Journal Sports Medicine*, 37(5), pp. 917–922.

Byrd, J., 2010. Femoroacetabular impingement in athletes, part 1: cause and assessment. *Sports Health*, 2(4), pp. 321–333.

Caneiro, JP., Smith, A., Rabey, M. et al., 2017. Process of change in pain-related fear: clinical insights from a single case report of persistent back pain managed with cognitive functional therapy. *Journal Orthopaedic Sports Physical Therapy*, (47), pp. 637–651.

Carsen, S., Moroz, P., Rakhra, K. et al., 2014. The Otto Aufranc Award. On the etiology of the cam deformity: a cross-sectional pediatric MRI study. *Clinical Orthopaedic Related Research*, 472(2), pp. 430–436.

Casartelli, N., Maffiuletti, N., Item-Glatthorn, S. et al., 2011. Hip muscle weakness in patients with symptomatic femoroacetabular impingement. *Osteoarthritis Cartilage*, 19, pp. 816–821.

Cholewicki, J., Panjabi, M. and Khachatryan, A., 1997. Stabilizing function of the trunk flexor/extensor muscles around a neutral spine posture. *Spine*, 22, pp. 2207–2212.

Cholewicki, J., Simons, A. and Radebold, A., 2000. Effects of external loads on lumbar spine stability. *Journal Biomechanics*, 33, pp. 1377–1385.

Cibere, J., Thorne, A., Bellamy, N. et al., 2008. Reliability of the hip examination in osteoarthritis: effect of standarization. *Arthritis and Rheumatism*, 59(3), pp. 373–381.

Clohisy, JC., Knaus, ER., Hunt, DM. et al., 2009. Clinical presentation of patients with symptomatic anterior hip impingement. *Clinical Orthopaedic Related Research*, 467, pp. 638–644. Available at: <https://doi.org/10.1007/s11999-008-0680-y> [accessed February 15, 2022].

Dankaerts, W., O'Sullivan, P., Burnett, A. et al., 2009. Discriminating healthy controls and two clinical subgroups of nonspecific chronic low back pain patients using trunk muscle activation and lumbosacral kinematics of postures and movements: a statistical classification model. *Spine*, 34, pp. 1610–1618.

Darlow, B., 2016. Beliefs about back pain: the confluence of client, clinician and community. *International Journal Osteopathic Medicine*, 20, pp. P53–61.

DeLeo, JA., Tanga, FY. and Tawfik, VL., 2004. Neuroimmune activation and neuroinflammation in chronic pain and opioid tolerance/hyperalgesia. *Neuroscientist*, 10, pp. 40–52.

Diamond, LE., Dobson, FL., Bennell, KL. et al., 2015. Physical impairments and activity limitations in people with femoroacetabular impingement: a systematic review. *British Journal Sports Medicine*, 49, pp. 230–242. Available at: <https://doi.org/10.1136/bjsports-2013-093340> [accessed February 15, 2022].

Downie, A., Williams, CM., Henschke, N. et al., 2013. Red flags to screen for malignancy and fracture in patients with low back pain: systematic review. *British Medical Journal*, 347, f7095. Available at: <https://doi.org/10.1136/bmj.f7095> [accessed February 15, 2022].

Edwards, S., Brooke, HC. and Cook, JL., 2017. Distinct cut task strategy in Australian football players with a history of groin pain. *Physical Therapy Sport*, 23, pp. 58–66. Available at: <https://doi.org/10.1016/j.ptsp.2016.07.005> [accessed February 15, 2022].

Epstein, N. and Epstein, J., 1991. Limbus lumbar vertebral fractures in 27 adolescents and adults. *Spine (Phila Pa 1976)*, 16(8), pp. 962–966.

Foster, NE., Hill, JC. and Hay, EM., 2011. Subgrouping patients with low back pain in primary care: are we getting any better at it? *Manual Therapy*, 16, pp. 3–8.

Frank, J., Gambacorta, P. and Eisner, E., 2013. Hip pathology in the adolescent athlete. *Journal American Academy Orthopaedic Surgery*, 21, pp. 665–674.

Franklyn-Miller, A., Richter, C., King, E. et al., 2017. Athletic groin pain (part 2): a prospective cohort study on the biomechanical evaluation of change of direction identifies three clusters of movement patterns. *British Journal Sports Medicine*, 51, pp. 460–468. Available at: <https://doi.org/10.1136/bjsports-2016-096050> [accessed February 15, 2022].

Freynhagen, R. and Baron, R., 2009. The evaluation of neuropathic components in low back pain. *Current Pain and Headache Reports*, 13, pp. 185–190.

Fryer, G., 2017. Integrating osteopathic approaches based on biopsychosocial therapeutic mechanism. Part 1: The mechanisms. *International Journal Osteopathic Medicine*, 25, pp. 30–41.

Ganz, R., Parvizi, J., Beck, M. et al., 2003. Femoroacetabular impingement: a cause for osteoarthritis of the hip. *Clinical Orthopaedics Related Research*, 417, pp. 112–120.

Gerrits, MM., van Marwijk, HW., van Oppen, P. et al., 2015. Longitudinal association between pain, and depression and anxiety over four years. *Journal Psychosomatic Research*, 78, pp. 64–70.

Gibbons, S., 2007. Clinical anatomy and function of psoas major and deep sacral gluteus maximus. In: Vleeming, A., Mooney, V. and Stoeckart, R., eds. *Movement, Stability & Lumbopelvic Pain*. London: Churchill Livingstone, pp. 95–102.

Goodman, D., Feighan, J., Smith, A. et al., 1997. Subclinical slipped capital femoral epiphysis: relationship to osteoarthrosis of the hip. *Journal Bone and Joint Surgery*, 79, pp. 1489–1497.

Griffin, D., Dickenson, E., O'Donnel, J. et al., 2016. The Warwick Agreement on femoroacetabular impingement syndrome (FAI syndrome): an international consensus statement. *British Journal Sports Medicine*, 50, pp. 1169–1176.

Guo, LH. and Schluesener, HJ., 2007. The innate immunity of the central nervous system in chronic pain: the role of Toll-like receptors. *Cell Molecular Life Science*, 64, pp. 1128–1136.

Hangai, M., Kaneoka, K., Okubo, Y. et al., 2010. Relationship between low back pain and competitive sports activities during youth. *American Journal Sports Medicine*, 38, pp. 791–796.

Hannibal, KE. and Bishop, MD., 2014. Chronic stress, cortisol dysfunction, and pain: a psychoneuroendrocrine rationale for stress management in pain rehabilitation. *Physical Therapy*, 94, pp. 1816–1825.

Harris-Hayes, M., Sahrmann, S. and Van Dillen, L., 2009. Relationship between the hip and low back pain in athletes who participate in rotation-related sports. *Journal of Sports Rehabilitation*, 18(1), pp. 60–75.

Haussler, K., 2012. *Functional Assessment and Rehabilitation of the Equine Axial Skeleton*. In ACVS Veterinary Symposium, National Harbor, Maryland, USA, November 1–3.

Hawkins, D. and Metheny, J., 2001. Overuse injuries in youth sports: biomechanical considerations. *Medicine Science Sports Exercise*, 33(10), pp. 1701–1707.

Henschke, M., Maher, CG., Refshauge, KM. et al., 2009. Prevalence of and screening for serious spinal pathology in patients presenting to primary care settings with acute low back pain. *Arthritis Rheumatology*, 60, pp. 3072–3080.

Hölmich, P., 2007. Long-standing groin pain in sportspeople falls into three primary patterns, a "clinical entity" approach: a prospective study of 207 patients. *British Journal Sports Medicine*, 41, pp. 247–252. Available at: <https://doi.org/10.1136/bjsm.2006.033373> [accessed February 15, 2022].

Hölmich, P., Hölmich, LR. and Bjerg, AM., 2004. Clinical examination of athletes with groin pain: an intraobserver and interobserver reliability study. *British Journal Sports Medicine*, 38, pp. 446–451. Available at: <https://doi.org/10.1136/bjsm.2003.004754> [accessed February 15, 2022].

Hölmich, P., Thorborg, K., Nyvold, P. et al., 2014. Does bony hip morphology affect the outcome of treatment for patients with adductor-related groin pain? Outcome 10 years after baseline assessment. *British Journal Sports Medicine*, 48, pp. 1240–1244.

Hoogendoorn, WE., van Poppel, MN., Bongers, PM. et al., 2000. Systematic review of psychosocial factors at work and private life risk factors for low back pain. *Spine (Phila Pa 1976)*, 25, pp. 2114–2125.

Hoy, D., Brooks, P., Blyth, F. et al., 2010. The epidemiology of low back pain. *Best Practice Research Clinical Rheumatology*, 24, pp. 769–781.

Huang, P., Anissipour, A., McGee, W. et al., 2016. Return to play recommendations after cervical, thoracic and lumbar spine injuries: a comprehensive review. *Sports Health*, 8(1), pp. 19–25.

Ito, K., Kahlnor, M., Leunig, M. et al., 2004. Hip morphology influences the pattern of femoroacetabular impingement. *Clinical Orthopaedics*, 429, pp. 262–271.

Iwamoto, J., Sato, Y., Takeda, T. et al., 2010. The return to sports activity after conservative or surgical treatment in athletes with lumbar disc herniation. *American Journal Physical Medicine Rehabilitation*, 89(12), pp. 1030–1035.

Janse van Rensburg, L., Dare, M., Louw, Q. et al., 2017. Pelvic and hip kinematics during single-leg drop-landing are altered in sports with long-standing groin pain: a cross-sectional study. *Physical Therapy in Sport*, 26, pp. 20–26.

Jónasson, P., Ekström, L., Hansson, HA. et al., 2015. Cyclical loading causes injury in and around the porcine proximal femoral physeal plate: proposed cause of the development of cam deformity in young athletes. *Journal Experimental Orthopaedics*, 2(6).

Jónasson, P., Thoreson, O., Sansone, M. et al., 2016. The morphologic characteristics and range of motion in the hips of athletes and non-athletes. *Journal of Hip Preservation Surgery*, 3(4), pp. 325–332.

Kapron, AL., Anderson, AE., Aoki, SK. et al., 2011. Radiographic prevalence of femoroacetabular impingement in collegiate football players. *Journal Bone Joint Surgery American*, 93(19), p. e111.

Kapron, AL., Anderson, S., Peters, C. et al., 2012. Hip internal rotation is correlated to radiographic findings of cam femoroacetabular impingement in collegiate football players. *Arthroscopy*, 28(11), pp. 1161–1170.

Kienle, K., Keck, J., Werlen, S. et al., 2012. Femoral morphology and epiphyseal growth plate changes of the hip during maturation: MR assessments in a 1-year follow-up on a cross-sectional asymptomatic cohort in the age range of 9–17 years. *Skeletal Radiology*, 41(11), pp. 1381–1390.

King, E., Ward, J., Small, L. et al., 2015. Athletic groin pain: a systematic review and meta-analysis of surgical versus physical therapy rehabilitation outcomes. *British Journal Sports Medicine*, 49, pp. 1447–1451. Available at: <https://doi.org/10.1136/bjsports-2014-093715> [accessed February 15, 2022].

Kivlan, BR., Nho, SJ., Christoforetti, JJ. et al., 2017. Multicenter outcomes after hip arthroscopy: epidemiology (MASH Study Group). What are we seeing in the office, and who are we choosing to treat? *American Journal Orthopedics (Belle Mead NJ)*, 46, pp. 35–41.

Kloskowska, P., Morrissey, D., Small, C. et al., 2016. Movement patterns and muscular function before and after onset of sports-related groin pain: a systematic review with meta-analysis. *Sports Medicine*, 46, pp. 1847–1867. Available at: <https://doi.org/10.1007/s40279-016-0523-z> [accessed February 15, 2022].

Koch, C. and Hansel, F., 2019. Non-specific low back pain and postural control during quiet standing – a systematic review. *Frontiers in Psychology*. Available at: <https://doi.org/10.3389/fpsyg.2019.00586> [accessed February 15, 2022].

Koes, BW., van Tulder, M., Lin, C. et al., 2010. An updated overview of clinical guidelines for the management of acute nonspecific low back pain in primary care. *European Spine Journal*, 19, pp. 2075–2094.

Kovacevic, D., Mariscalco, M., Goodwin, RC., 2011. Injuries about the hip in the adolescent athlete. *Sports Medicine Arthroscopy*, 19(1), pp. 64–74.

Lamontagne, M., Kennedy, M. and Beaule, P., 2008. The effect of cam FAI on hip and pelvic motion during maximum squat. *Clinical Orthopaedics Related Research,* 467(3), pp. 645–650.

Laslett, M., Aprill, CN., McDonald, B. et al., 2005. Diagnosis of sacroiliac joint pain: validity of individual provocation tests and composites of tests. *Manual Therapy,* 10, pp. 207–218.

Laslett, M., McDonald, B., Aprill, CN. et al., 2006. Clinical predictors of screening lumbar zygapophyseal joint blocks: development of clinical prediction rules. *Spine Journal,* 6, pp. 370–379.

Lee, D., and Lee, LJ., 2011. An integrated approach to assessment and treatment of the lumbopelvic-hip region. In D. Lee, *The Pelvic Girdle.* 4th ed. Edinburgh: Churchill Livingstone/Elsevier.

Liebenson, C., 2006. *Rehabilitation of the Spine: A Practitioner's Manual.* 2nd ed. Philadelphia: Lippincott Williams & Wilkins.

Lundin, O., Hellstrom, M., Nilsson, I. et al., 2001. Back pain and radiological changes in the thoraco-lumbar spine of athletes: a long-term follow-up. *Scandanivan Journal Medicine Science Sports,* 11(2), pp. 103–109.

Main, C. and Watson, P., 1999. Psychological aspects of pain. *Manual Therapy,* 80, pp. 113–119.

Majlesi, J., Togay, H., Unalan, H. et al., 2008. The sensitivity and specificity of the slump and the straight leg raising tests in patients with lumbar disc herniation. *Journal Clinical Rheumatology,* 14(2), pp. 87–91.

Martin, R. and Philippon, M., 2007. Evidence of validity for the hip outcome score in hip arthroscopy. *Arthroscopy,* 23(8), pp. 882–826.

Martin, R. and Sekiya, J., 2008. The interrater reliability of 4 clinical tests used to assess individuals with musculoskeletal hip pain. *Journal Orthopaedic Sports Physical Therapy,* 38(2), pp. 71–77.

Maslowski, E., Sullivan, W., Forster Harwood, J. et al., 2010. The diagnostic validity of hip provocation maneuvers to detect intra-articular hip pathology. *Journal Injury, Function and Rehabilitation,* 2(3), pp. 174–181.

McCullough, BJ., Johnson, GR., Martin, BI. et al., 2012. Lumbar MR imaging and reporting epidemiology: do epidemiologic data in reports affect clinical management? *Radiology,* 262, pp. 941–946.

McGill, S., 2004. *Ultimate Back Fitness and Performance.* Waterloo, Ontario: Wabuno.

Mendis, M., Wilson, S., Hayes, D. et al., 2014. Hip flexor muscle size, strength and recruitment patterns in patients with acetabular labral tears compared to healthy controls. *Manual Therapy,* 19, pp. 405–410.

Mens, J., Vleeming, A., Snijders, C. et al., 1999. The active straight leg raise test and mobility of the pelvic joints. *European Spine Journal,* 8, pp. 468–473.

Mens, JM., Vleeming, A., Snijders, CJ. et al., 2001. Reliability and validity of the active straight leg raise test in posterior pelvic pain since pregnancy. *Spine,* 26, pp. 1167–1171.

Mens, JM., Vleeming, A., Snijders, CJ. et al., 2002. Validity of the active straight leg raise test for measuring disease severity in patients with posterior pelvic pain after pregnancy. *Spine,* 27, pp. 196–200.

Merskey, H., and Bogduk, N., 1994. *Classification of Chronic Pain: Description of Chronic Pain Syndromes and Definitions of Pain Terms.* 2nd ed. Seattle: IASP Press, pp. 209–214.

Meyer, RA., Campbell, IT. and Raja, SN., 1995. Peripheral neural mechanisms of nociception. In: Wall, PD. and Melzack, R. (eds). *Textbook of Pain.* 3rd ed. Edinburgh: Churchill Livingstone, pp. 13–44.

Mortazavi, J., Zebardast, J. and Mirzashahi, B., 2015. Low back pain in athletes. *Asian Journal Sports Medicine,* 6(2), p. e24718.

Naito, H., Yoshihara, T., Kakigi, R. et al., 2012. Heat stress-induced changes in skeletal muscle: heat shock proteins and cell signalling transduction. *Journal Physical Fitness,* 1, pp. 125–131.

Naugle, KM., Fillingim, RB. and Riley, JL., 2012. A meta-analytic review of the hypoalgesic effects of exercise. *Journal Pain,* 13, pp. 1139–1150.

Ng, L., Campbell, A., Burnett, A. et al., 2015. Spinal kinematics of adolescent male rowers with back pain in comparison with matched controls during ergometer rowing. *Journal Applied Biomechanics,* 31, pp. 459–468.

Nicotra, L., Loram, LC., Watkins, LR. et al., 2012. Toll-like receptors in chronic pain. *Experimental Neurology,* 234, pp. 316–329.

Nijs, J., Van Houdenhove, B. and Oostendorp, RA., 2010. Recognition of central sensitization in patients with musculoskeletal pain: application of pain neurophysiology in manual therapy practice. *Manual Therapy,* 15, pp. 135–141.

Nijs, J., Torres-Cueco, R., van Wilgen, CP. et al., 2014. Applying modern pain neuroscience in clinical practice: criteria for the classification of central sensitization pain. *Pain Physician,* 17, pp. 447–457.

Nijs, J., Apeldoorn, A., Hallegraeff, H. et al., 2015. Low back pain: guidelines for the clinical classification of predominant neuropathic, nociceptive or central sensitization pain. *Pain Physician,* 18, pp. E333–E346.

O'Keefe, M., Maher, CG. and O'Sullivan, K., 2017. Unlocking the potential of physical activity for back health. *British Journal Sports Medicine*, 51, pp. 760–761.

O'Sullivan, P., 2000. Lumbar segmental "instability" clinical presentation and specific stabilizing exercise management. *Manual Therapy*, 5(1), pp. 2–12.

O'Sullivan, P., Caneiro, JP., O'Keefe, M. et al., 2018. Cognitive functional therapy: an integrated behavioural approach for the targeted management of disabling low back pain. *Physical Therapy*, 98(5), pp. 408–423.

Owen, P., Miller, C., Mundell, N. et al., 2019. Which specific modes of exercise training are most effective for treating low back pain? Network meta-analysis. *British Journal Sports Medicine*, 0, pp. 1–12. DOI:10.1136/bjsports-2019-100886.

Pezet, S. and McMahon, S., 2006. *Neurotrophins: Mediators and Modulators of Pain*. London: London Pain Consortium, King's College.

Prather, H., Harris-Hayes, M., Hunt, D. et al., 2010. Reliability and agreement of hip range of motion and provocative physical examination tests in asymptomatic volunteers. *Journal Injury, Function, and Rehabilitation*, 2(10), pp. 888–895.

Ratzlaff, C., Simatovic, J., Wong, H. et al., 2013. Reliability of hip examination tests for femoroacetabular impingement. *Arthritis Care & Research*, 65(10), pp. 1690–1696.

Reiman, MP., Goode, AP., Cook, CE. et al., 2015. Diagnostic accuracy of clinical tests for the diagnosis of hip femoroacetabular impingement/labral tear: a systematic review with meta-analysis. *British Journal Sports Medicine*, 49, p. 811. Available at: <https://doi.org/10.1136/bjsports-2014-094302> [accessed February 15, 2022].

Rice, D. and McNair, P., 2010. Quadriceps arthrogenic muscle inhibition: neural mechanisms and treatment perspectives. *Seminars Arthritis Rheumatism*, 40, pp. 250–66.

Richardson, C., Snijders, C., Hides, J. et al., 2002. The relation between the transversus abdominis muscles, sacroiliac joint mechanics and low back pain. *Spine*, 27, pp. 399–405.

Rosenberg, K. and DeSilva, J., 2017. Evolution of the human pelvis. *Anatomy Record*, 300(5), pp. 789–797.

Roussouly, P., Berthonnaud, E. and Dimnet, J., 2003. Geometrical and mechanical analysis of lumbar lordosis in an asymptomatic population: proposed classification. *Revue de Chirurgie Orthopédique et Réparatrice de l'Appareil Moteur*, 89, pp. 632–639.

Sahrmann, S., 2002. Chapter 3. In: *Diagnosis and Treatment of Movement Impairment Syndromes*. Philadelphia: Mosby, p. 63.

Sansone, M., Ahldén, M., Jonasson, P. et al., 2014. Can hip impingement be mistaken for tendon pain in the groin? A long-term follow-up of tenotomy for groin pain in athletes. *Knee Surgery Sports Traumatology Arthroscopy*, 22, pp. 786–792. Available at: <https://doi.org/10.1007/s00167-013-2738-y> [accessed February 15, 2022].

Sassmannshausen, G. and Smith, BG., 2002. Back pain in the young athlete. *Clinical Sports Medicine*, 21(1), pp. 121–132.

Schilder, A., Hoheisel, U., Magerl, W. et al., 2014. Sensory findings after stimulation of the thoracolumbar fascia with hypertonic saline suggest its contribution to low back pain. *Pain*, 155, pp. 222–231.

Schuett, J., Bomar, J. and Pennock, A., 2015. Pelvic apophyseal avulsion fractures: a retrospective review of 228 cases. *Journal Pediatric Orthopaedics*, 35(6), pp. 617–623.

Serner, A., Weir, A., Tol, JL. et al., 2016. Can standardized clinical examination of athletes with acute groin injuries predict the presence and location of MRI findings? *British Journal Sports Medicine*, 50, pp. 1541–1547. Available at: <https://doi.org/10.1136/bjsports-2016-096290> [accessed February 15, 2022].

Severin, A., Burkett, B., McKean, M. et al., 2017. Quantifying kinematic differences between land and water during squats, split squats, and single-leg squats in a healthy population. *PloS One*, 12(8), e0182320. Available at: <https://doi.org/10.1371/journal.pone.0182320> [accessed February 15, 2022].

Shan, G. and Westerhoff, P., 2005. Full-body kinematic characteristics of the maximal instep soccer kick by male soccer players and parameters related to kick quality. *Sports Biomechanics*, 4(1), pp. 59–72.

Siebenrock, K., Wahab, K., Werlen, S. et al., 2004. Abnormal extension of the femoral head epiphysis as a cause of cam impingement. *Clinical Orthopaedic Related Research*, 418, pp. 54–60.

Siebenrock, K., Ferner, F., Noble, P. et al., 2011. The cam-type deformity of the proximal femur arises in childhood in response to vigorous sporting activity. *Clinical Orthopaedic Related Research*, 469(11), pp. 3229–3240.

Siebenrock, KA., Kaschka, I., Frauchiger, L. et al., 2013. Prevalence of cam-type deformity and hip pain in elite ice hockey players before and after the end of growth. *American Journal Sports Medicine*, 41(10), pp. 2308–2313.

Sink, E., Gralla, J., Ryba, A. et al., 2008. Clinical presentation of the femoroacetabular impingement in adolescents. *Journal Pediatric Orthopaedics*, 28(8), pp. 806–811.

Smart, KM., Blake, C., Staines, A. et al., 2010. Clinical indicators of "nociceptive", "peripheral neuropathic" and "central" mechanisms of musculoskeletal pain. A Delphi survey of expert clinicians. *Manual Therapy*, 15, pp. 80–87.

Smith, B., Hendrick, P., Bateman, M. et al., 2019. Musculoskeletal pain and exercise – challenging existing paradigms and introducing new. *British Journal Sports Medicine*, 53(4), pp. 907–912.

Snijders, C., Vleeming, A. and Stoeckart, R., 1993. Transfer of lumbosacral load to iliac bones and legs. Part 1: Biomechanics of self-bracing of the sacroiliac joints and its significance for treatment and exercise. *Clinical Biomechanics (Bristol, Avon)*, 18(6), pp. 285–294.

Spencer, J., Hayes, K. and Alexander, I., 1984. Knee joint effusion and quadriceps reflex inhibition in man. *Archives Physical Medicine Rehabilitation*, 65, pp. 171–177.

Steffens, D., Hancock, M., Maher, C. et al., 2014. Does magnetic resonance imaging predict future low back pain? A systematic review. *European Journal Pain*, 18, pp. 755–765.

Steffens, D., Ferreria, ML., Latimer, J. et al., 2015. What triggers an episode of acute low back pain? A case-crossover study. *Arthritis Care Research (Hoboken)*, 67, pp. 403–410.

Stokes, M. and Young, A., 1984. The contribution of reflex inhibition to arthrogenous muscle weakness. *Clinical Science*, 67, pp. 7–14.

Stubbs, B., Koyanagi, A., Thompson, T. et al., 2016. The epidemiology of back pain and its relationship with depression, psychosis, anxiety, sleep disturbances, and stress sensitivity: data from 43 low and middle income countries. *General Hospital Psychiatry*, 43, pp. 63–70.

Sward, L., Hellstrom, M., Jacobsson, B. et al., 1990. Back pain and radiologic changes in the thoracolumbar spine of athletes. *Spine (Phila Pa 1976)*, 15(2), pp. 124–129.

Sward, L., Hellstrom, M., Jacobsson, B. et al., 1991. Disc degeneration and associated abnormalities of the spine in elite gymnasts: a magnetic resonance imaging study. *Spine (Phila Pa 1976)*, 16(4), pp. 437–443.

Tak, I., Weir, A., Langhout, R. et al., 2015. The relationship between the frequency of football practice during skeletal growth and the presence of a cam deformity in adult elite football players. *British Journal Sports Medicine*, 49, pp. 630–634.

Thomson, O. and Collyer, K., 2017. "Talking a different language" a qualitative study of chronic low back pain patients' interpretation of the language used by osteopathic students. *International Journal Osteopathic Medicine*, 24, pp. 3–11.

Thorborg, K., Branci, S., Nielsen, MP. et al., 2014. Eccentric and isometric hip adduction strength in male soccer players with and without adductor-related groin pain: an assessor-blinded comparison. *Orthopaedic Journal Sports Medicine*, 2(2), p. 2325967114521778.

Thorborg, K., Bandholm, T., Zebis, M. et al., 2015. Large strengthening effect of a hip-flexor training programme: a randomized controlled trial. *Knee Surgery Traumatology Arthroscopy*, 24, pp. 2346–2352.

Thorborg, K., Reiman, M., Weir, A. et al., 2018. Clinical examination, diagnostic imaging and testing of athletes with groin pain: an evidence-based approach to effective management. *Journal Orthopaedic Sports Physical Therapy*, 48(4), pp. 239–249.

Thoreson, T., Svensson, K., Jonasson, P. et al., 2015. Back pain and MRI abnormalities in the thoracolumbar spine of elite long-distance runners: a cross sectional study. *Medical Research Archives*, 2(4), pp. 22–28.

Todd, C., Kovac, P., Sward, A. et al., 2015. Comparison of radiological spino-pelvic sagittal parameters in skiers and non-athletes. *Journal Orthopaedic Surgery and Research*, 162. Erratum 2016 11, 148.

Todd, C., Wiswam, W., Kovac, P. et al., 2016. Pelvic retroversion is associated with flat back and cam type femoro-acetabular impingement in young elite skiers. *Journal Spine*, 5, p. 326. DOI:10.4172/2165-7939.1000326.

Todd, C., Karlsson, J. and Baranto, A., 2020. Resolving anterior hip pain in a young male footballer following arthroscopic surgery for femoroacetabular impingement syndrome: a case report. *Journal Bodywork and Movement Therapies*, 24, pp. 63–68.

Tsao, H., Tucker, KJ., Coppieters, MW. et al., 2010. Experimentally induced low back pain from hypertonic saline injections into lumbar interspinous ligament and erector spinae muscle. *Pain*, 150, pp. 167–172.

Tschudi-Madsen, H., Kjeldsberg, M., Natvig, B. et al., 2011. A strong association between non-musculoskeletal symptoms and musculoskeletal pain symptoms: results from a population study. *BMC Musculoskeletal Disorders*, 12, p. 285.

Van Tulder, M., Becker, A., Bekkering, T. et al., 2006. Chapter 3. European guidelines for the management of acute nonspecific low back pain in primary care. *European Spine Journal*, 1, pp. S169–191.

Vardeh, D. and Naranjo, JF., 2017. Peripheral and central sensitization. In: Yong, R., Nguyen, M., Nelson E. et al. (eds), *Pain Medicine*. Cham, Switzerland: Springer.

Vleeming, A., Mooney, V., Stoeckart, R., 2007. *Movement, Stability & Lumbopelvic Pain, Integration of Research and Therapy*. Edinburgh: Churchill Livingstone/Elsevier.

Waddell, G., 1987. Volvo Award in clinical sciences: a new clinical model for the treatment of LBP. *Spine*, 12(7), pp. 632–644.

Waicus, KM. and Smith, BW., 2002. Back injuries in the pediatric athlete. *Current Sports Medicine Reports*, 1(1), pp. 52–58.

Walden, M., Hagglund, M. and Ekstrand, J., 2015. The epidemiology of groin injury in senior football: a systematic review of prospective studies. *British Journal Sports Medicine*, 49(12), pp. 792–797.

Weir, A., Brukner, P., Delahunt, E. et al., 2015. Doha agreement meeting on terminology and definitions in groin pain in athletes. *British Journal Sports Medicine*, 49, pp. 768–774. Available at: <https://doi.org/10.1136/bjsports-2015-094869> [accessed February 15, 2022].

Witwit, W., Kovac, P., Sward, A. et al., 2018. Disc degeneration on MRI is more prevalent in young elite skiers compared to controls. *Knee Surgery Sports Traumatology Arthroscopy*, 6(1), pp. 325–332.

Witwit, W., Thoreson, O., Sward Aminoff, A. et al., 2020. Young football players have significantly more spinal changes on MRI compared to non-athletes. *Translational Sports Medicine*, 3, pp. 288–295.

Woolf, C., 2011. Central sensitization: implications for the diagnosis and treatment of pain. *Pain*, 152, pp. S2–S15.

Chapter 5 structure

Introduction   123

Clinical reasoning   125

EducATE   126

Functional evaluation   127

Techniques for functional evaluation   128

Positional and passive evaluation   138

Techniques for positional and passive evaluation   139

Articular evaluation   142

Techniques for articular evaluation   143

Muscular evaluation   146

Techniques for muscular evaluation   149

Neural sensitivity evaluation   155

Techniques for neural sensitivity testing   157

Muscle strength and capacity evaluation   160

Techniques for muscle strength and capacity testing   161

Conclusion   163

Introduction

 In Chapter 1, I proposed the "five 'ATEs" model, designed to help clinicians integrate current biomedical (functional and clinical) and bio-psychosocial approaches. This is based on my clinical experience and is a reflection on patient outcomes, across the course of my professional practice. It may be used to formulate a plan of action for approaching or managing complex musculoskeletal (MSK) issues. I described the framework as the supporting structure, based on a system of concepts, which are the "five 'ATEs." One of the strengths of this framework is the potential for flexibility, highlighting how interchangeable the "five 'ATEs" are, depending on the presenting complaint or clinical situation under observation.

I use this framework to guide the clinical management of each patient. I also find it helps with patient education, which I think is the key to the successful resolution of patient MSK issues. In the course of mentoring colleagues during the consultation and treatment of a patient, they have commented on how often I re-evaluate the patient throughout the session. For example, I always re-evaluate after performing a manual therapy technique, whether it is used to restore tissue compliance or to address a control deficit following a motor control exercise. This approach is very different to the way many practitioners have been trained. I am not advocating that anyone, practitioner or trainee, should disregard their training or discard their own particular approach. However, it is my hope that if I describe the model in detail, it will be evident how it flows continually alongside the treatment journey, during every clinical condition a practitioner may encounter.

In this chapter, I will discuss the first two components of this approach: *evaluATE* and *educATE*. To begin with, the central component of patient-centered care is the development of the therapeutic relationship (MacLeod and McPherson, 2007; Mead and Bower, 2000). Research highlights the positive association between better therapeutic relationships and increased patient satisfaction (Hush et al., 2007), adherence to treatment (Schönberger et al., 2006) and improved clinical outcomes (Fuentes et al., 2014; Ferreria et al., 2013; Hall et al., 2010). A fundamental component that is influential for the therapeutic relationship is patient engagement (Higgins et al., 2017). Historically, discussion of this concept appears to have been more focused on clinician perspectives; however, it is now understood that patient contributions are essential for the development of the therapeutic relationship (Miciak et al., 2018).

To evaluate, the clinician must begin to build a subjective case history, by interviewing the patient. This would normally begin by asking the patient to describe the reason for their visit: for example, by simply asking: "What has brought you here today?" This invites the patient to narrate their story and must be encouraged because it provides information about what caused the initial injury and, importantly, provides an insight into other factors that may have an impact on the patient from a bio-psychosocial perspective. The clinician must take control and guide this narrative process; however, it is important for the patient to be heard, and therefore the clinician must ask open-ended questions, listen for cues, observe body language, be receptive, be empathetic to their needs, and appear genuine and involved "in the moment" (Miciak et al., 2018).

Making a connection, in order to build a therapeutic relationship, helps to develop reassurance (Pincus et al., 2013). Reassurance can be viewed as a continuum. At one end there is the affective element: this is the part where we, as clinicians, build a rapport and show a real concern for our patient. At the other end there is the cognitive element: this is where we might act as educators, provide explanations, and help explore and develop coping strategies with the patient. Somewhere in the middle is where, from my years of clinical practice and experiences, I consider the art of being a good practitioner develops. A word of caution, though: cognitive reassurance may be more beneficial than affective, as too much empathy can be detrimental to the patient's outcome and render the patient's role redundant, leaving them with few or no coping strategies to self-manage effectively (Pincus et al., 2013).

The clinician must recognize and consider any potential red flags and the possibility of organizing other clinical investigations if required. It is extremely important, at this stage, to determine what goals the patient would like to achieve from undergoing treatment and completing a rehabilitation plan. The collaborative process sets the tone at this early stage, with realistic aims developed through a therapeutic alliance (Miciak et al., 2018; Schönberger et al., 2006) between both parties.

During the case history conversation, I would suggest you discuss with the athlete or patient the method of injury and onset of symptoms. Was this insidious, acute/chronic or acute on chronic? Encourage them to talk about the type and location of pain, referral patterns, aggravating and relieving factors, and whether there is distal pain away from the location of injury. The use of screening questionnaires may be beneficial at this stage. For example, I often use the following in clinical practice:

- The Back Pain Functional Scale (BPFS; see Appendix 1 at the end of this book): this is a useful tool to evaluate functional ability in patients with back pain (Stratford et al., 2000), and is extremely helpful for showing evidence of outcomes, especially for medicolegal requirements.

- The STarT Back Screening Tool (Appendix 2): this is a validated questionnaire that helps match patients to a particular treatment plan by stratifying them according to poor outcomes (Hill et al., 2008; 2011).

- The Copenhagen Hip and Groin Outcome Score (HAGOS; Appendix 3): this provides a quantitative

measure in young or middle-aged, physically active patients with hip and/or groin disability (Thorborg et al., 2011a).

This information needs to be collated by the practitioner taking stock of the situation. Try to create a working hypothesis and then test it. Re-evaluate but do not let your education – that is, what you expect to see – get in the way of your learning and distract you from the information in front of you.

Case study: Patient H

 Patient H is an 18-year-old amateur rugby player, who presented with a 9-month history of lower back pain (LBP). Symptoms appeared vague, with pain being reported only when he was standing and sitting, but not with any particular movement. He had participated in rugby for most of his teenage years and throughout this period had never reported any LBP issues. Rugby had ceased during the last 9 months due to Covid restrictions and he admitted becoming less active. His family doctor (GP) had organized blood tests and a magnetic resonance imaging (MRI) scan; however, nothing had been reported after either investigation. Previous management involved sports massage and chiropractic manipulation, and he had been told that he had a leg length inequality and should wear orthotic insoles.

Evaluation highlighted the fact that Patient H could perform full spinal range of movement (ROM) pain-free; furthermore, no apparent leg length inequality was noted. At this stage, I asked Patient H how he felt and he reported that, as he was standing talking to me, he was becoming more aware of his LBP. I sat Patient H down and I spoke to him about the fact that his spine must have been very robust to play rugby from a young age without any issues. He had undergone a series of investigations that failed to find anything wrong and a course of chiropractic manipulation had not helped; wearing orthotics appeared to be making no difference to his symptoms.

 He appeared quite uptight and anxious, and as he was talking to me his posture changed, as he began tensing his abdominal muscles. I asked why he was doing this and he explained that he had been told he should sit upright, with his core contracted. When he was asked what he would like to gain from seeing me, his response was "to get my fitness back." I asked if he could complete the STarT Back screening tool (Hill et al., 2008). This is a risk stratification questionnaire to empower clinicians to manage patients with chronic LBP. Patient H scored 2, highlighting that he was at low risk (unlikely to require a course of manual therapy) and therefore cognitive coping strategies and exercise could be influential (O'Sullivan et al., 2018). I explained to Patient H that the only person who would get him better would be himself. We discussed the possibility of breathing and relaxation exercises to help down-regulate his nervous system, especially when sitting at his desk, and, once he felt better, an exercise plan to challenge his muscle capacity and help him regain his fitness. I explained the benefits of not having his core muscles constantly in a state of contraction. I used an analogy to describe how, if he held a dumbbell at arm's length for any length of time, his shoulder would become fatigued and painful, and I pointed out that his core muscles were no different. Something I said seemed to resonate with Patient H: he appeared to have a "light bulb moment" and agreed with this approach. An alliance was thus formed between us, with him as patient and me as practitioner, and we were able to set realistic goals, which has been shown to be a key component in building positive clinician–patient alliances (Miciak et al., 2018).

The value of this case is that it highlights how both patient and clinician reached a decision together. Patient engagement promotes better outcomes, and in this particular case proved to be highly influential. The approach I used with Patient H is an example of reflection in action; by understanding what was required, in this instance, I was able to offer reassurance and provide cognitive strategies to help him regain his fitness. By choosing not to adopt a passive approach – for example, using solely manual therapy – I was demonstrating my intention of not falling into a similar pattern of treatment/therapeutic approach to the one his previous management practitioners/healthcare professionals had chosen. If he had scored 4 or more on the STarT Back screening tool, I might have taken the decision to refer him to another more experienced healthcare professional for further psychosocial support. However, in Patient H's case, he scored 2 and was stratified as low risk. I reasoned, based on the questionnaire score and my clinical evaluation of him, that the situation could be managed conservatively "in house." This is a clear example of how a questionnaire such as the StarT Back can be incorporated into clinical practice.

Clinical reasoning

I previously described clinical reasoning (Chapter 1) as incorporating the thinking skills and knowledge used to make clinical decisions (Jones, 1992).

Case study: more on Patient A

 I used an example in Chapter 2 to highlight how pattern recognition may have led the clinician to follow the path of releasing the deep hip flexor muscle to alleviate LBP. Deep tissue release techniques might have helped other athletes presenting similarly on previous occasions but what happens when the patient continues to report pain? Should the clinician assume the athlete needs even more myofascial release work? Let's find out.

Developing a number of hypotheses is important, the best evaluation of any hypothesis results from it being tested against others. Using a combination of the clinical reasoning models from Chapter 1 will help you to do this. Of course, a clinician may have a preference for one particular model: for example, hypothetical deductive or diagnostic reasoning. The particular model used does not necessarily matter, as long as it involves the processes of data collection, hypothesis generation and hypothesis testing. Hypotheses are developed from the observation and acquisition of clues the patient provides during the subjective evaluation. The clinician can then apply this information to test their hypotheses. Symptom modification techniques (SMTs) are a useful tool to help test and validate hypotheses. Although they are essentially a mini-treatment, the real power of using SMTs is their effectiveness in educating the patient.

Case study: more on Patient A

Let's recap the information about our athlete from the case study in Chapter 2, Patient A. He is still reporting LBP and anterior and groin pain, despite having manual therapy involving deep tissue release and stretching techniques. Using pattern recognition, the clinician might assume that the tissues needed to be released and stretched. However, we should also consider an alternative option, requiring a more flexible, open-minded approach: in this case, for instance, the hip flexors may not actually be tight and shortened. With effective clinical reasoning used to validate the hypotheses, it could be concluded that the deep hip flexor tissues may, in fact, be inhibited and, as a result, susceptible to fatigue (Hodges et al., 2003; 2002). In my experience, evaluation of hip flexor weakness is not routinely performed. This will be covered in greater detail later in this chapter. Considering the function of the deep hip flexors across the hip joint, pelvic girdle and lumbar spine can help in generating a working hypothesis: loss of acetabular compression and axial spinal stabilization, associated with increased levels of LBP and anterior hip and groin pain (Gibbons,

2007). The appropriate management in this scenario would be to restore function to the deep hip flexors by activation techniques and appropriate loading, by prescribing functional movement/exercise. This concept will be discussed in Chapter 7.

EducATE

Patients need to own their issue and the clinician must try to be sympathetic, while being realistic about their patient's concerns. Education will build the patient's self-confidence, offer reassurance and help to dispel any mistrust, skepticism and negative beliefs and attitudes that stem from poor previous experiences that they may have had. I advocate using SMT to start their education, and to reduce pain and improve ROM and function. You evaluate … then you re-evaluate! This serves to improve patient self-confidence and drives the correct management strategy. I have found the SMT approach to be an excellent starting point in the education of a patient or athlete, even while I am still performing my evaluation. The aim of SMT is to modify symptoms and improve function, using manual techniques or low-threshold exercises. These may help to reposition, and to increase or decrease the movement of, a structure with the goal of improving function and reducing pain. This acts a learning tool for the patient; if pain is modulated and/or function improves, it helps to reduce fear and anxiety, dispel old habits and beliefs, improve self-confidence and, above all, increase patient compliance. As a consequence, education becomes the way to manage patients back to their valued activities. As clinicians, we start to develop our clinical reasoning skills and develop working hypotheses, based on verifying, rejecting and refining our hypothesis testing.

I am now going to focus on evaluations that relate specifically to the spino-pelvic-hip complex. Clinical relevance must be established before a decision is taken to carry out any objective test. Evidence-based studies of clinical tests have shown that sensitivity and specificity

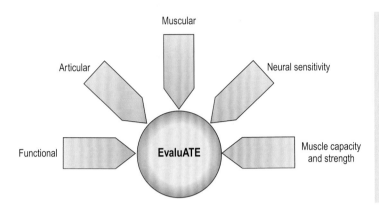

vary significantly, depending on the test. The value of many of the clinical tests proposed in orthopedic texts has also been questioned, due to their poor level of reproducibility and validity (Hegedus et al., 2008; Rubinstein and van Tulder, 2008). Sadly, this has led to a decline in the capability of some clinicians to perform effective clinical evaluations (Feddock, 2007), and has fostered a reliance on laboratory tests and clinical imaging instead. It must be stressed that the subtleness, precision and palpation awareness required for performing any clinical test must be of the highest caliber, with proper attention paid to detail. The components illustrated in Figure 5.1 are the clinical skills that I use daily and present in lectures, when delivering my courses for students and clinicians. I have excluded many tests in order to focus on those that, as I have learned through clinical experience, enable me to make effective and efficient decisions when managing the spino-pelvic-hip complex. I have broken them down into five evaluation phases: functional, articular and muscular imbalance, neural sensitivity, and muscle strength and capacity.

Functional evaluation

 The concept of using functional testing helps with the evaluation of the many constructs that relate to a patient/athlete's presenting complaint. For functional movement to be optimal, numerous factors are simultaneously required, such as neuromuscular coordinated motor control,

sensory feedback and processing within the central nervous system (CNS). These factors need to be evaluated to include examination of the MSK system and evaluation of the CNS. Essentially, this provides an opportunity for the clinician to observe the interdependence of all the structures in the MSK system and CNS, for enabling screening of movement limitations, restrictions and asymmetries. Dysfunction in either system (MSK or CNS), or in both, will result in aberrant muscle patterns, hyper-/hypotonicity, muscular imbalance and poorly coordinated movement patterns that may ultimately affect performance. As stated in Chapter 2, there is no such thing as perfect posture or normal movement. Observing the quality of movement (mobility) versus control (stability) and including the ability of an individual to dissociate one limb independently of another can be an extremely useful and important clinical tool. Therefore, clinical observation tools will normally be extensively utilized during the initial functional evaluation.

There is evidence of good inter-tester reliability (that is, between one individual and another) for clinician assessment of how a patient performs a movement test (Van Dillen et al., 2009; Roussel et al., 2009). In addition, attempts have been made to quantify functional testing. For example, clinician observation has been shown to correlate closely with 3-D motion analysis, using a camera-based system. Notwithstanding, I believe clinician observation and functional testing predominantly constitute a qualitative evaluation process. Unfortunately, because access to cameras and motion-testing laboratories is not universal, attention to detail is critical for the clinician's observation to be effective.

Techniques for functional evaluation

Standing

- Malalignment, as judged against clinical markers, may not necessarily be an indication of pathology.

- The clinician should observe and palpate for asymmetries, such as scoliosis, or biomechanical issues within the spino-pelvic complex or spino-pelvic canister (Figure 5.2).

- Observe for evidence of pelvic tilt, femoral head position, hip anteversion/retroversion, leg length inequalities that may be structural/functional and knee joint valgus/varus.

- Examine foot biomechanics, such as position of talus, pes planus (absence of arch/flat foot) or pes cavus (a high arch).

Spinal flexion

- The clinician palpates the posterior superior iliac spine (PSIS) and instructs the patient to bend forwards (Figure 5.3), observing to see if movement/structures are symmetrical, and then to flex forward without bending the knees. If the PSIS on one side moves more cephalically and ventrally, the test is positive. False-positive tests from standing flexion can be the result of asymmetries – that is, the ipsilateral quadratus lumborum muscle is relatively stiff – or contralateral hamstring shortening.

- The muscles should work synergistically to allow for controlled and balanced movement to occur within the kinetic chain, demonstrating no restriction or loss of segmental or multi-segmental motion, or translation, in the lumbar spine. Note if painful and observe for ROM, for loss of motion (hypomobility) restriction and for asymmetries between the pelvis and thoracic spine.

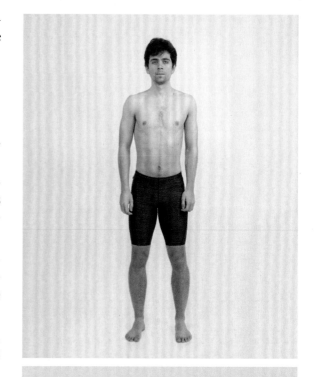

Figure 5.2

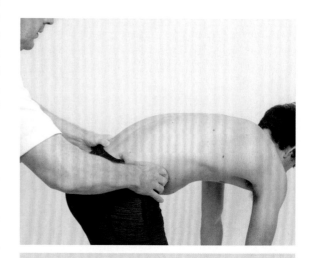

Figure 5.3

- The clinician palpates the interspinous spaces and observes for lumbar intersegmental translation between levels (hypermobility); if present, reduced hip joint flexion is often observed alongside increased lumbar accessory translation (Figure 5.4).

- There should be no rotation or lateral flexion occurring within the spine during sagittal movement. If the patient reports that symptoms are increased in a sustained position, such as flexion, the clinician should ask them to maintain this position at end of range to ascertain if symptoms increase. A word of caution: in instances when patients present with acute LBP, it is not advisable, in my opinion, to ask them to maintain spinal flexion at end of range.

Spinal extension

- The clinician palpates the innominates and PSIS and instructs the patient to bend backwards (Figure 5.5). Note if this is painful and observe and palpate to assess whether posterior innominate motion and anterior pelvic sway are present (they would not be expected and therefore indicate a positive test).

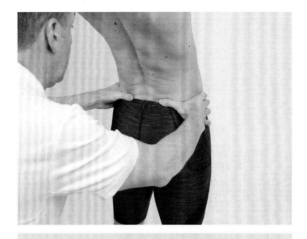

Figure 5.5

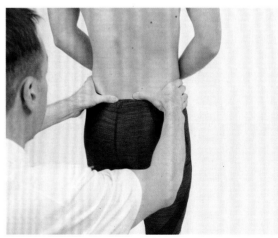

Figure 5.6

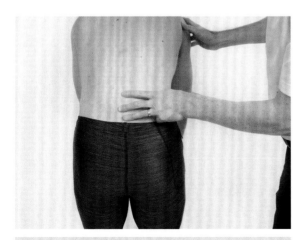

Figure 5.4

- The clinician palpates the innominate and sacrum (level with S2 or the inferior lateral angle) with both hands (Figure 5.6). The patient is instructed to bend backwards while the clinician palpates and observes for symmetrical motion in both bones.

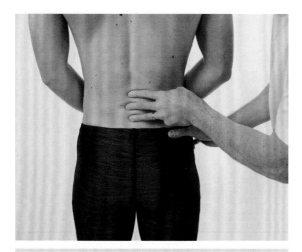

Figure 5.7

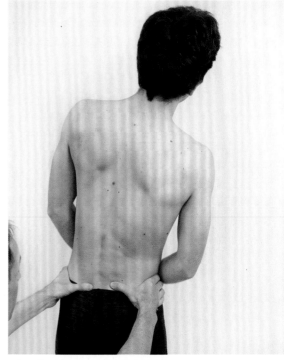

Figure 5.8

- The clinician palpates the interspinous spaces and observes for lumbar intersegmental translation ("hinging") between levels; loss of hip joint extension motion often increases lumbar accessory translation (Figure 5.7).

- The muscles should work synergistically to allow for controlled and balanced movement to occur within the kinetic chain, demonstrating no restriction in relation to the test, the pathological implication impacting loss of segmental or excessive motion or translation in the lumbar spine.

- There should be no rotation or lateral flexion occurring within the spine during sagittal movement.

Spinal lateral flexion

- The clinician palpates the innominate and sacrum, and instructs the patient to perform side bending away from the hand placed on the innominate (Figure 5.8).

- Note any pain or reduced motion into side bending in all, or any, lumbar segments, and observe for pelvic sway/pelvic tilt on both sides of the pelvis. The muscles should work synergistically to allow for controlled and balanced movement to occur within the kinetic chain, demonstrating no restriction in relation to the test, the pathological implication impacting loss of segmental or excessive motion or translation in the lumbar spine.

- Palpation of both PSISs in the presence of no pathology will highlight, during spinal lateral flexion to the right, a left posterior innominate rotation relative to the right, which should also be similar for the sacrum.

- Similarly, specific attention should be paid during the assessment to the normal accessory motion of lateral tilt that occurs within the pelvic girdle, resulting in abduction of the right femur and adduction of the left femur.

Spinal rotation

- The clinician stabilizes the pelvic girdle and instructs the patient to perform spinal rotation, independently of pelvic or hip motion (Figure 5.9).

- Attention should be paid to the movement and timing of rotation that occurs in the thoracic and lumbar spine.

- The muscles should work synergistically to allow for controlled and balanced movement to occur within the kinetic chain, demonstrating no restriction in relation to the test, the pathological implication impacting loss of segmental or excessive motion or translation in the lumbar spine.

- Spinal rotation to the right should highlight a posterior rotation of the right innominate, relative to the left. Note for pain and observe for loss of trunk rotation and segmental or multi-segmental restrictions in motion.

- If trunk rotation on one side is reduced, the clinician should palpate the tone of the tensor fasciae latae (TFL) and adductor muscles (for example, for increased tone in these muscles) on the ipsilateral side, as the hip joint may be in relative internal rotation, which would result in increased spinal rotation to maintain an upright stance.

Spinal rotation with glenohumeral joint (GHJ) internal/external rotation

- This is a modification of the spinal rotation test to evaluate what influence the scapular and glenohumeral muscles have on spinal mechanics.

- The patient is instructed to perform this test again with the GHJ in internal rotation (Figure 5.10A) and external rotation (Figure 5.10B), to assess whether specific upper-extremity myofascial tension is reducing spinal rotation.

Squat

- Evidence has shown that patients with intra-articular hip pain demonstrate reduced squat depth compared to those without pain, who were able to demonstrate an increased squat depth (Lamontagne et al., 2009).

- The clinician palpates for pelvic control with one hand on the innominate and one on the sacrum. The patient is instructed to squat, and movement should occur simultaneously through active anterior pelvic tilt over the lower limbs (Figure 5.11A).

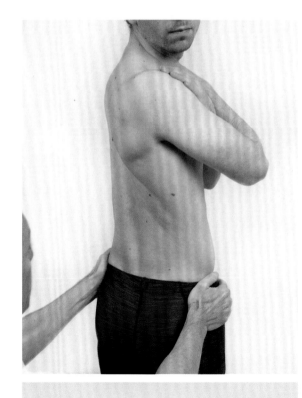

Figure 5.9

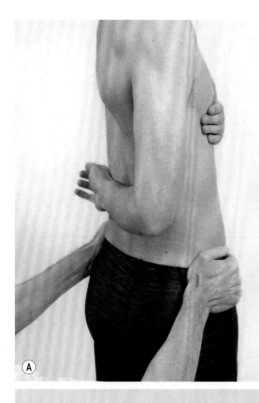
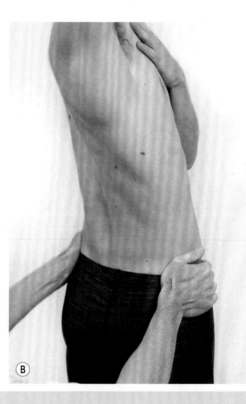

Figure 5.10

- The clinician palpates the greater trochanter, noting any asymmetry. The patient is instructed to perform a squat while the clinician observes and palpates for loss of femoral head centration, resulting in excessive (anterior tilt) rotation of the pelvis.

- The squat may be used to assess overall mobility in a sagittal plane for the spine, pelvis, hips, knees and ankle joints. The spine should remain in a neutral position throughout the squat movement.

Squat with arms overhead

- The clinician instructs the patient to raise their arms above head height, to maximum elevation (Figure 5.11B).

- If they are unable to keep their arms above their head, it could indicate a lack of thoracic spine and GHJ mobility and increase extension "hinging" that is palpable in thoracolumbar region.

- A reduction in ROM may be due to lack of iliopsoas, quadriceps, hamstring and adductor flexibility.

- Excessive lifting of the heels off the floor could be an indication of lack of triceps surae flexibility or a reduction in ankle dorsiflexion ROM.

Single-leg (SL) stance test

- This test involves a 30 second hold in SL stance and is used to evaluate an individual's ability to transfer load through one leg. The diagnostic accuracy of this

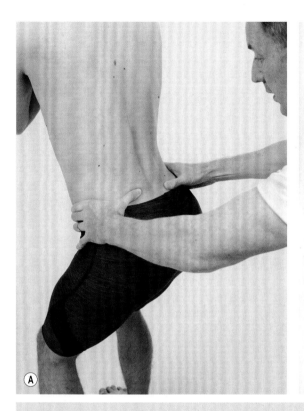 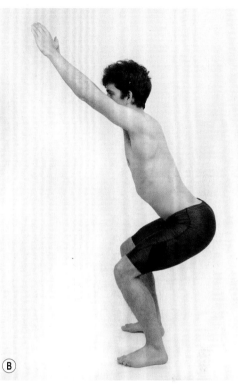

(A) (B)

Figure 5.11

test, to detect pain that could be related to lateral gluteal tendinopathy, sacroiliac joint (SIJ) pain and/or LBP, or hip joint intra-articular pain, is high (sensitivity 100 percent and specificity 97 percent) (Lequesne et al., 2008).

- Assess for excessive pelvic anterior/posterior/lateral tilt or rotation motion, occurring when the pelvis is positioned over the weight-bearing leg. Hip abductor non-pathological function should maintain the pelvis almost perpendicular to the femur in the SL stance position (Youdas et al., 2007).

- The clinician palpates the innominate and S2, using both hands. The patient is instructed to raise their contralateral leg and the clinician palpates and observes for anterior rotation of the innominate on the weight-bearing leg (Figure 5.12A).

- The clinician stands behind the patient and palpates the spinous process of S2 and the PSIS. The patient is instructed to lift the involved leg by raising their knee (Figure 5.12B). During optimal coupling of the spino-pelvic-hip complex, the PSIS moves caudally in relation to the spinous process of S2. A positive test is noted (indicated) when the PSIS moves cephalically, often with a lateral pelvic tilt towards the side of the weight-bearing leg. Comparison must be made with the contralateral side. This evaluation has been shown to have moderate (left 0.59, right 0.59) to good (left 0.67, right 0.77) levels of inter-tester

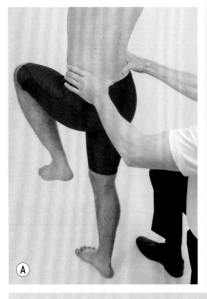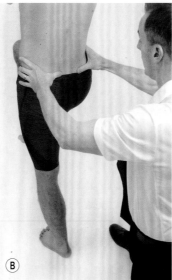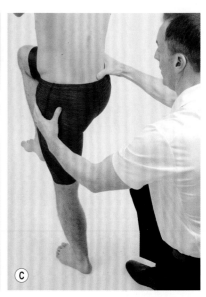

Figure 5.12

reliability, depending on which measurement scale is used (Hungerford et al., 2007).

- The clinician palpates the greater trochanter and innominate of the weight-bearing leg and instructs the patient to raise their contralateral leg (Figure 5.12C). The clinician palpates and observes for loss of femoral head centration. The femoral head may glide anteriorly and/or rotate internally or externally, indicating loss of hip joint control in weight-bearing.

Single-leg stance with small knee bend (SKB)

- The clinician palpates the innominate and greater trochanter on the weight-bearing leg. The patient is instructed to perform an SKB in SL stance (Figure 5.13A).

- The clinician observes for loss of pelvic–hip control, resulting in rotation of the innominate, femoral rotation, and associated knee joint valgus and varus, and increased subtalar pronation.

- In SKB, the patient may be instructed to perform femoral internal (Figure 5.13B) and external rotation (Figure 5.13C), while the clinician observes the capacity for dissociation between the pelvis and hips.

Thoracic spine rotation in heel-sit position

- The patient is in quadruped position (Figure 5.14), sitting back on their heels and placing the lumbar spine and hips in maximum flexion to minimize lumbar motion.

- The patient's ipsilateral hand is placed behind their neck, maintaining elbow flexion and GHJ external rotation.

- Keeping the head aligned with the thoracic spine, the patient is instructed to rotate the thoracic spine to end of range by taking the elbow behind their neck, away from the supporting elbow.

- This has been shown to have strong validity as a predictor of thoracic rotation range, in a study

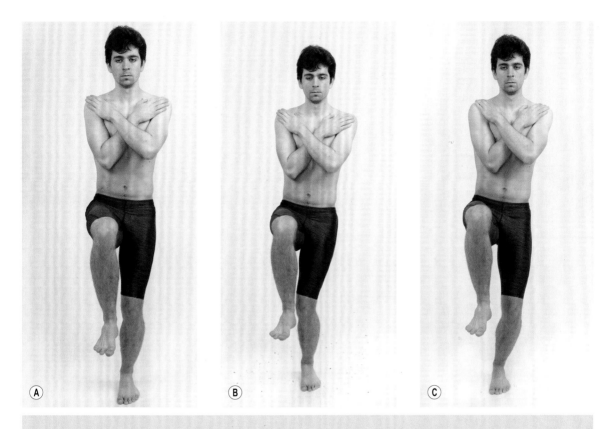

Figure 5.13

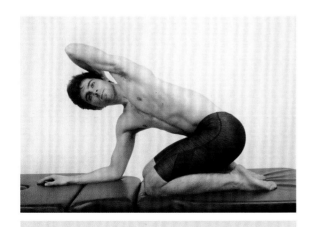

Figure 5.14

which compared motion analysis performed with ultrasound with measurements from a digital inclinometer (0.88) and an iPhone (0.88), with the latter methods demonstrating high concurrent validity (0.98) (Buckle et al., 2017).

Seated flexion

- This test may be used to evaluate the ability of the sacrum to move when the pelvis is fixed. The patient is seated with knees apart and feet placed on the floor.

- The clinician palpates the PSIS and the patient is instructed to flex forward with arms hanging between their legs as the clinician follows the movement of each PSIS (Figure 5.15).

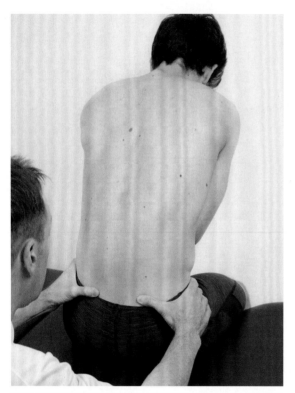

Figure 5.15

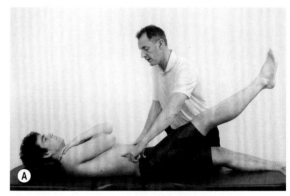

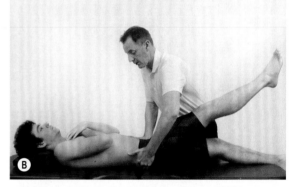

Figure 5.16

- Observe and palpate for movement of the PSIS. A positive test is indicated if, on one side, the PSIS shows more cephalic and ventral movement.

Active straight leg raise (ASLR) in supine

- The patient lies supine; the clinician instructs the patient to perform an ASLR (Figure 5.16A).

- Observe for pain or discomfort over the pubic and lower abdominal regions, hip flexor inhibition, or over-activity of the oblique muscles which may lead to increased translatory motion around the thoracolumbar junction.

- The evidence suggests this test is highly accurate diagnostically (87 percent sensitivity, 94 percent specificity) and demonstrates good intra- and inter-tester reliability (ICC 0.83 and 0.87, respectively) (Mens et al., 2006).

ASLR in supine with pelvic reinforcement

- The clinician provides external compression to the pelvic girdle in different positions, using symptom modification techniques, either to modify pain or to improve function, as the patient performs an ASLR in hip flexion (Figure 5.16B) (Vleeming et al., 1990ab).

ASLR in prone

- The patient lies in the prone position and the clinician instructs the patient to perform an active straight leg hip extension (Figure 5.17A).

- Observe for pain or discomfort over the sacral region or lower lumbar spine, inefficiency of the gluteus maximus in performing the movement, or knee joint flexion as a result of hamstring over-recruitment (Lee, 2011).

ASLR in prone with pelvic reinforcement

- The clinician provides external compression to the pelvic girdle in different positions, using symptom modification techniques either to modify pain or to improve function while the patient performs an ASLR in hip extension (Figure 5.17B).

Influence of psoas on spinal control

- The patient is prone-lying, with one knee flexed to 90° and a towel under it, to encourage a small degree of hip extension (Figure 5.18).

- The clinician palpates either side of the lower lumbar paravertebral muscles to assess whether there is increased/decreased tone, and instructs the patient to perform hip flexion by contracting their thigh into the couch.

- The clinician palpates and examines for any loss of axial spinal control during the phase of contraction, which is an indication of an inhibited psoas muscle (Gibbons, 2007).

Seated hip flexion test

- The patient is seated in a neutral position, with one hand placed on the xiphoid process and the other hand placed on the lumbar spine.

- With the pelvis in a neutral position, the patient is instructed to raise their knee, by performing hip flexion to approximately 120°, and to hold this position for 10 seconds (Figure 5.19).

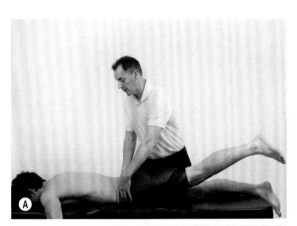

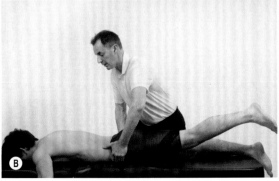

Figure 5.17

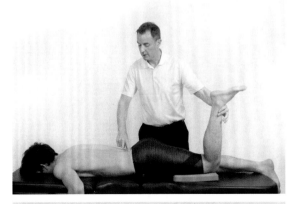

Figure 5.18

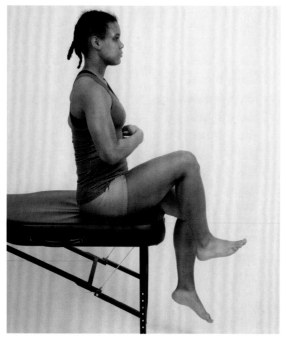

Figure 5.19

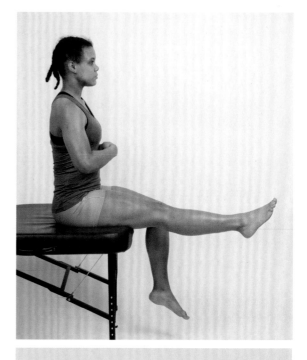

Figure 5.20

- The clinician observes for hip joint external rotation, lateral spinal shift away from the tested side, excessive lumbar extension or anterior hip cramping, indicating an overactive TFL.

- The clinician observes for loss of active hip joint control due to fatiguability of the deep hip flexors, such as psoas major. Handheld dynamometer (HHD) testing can be used to provide a more specific measurement of force.

Seated hamstring test

- The patient is seated in a neutral position, with one hand placed on the xiphoid process and the other hand placed on the lumbar spine.

- The leg is actively extended and the ankle can be either relaxed or in dorsiflexion, to observe posterior chain length (Figure 5.20) (Lee, 2011).

Positional and passive evaluation

Particular attention should be paid to any lack of mobility or increased translatory motion exhibited by one side when compared to the other side of the pelvis. Essentially, these tests are used to determine symmetry or asymmetry (Lee, 2011). Performing them can help to eliminate muscle tension which may contribute to stiffness across the pelvic girdle (Lee, 2011). Table 5.1 highlights positional evaluation in supine and prone. Specific attention should be paid to the quality and end-feel of the tissues with palpation.

These tests help the clinician form an impression of what is causing an individual to experience reduced levels of mobility. For example, anterior innominate rotation relative to the sacrum might influence hip flexion ROM and any reduction in hip joint flexion could be

Table 5.1 Highlighting positional evaluation supine and prone

Position	Anterior superior iliac spine supine	Medial malleolus	Pubic tubercle (PTu) Inferior lateral angle (ILA)	Posterior superior iliac spine prone
Anterior right	Inferior	Long	PTu inferior	Superior
Anterior left	Inferior	Long	PTu inferior	Superior
Posterior right	Superior	Short	ILA inferior	Inferior
Posterior left	Superior	Short	ILA inferior	Inferior

the result of the positional alignment of the innominate, increasing hip joint over-coverage, rather than a specific issue with the hip joint (Swärd-Aminoff et al., 2018). Individually, provocative tests for the pelvic girdle are not reliable enough and so a combination should always be used, with two positive tests out of the four suggesting the predictive outcome is enhanced (Laslett et al., 2005).

Techniques for positional and passive evaluation

Supine spino-pelvic alignment

- The patient is instructed to bend the knees, raise the hips up and down on the couch and extend their legs again.

- The clinician examines the inferior aspect of each medial malleolus and any difference between them, in terms of whether one leg is presenting as shorter or longer than the other at the level of the malleolus (Figure 5.21A).

- The clinician examines the levels of the anterior superior iliac spine (ASIS) in the frontal plane; any difference in height should be noted. Compression through each innominate can be applied to test the quality of the motion or to provoke pain (Figure 5.21B) (Laslett et al., 2005).

- The clinician examines the levels of the symphysis pubis by placing the heel of their hand on the lower abdominal muscles until the pubic bones are palpated.

- The clinician replaces their thumbs over the pubic bones and moves them slightly laterally until the superior tubercle is palpated (Figure 5.21C).

- During examination of the pubic tubercles in the frontal plane, any difference in height, tension or pain in the inguinal ligaments should be noted.

Prone spino-pelvic alignment

- The clinician palpates the levels of the PSIS, the depths of the sacral sulcus and the inferior lateral angles of the sacrum, noting any difference in depth or shallowness.

- Palpation of the sacral sulcus can be achieved by a gentle springing motion at the opposite ilium (Figure 5.22A). Particular attention should be paid to the lack, or degree, of mobility exhibited. Pain on palpation of the sacral sulcus has been confirmed to occur in 89 percent of SIJ patients (Dreyfuss et al., 1996; 1994).

- The clinician palpates the spinous process of L5 and applies pressure. If motion is observed, the lumbar spine should be freely moving. If lack of motion is noted, this is an indication of a rigid lumbar spine (Figure 5.22B).

Supine SIJ evaluation

- The patient lies in supine. Both knees are bent to flex the lumbar spine and hip joints and to place the SIJ in a relaxed, packed position.

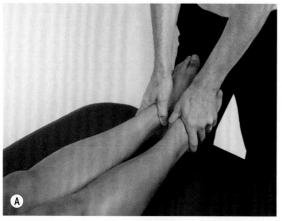

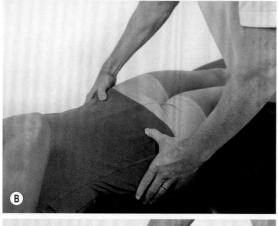

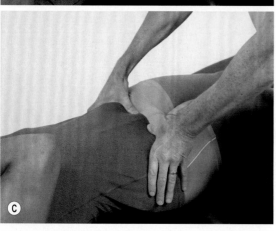

- The clinician palpates the PSIS for quality of movement by springing gently on the ilia (Figure 5.23). The clinician should be mindful of using too much pressure to palpate for SIJ translation.

- Clinicians should be aware that an SIJ that exhibits increased translation may be the source of pain, and it should be compared with the contralateral side.

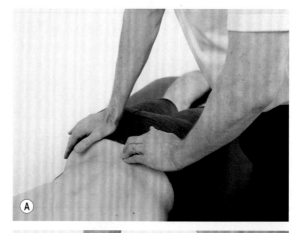

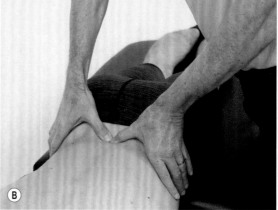

Figure 5.21

Figure 5.22

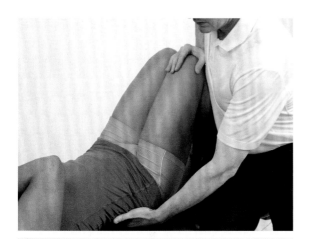

Figure 5.23

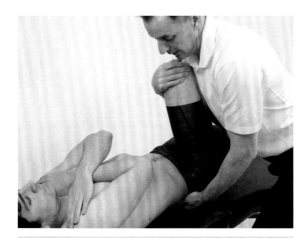

Figure 5.24

Thigh thrust test

- The patient is supine and the clinician flexes the hip to 90°.

- One hand palpates the SIJ joint as the clinician thrusts down through the knee and hip joint on the tested side (Figure 5.24).

- Evidence suggests that that this test is both specific (75 percent) and sensitive (63 percent) for provoking pain in the SIJ (Laslett et al., 2005).

Respiration control supine

- Respiratory dysfunction, although often painless, can lead to musculoskeletal dysfunction that contributes to persisting and recurring compensation issues within the thoracic spine (Lewit, 1999; Greenman, 1996).

- The patient is supine and the clinician palpates for mobility and translation in the ribcage (Figure 5.25). Loss of translation may be an indication of a poor respiratory mechanism.

- Respiratory motor control is observed while the patient is instructed to perform deep inhalation/exhalation.

- Note any loss of rib expansion and tenderness on palpation around the diaphragm and oblique region.

- The clinician palpates for loss of rib motion. Normal rib mechanics are examined for pump handle motion in the upper ribs, bucket handle motion in the middle ribs and a pincer mechanism in the lower ribs (Greenman, 1996).

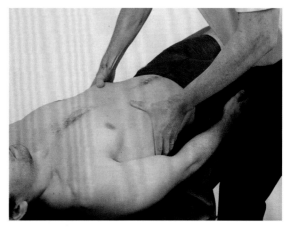

Figure 5.25

Articular evaluation

 The articular evaluation should always comprise a structural and a passive component. For example, why would we want to test a particular joint if we haven't first observed it in a resting or relaxed position? It would be easy to comment on an individual presenting with a posterior pelvic tilt but the true cause may actually relate to the hip joint being affected by symptoms of femoroacetabular impingement (FAI) syndrome. This would suggest that the posterior pelvic tilt may be purely compensatory, as the pelvis may have rotated posteriorly to accommodate the development of increased hip joint cam-type morphology. Special care should be taken with palpation skills, especially with regard to the passive evaluation, in terms of joint play, neutral and elastic zones, increased or decreased laxity, and increased or decreased stiffness. Remember: only small degrees of motion are readily available at the pelvic girdle and lumbar spine.

With passive evaluation, the clinician must be comfortable with the concept of normal and abnormal barriers, especially in relation to the anatomical and physiological barriers (Figure 5.26). The limitation of any end-of-range position is controlled by the anatomical congruity of the articular surfaces and the ligaments, muscles and fascia that support it. Moving beyond this anatomical barrier will only lead to tissue disruption and injury. Clinicians should be capable of evaluating any joint and comfortable with the limitations of passive movement and the feeling of an elastic barrier.

The physiological barrier is the end point of active range of motion, and the ROM is normally less than that of passive testing. In most cases, a reduction in the physiological barrier is due to myofascial shortening, especially in athletes or individuals who exercise regularly. This will be considered in more detail when we discuss muscular evaluation. Every barrier will have a palpable end-feel. This end-feel can be normal or abnormal. For example, soft tissue contracture, leading to a reduced ROM exhibited at the physiological barrier, will have an elastic end-feel, compared to that of an abnormal bony end-feel that is caused by a pathological mechanism, such as osteoarthritis.

Unfortunately, this is where palpation skills are often criticized. Reproducibility, and what we can detect by palpation with our hands, can vary tremendously between clinicians. This is true for locating anatomical landmarks and applying compression and distraction forces through the various joint planes of motion. It

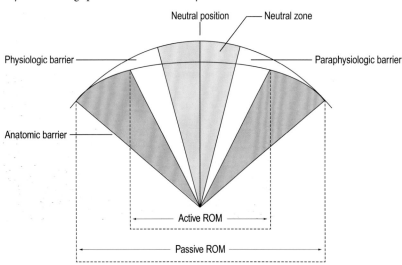

Figure 5.26
The barrier concept.
ROM: range of movement.

is not unusual for two clinicians on a course (both having a similar level of postgraduate degree training) to perform the same test but produce a different set of results. So, what is the answer? Should we not rely on palpation skills or dismiss clinical evaluations because they show poor levels of sensitivity and specificity?

I believe that every piece of information helps to build the jigsaw puzzle. If that comes down to using structural and clinical evaluations to help construct part of that puzzle, then so be it. Radiological investigations are seen as a "gold standard" evaluation but perhaps we should not be too dismissive of our palpation skills. What about the patient or athlete complaining of pain who undergoes a radiological investigation that produces a negative report? No significant correlations have been shown for comparing radiological investigations and clinical tests (Quack et al., 2007). In addition, this is similar to comparing the results from radiological investigations

and correlating them with clinical presentations (Yong et al., 2003). Consequently, clinical expertise should encompass all aspects of the knowledge and skills we have developed, and will continue to develop, through refining our illness scripts. This is our experience of the narrative of injury and healing that we gain over years of clinical practice and exposure to patient presentations.

Techniques for articular evaluation

Lumbar segmental passive evaluation

- The patient is placed in a side-lying position, with spine in neutral and knees bent.

- Passive physiological intervertebral motion (PPIVM) is applied in all spinal ROMs to move one vertebra through its physiological ranges in relation to another adjacent vertebra as shown using lateral flexion (Figure 5.27).

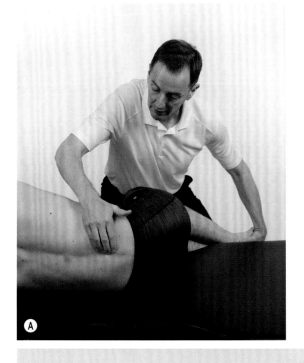
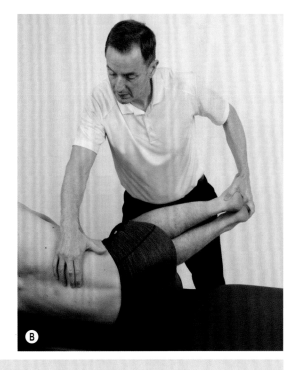

Figure 5.27

- Passive accessory intervertebral motion palpation (PAIVM) is applied to assess segmental mobility through evaluating the translatory motions which are associated with physiological motions (Haneline et al., 2008).

- Passive segmental evaluation appears to be heavily dependent on the skill and expertise of the clinician. A moderate inter-rater reliability for this evaluation has previously been shown (Panzer, 1992; Inscoe et al., 1995).

Thoracic segmental extension/flexion passive evaluation

- The patient is in sitting position with their arms folded across the chest; the clinician stabilizes the patient's opposite shoulder.

- Segmental motion is palpated through flexion (Figure 5.28A) and extension ROM (Figure 5.28B).

- This may be used as an articular technique or as a muscle energy technique (MET), or as a myofascial stretch technique.

Thoracic segmental lateral flexion passive evaluation

- The patient is in sitting position with their arms folded across the chest; the clinician stabilizes the patient's opposite shoulder.

- Segmental motion is palpated by introducing a side-bending component through the thoracic spine (Figure 5.29).

- This evaluation technique may be used as an articular MET or a myofascial stretch technique.

Thoracic segmental rotation passive evaluation

- The patient is in sitting position with their arms folded across the chest; the clinician stabilizes the patient's opposite shoulder.

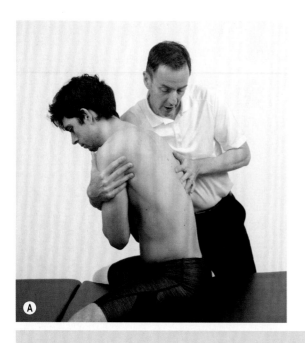

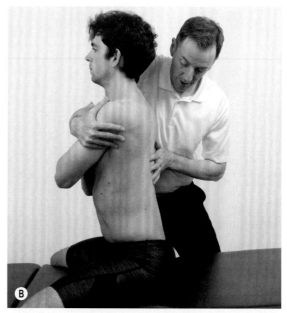

Figure 5.28

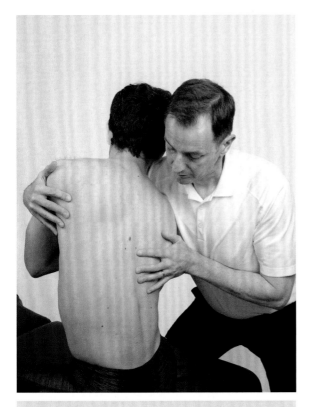

Figure 5.29

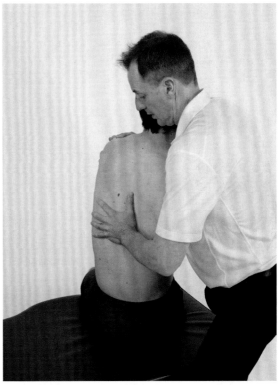

Figure 5.30

- Segmental motion is palpated by introducing a rotational component through the thoracic spine (Figure 5.30).

- This may be used as an articular MET or a myofascial stretch technique.

Hip joint passive flexion, adduction and internal rotation (FADIR)

- The patient lies in supine and the clinician encourages passive hip joint flexion to 90°, followed by hip adduction and internal rotation (Figure 5.31).

- Reproduction of symptoms may suggest a positive test.

- This evaluation has been shown to have high sensitivity (94 percent) but low specificity (11 percent) for investigating intra-articular hip joint pathology (Ranawat et al., 2017; Reiman et al., 2015).

Hip joint passive flexion, abduction and external rotation (FABER)

- The patient lies in supine and the clinician encourages passive hip joint flexion, abduction and external rotation (Figure 5.32).

- The lateral malleolus of the examined hip is placed superiorly to the patella and the hip is further abducted, while the pelvis is stabilized with the clinician's other hand.

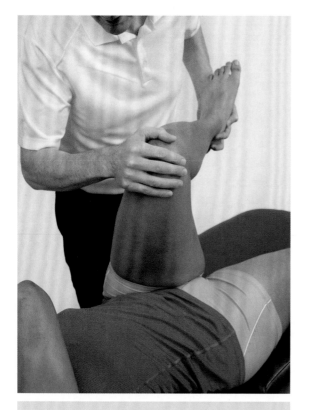

Figure 5.31

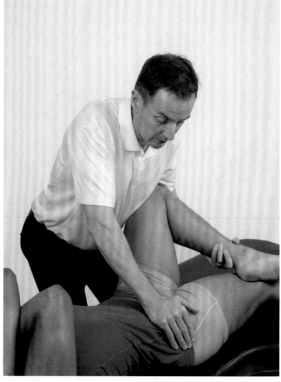

Figure 5.32

- Reproduction of symptoms may suggest a positive test.

- The angle between the treatment couch and the lower leg can be measured as an indication of ROM.

- Excellent intra-rater reliability (0.87) has been shown for this test (Cibulka et al., 2009).

Muscular evaluation

 The health of any joint is dependent on the strength of the opposing muscle groups (Janda, 1998). Therefore, if muscle imbalance arises, this may give rise to dysfunctional movement, pain and eventually degeneration. Previously I mentioned that every athlete or every patient has a

functional asymmetry that they can generally cope with. However, if the professional athlete or recreational fitness enthusiastic is exposed to an increased spike in loading, then the muscular system may be more vulnerable to injury. If we consider the evaluation of our patient or athlete from a holistic standpoint, we need to apply a similar approach to evaluating the muscular system. So, in this instance, muscular overload and imbalances would affect the whole muscular system and not just one individual muscle (Janda, 1998). A common mistake that I often observe is clinicians over-stretching the hamstring muscles to improve flexibility. Of course, there is nothing wrong with this if the hamstrings are shortened, but if the hamstrings were actually lengthened and under increased tension, this would only increase the athlete's susceptibility to potential injury. In this instance, addressing the opposing hip flexor muscle group would help to restore hamstring length.

Clinically, muscle tone presents as a combination of the viscoelastic properties of the soft tissues surrounding, and associated with, the muscle, and of the levels of contractility or activation associated with the muscle (Johansson et al., 1991). Viscoelastic properties are derived from the material properties of the components of the muscle tissues which have been shown to influence the capacity to develop maximal tension and relaxation (Meyer et al., 2011). If we consider the contractile capability of a muscle, we are specifically talking about the force generated by a muscle related to an increase in activity. This is determined by the numbers of actin–myosin cross-bridges that are formed: a majority of the fibers contracting (higher force) could result in muscle spasm, whereas only a few fibers contracting could create a trigger point (TrP).

Electromyography (EMG) has been used for measuring contractile muscle activity (Elkstrom et al., 2020); it is similar to sonoelastography, which has been proposed for measuring muscle's viscoelasticity properties (Hoyt et al., 2008). However, muscle testing and palpation skills, subjective as they may be, are fundamental clinical tools for evaluating the types of muscle tone that a patient may present with. Early development of an upright posture in infants is maintained by a "tonic" muscular system. As subsequent development occurs, coactivation of the "phasic" muscles combines with activation of the "tonic" muscles to maintain an upright posture. Therefore, optimal muscle balance could be viewed as the relationship between the length and tension of the "tonic" and "phasic" muscles (Table 5.2).

It is my opinion, based on my clinical experience, that muscle imbalance often develops as a response to over-training or under-training. The end result is that the "tonic" muscles begin to develop tightness and the "phasic" muscles develop inhibition. Such a functional

Table 5.2 Examples of "tonic" and "phasic" muscles

Predominantly "tonic" muscles	Predominantly "phasic" muscles
Pectoralis major	Rhomboids
Pectoralis minor	Deep cervical stabilizers
Trapezius (upper fibers)	Trapezius (lower and mid fibers)
Biceps brachii	Triceps brachii
Scalenes	Posterior deltoid
Levator scapulae	Teres minor
Sternocleidomastoid	Serratus anterior
Anterior deltoid	Thoracic erector spinae
Cervical and lumbar erector spinae	Subscapularis
Latissimus dorsi	Deep erector spinae
Teres major	Rectus abdominis
Quadratus lumborum	External oblique
Multifidus	Internal oblique
Hamstrings	Transversus abdominis
Psoas major (and minor, if present)	Gluteus maximus
Iliacus	Gluteus medius
Rectus femoris	Gluteus minimus
Adductors	Vastus medialis
Piriformis	Vastus lateralis
Tensor fasciae latae	Tibialis anterior
Tibialis posterior	Peroneals
Gastrocnemius	
Soleus	

inefficiency will reduce the ability of a muscle to contract and generate tension. In the mid-range position, a muscle is more efficient at generating force; however, this changes significantly in both the inner and outer ranges, with muscles appearing to become less efficient. Muscle contraction in the inner range is less efficient (Figure 5.33). Classed as physiological insufficiency, this results from the shortened position, which increases the overlapping of actin filaments with myosin filaments; this, in turn, reduces the number of cross-bridges that can be formed.

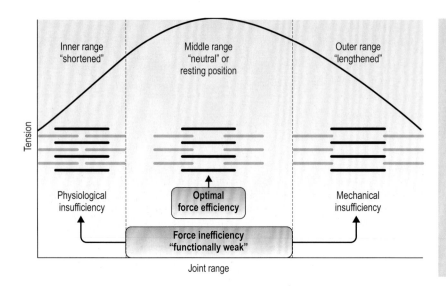

Figure 5.33
Functional efficiency and physiological and mechanical insufficiency.

Case study: Patient I

Let's consider another case. Patient I is a 28-year-old runner who had developed lateral gluteal tendon pain after an increased load in mileage. She had been referred from another clinician who had come to standstill with her management. Previous rehabilitation had focused on exercises for her hip abductors, working on the hypothesis that if these muscles became stronger, then the lateral gluteal pain would modulate. It became clear, on evaluation, that in a neutral and outer-range position the hip abductor muscles tested strong; however, inner-range testing highlighted that this woman was unable to generate optimal muscle contraction of the gluteus medius muscle and, therefore, tested weak in this position. Clinically, I was able to reproduce her symptoms.

The significance of this case lies in the length–tension relationship and physiological insufficiency I described previously, highlighting the necessity to be mindful of position in range during clinical evaluation of force production. Chapter 7 will provide examples of exercise strategies for managing this case.

Muscle contraction in the outer range is less efficient (see Figure 5.33). Classed as mechanical inefficiency, this results from muscle contraction taking place in a lengthened position, which gives rise to inadequate overlapping of actin filaments and myosin filaments and therefore reduces the formation of actin–myosin cross-bridges.

Case study: Patient J

Let's consider another case example: Patient J, a 22-year-old male rugby player with ongoing groin pain. He had been referred to me from another clinician, as both patient and clinician had reached a point where there was no further progression with his management and the patient had stagnated. Much of his previous rehabilitation had biased gluteal exercises. In a frontal plane adductor squeeze test, he was capable of generating sufficient force, tested strong (Verrall et al., 2005) and was pain-free. When the test was performed with a single-leg in an inner and mid-range position, this was similar. However, when he was taken into an outer range and retested, we observed mechanical insufficiency and a reproduction of his symptoms (Verrall et al., 2005).

 Once again, this case illustrates the significance of being mindful of the testing position in range during clinical evaluation of force production. Chapter 7 will provide examples of exercise strategies for managing this case.

Techniques for muscular evaluation

Adductors

- To test adductor flexibility, the clinician places the test leg in a neutral position with no hip joint lateral rotation; the clinician places one hand on the ASIS on the non-test side and passively abducts the tested leg (Figure 5.34A).

- Movement inferiorly of the ASIS on the non-tested side, before the abducted leg reaches 45°, indicates hypertonic adductors. If the abducted leg is flexed at the knee and further abduction is achieved, then short adductors are eliminated. Evidence suggests that this test has moderate to good intra-tester (ICC 0.67) and inter-tester (ICC 0.74) reliability (Hölmich et al., 2004).

- Adductor strength is tested with manual resistance in straight leg neutral, emphasizing the symphysis pubis (Figure 5.34B) (intra-tester ICC 0.79, inter-tester ICC 0.79; Mens et al., 2002), bent knee 60° emphasizing adductor longus (Figure 5.34C) (43 percent sensitivity, 91 percent specificity; Verrall et al., 2005), bent knee 90°, emphasizing lower abdominals

(Figure 5.34D), and single-leg outer range (Figure 5.34E) (30 percent sensitivity, 91 percent specificity; Verrall et al., 2005).

- Adductors can be tested in side lying for inner-range control (Figure 5.34F) in neutral: for external rotation, emphasizing adductor magnus; for internal rotation, emphasizing the short adductors, adductor brevis and pectineus.

- Side-lying assessment of the adductors (Figure 5.34G), using palpation, has shown good sensitivity (intra-tester ICC 0.89, inter-tester ICC 0.94 reliability) (Hölmich et al., 2004) in detection of adductor muscle injuries. Absence of adductor pain on palpation has a high probability of predicting a negative MRI (Serner et al., 2016).

- HHD testing could be performed to provide a measurement of force.

Psoas and rectus femoris
Adapted Thomas test (Figure 5.35)

- The patient is instructed to stand at the end of the couch, resting their bottom on the edge of the couch, and to bring one knee to their chest (hip flexion).

- The clinician then instructs the patient to rock back onto the couch until they are lying supine, while maintaining their knee tight to their chest, with the other leg hanging off the edge of the couch.

- The clinician assists with stabilizing the patient in this position while clinically evaluating the following.

- Failure of the thigh to remain flat on the couch is an indication that the deep hip flexors are hypertonic.

- A knee that does not flex to approximately 90° is an indication that rectus femoris is hypertonic.

- Excessive lateral rotation at the hip joint is an indication that the TFL is hypertonic.

- Observe for innominate anterior translation.

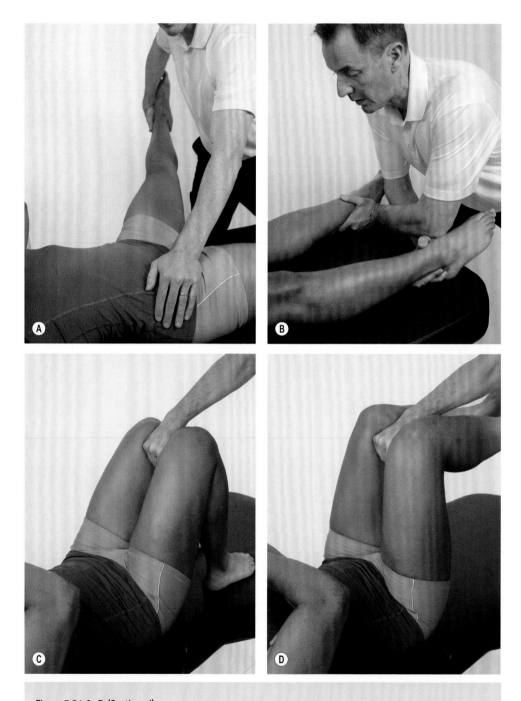

Figure 5.34 A–D *(Continued)*

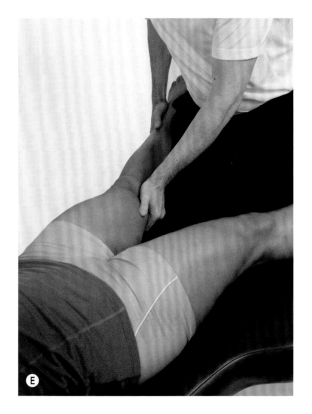

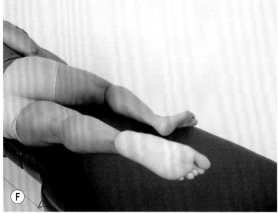

- The Thomas test has been shown to be highly sensitive (89 percent) and specific (92 percent) diagnostically (Reiman et al., 2015).

- Assessment of strength can be performed for testing the hip flexors in an outer-range position.

Prone knee bend (PKB)

- A correlation has been shown between the Thomas test and the PKB (Anloague et al., 2015), suggesting

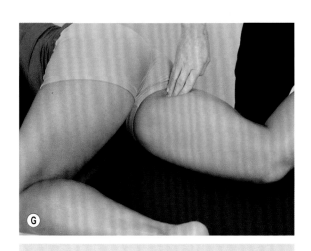

Figure 5.34 E–G

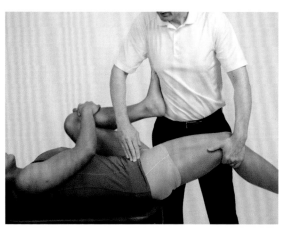

Figure 5.35

151

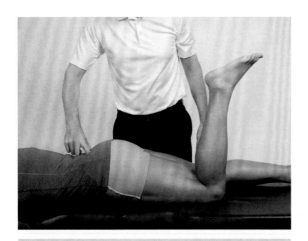

Figure 5.36

both tests can be useful for clinically evaluating anterior hip flexibility.

- The patient lies in prone and the clinician instructs them to actively perform knee joint flexion (Figure 5.36).

- The clinician observes for excessive "hitching" (elevation the of ilium in the frontal plane/lateral pelvic tilt) of the hip, indicating hypertonic anterior hip flexors. Evidence suggests that this test has poor reliability (inter-rater ICC 0.26) (Riddle and Freburger, 2002).

- The clinician performs passive evaluation, noting any change in symptoms, and measures the distance from the patient's heel to their ischial tuberosity; a comparison is then made with the contralateral side.

Psoas

- Psoas strength testing (Figure 5.37A) can be performed in supine in the inner range (90°), mid-range (45°) or outer range (greater than 45°) in Thomas's test position (Figure 5.37B).

- To assess whether muscle hypertonicity or injury is present, the deep hip flexors are palpated in supine lying (Figure 5.37C).

Hamstrings

- To test hamstring flexibility, the clinician passively raises the test leg; failure to achieve 80° SLR indicates hypertonic hamstrings (Figure 5.38A). Performing the same test with the hip in medial rotation will emphasize biceps femoris; with the hip in lateral rotation, it will emphasize the medial hamstrings.

- To test hamstring strength, the patient's leg is placed on the clinician's shoulder. The leg is tested in straight position (Figure 5.38B) and then with the knee flexed (Figure 5.38C).

Abdominals

- The patient is supine, arms crossed over the chest, and is instructed to perform a sit-up.

- The clinician observes for quality of movement and report of symptoms; the clinician may add resistance by applying pressure centrally against the patient's chest (Figure 5.39). This would emphasize more activity in the rectus abdominis muscle. Evidence suggests this test is moderately reliable (intra-tester ICC 0.63 and inter-tester ICC 0.57) for evaluation of abdominal strength (Hölmich et al., 2004).

- The patient performs an oblique crunch and the clinician observes the quality of movement and report of any symptoms.

- The clinician may add resistance by applying pressure through the shoulder as the patient performs the oblique crunch, to generate more activity in the oblique muscles (Figure 5.39). Evidence suggests this test has moderate to poor reliability (intra-tester ICC 0.51, inter-tester ICC 0.41) for evaluating the obliques (Hölmich et al., 2004).

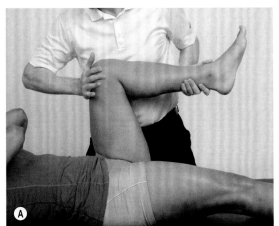

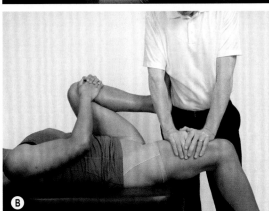

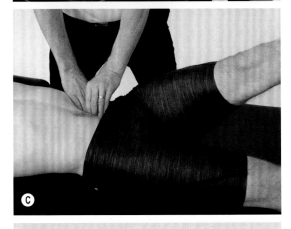

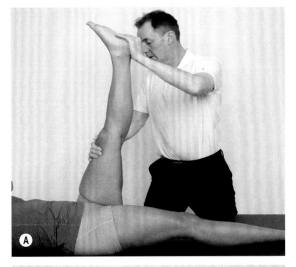

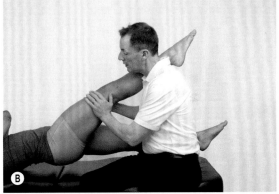

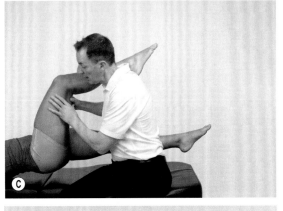

Figure 5.37

Figure 5.38

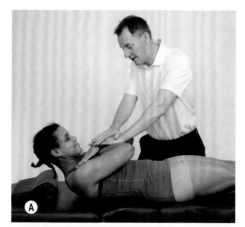

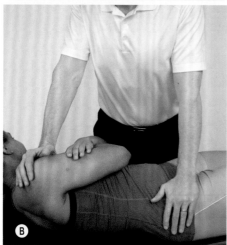

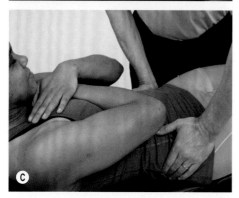

Figure 5.39

Abdominals with pelvic reinforcement

- The clinician provides external compression to the pelvic girdle, using symptom modification techniques in different positions, either to modify pain or to improve function, while the patient performs an abdominal or oblique crunch (Figure 5.39C).

Seated piriformis evaluation

- The patient is seated, in 90° of hip flexion; the clinician extends the knee (tensioning the sciatic nerve) and passively moves the flexed hip into adduction and internal rotation, while palpating 1cm laterally to the ischium and proximally at the sciatic notch (Figure 5.40A).

- A positive test is indicated on recreation of posterior hip pain at the level of piriformis.

- The test has been shown to have moderate sensitivity (0.52) and specificity (0.53) (Martin et al., 2014) for detecting posterior hip pain attributed to the piriformis muscle.

Active side-lying piriformis evaluation

- The patient is side-lying and pushes their heel down into the table, actively abducting the hip, in external rotation, against resistance (Figure 5.40B).

- The clinician palpates at the level of piriformis and notes whether pain or lack of strength is present.

- Evidence suggests that this test has been shown to have good levels of sensitivity (0.78) and specificity (0.80) (Martin et al., 2014); however, when combined with the seated piriformis test, excellent levels of sensitivity (0.91) and specificity (0.80) are produced (Martin et al., 2014).

Inner-range hip abduction side-lying

- The patient is side-lying and the clinician takes the tested leg passively into hip abduction and slight hip extension (Figure 5.41).

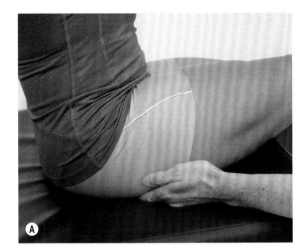

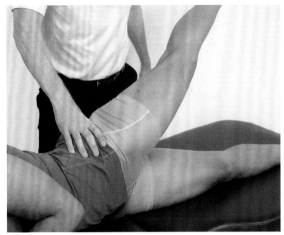

Figure 5.41

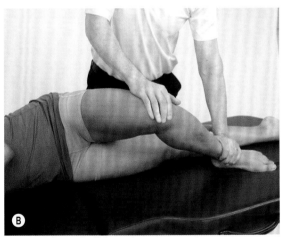

Figure 5.40

- The patient is instructed to hold this position against gravity. Failure to hold the leg against gravity is often observed clinically in patients with tendon-related gluteal pain.

- The clinician observes for any anterior drift of the leg, which could be indicative of over-recruitment of the TFL.

- HHD testing could be performed to provide a specific measurement of force.

Tensor fasciae latae (TFL)/iliotibial band (ITB) evaluation (adapted Ober's test)

- The clinician abducts and extends the patient's test leg, while supporting the knee (Figure 5.42).

- Maintaining the knee at 90°, the clinician lowers the leg towards the couch.

- Failure of the leg to reach the couch indicates a hypertonic TFL/ITB and palpation of this structure will cause tenderness.

- This test (adapted Ober's) has demonstrated excellent intra-rater reliability (ICC 0.91) for the assessment of iliotibial band flexibility using an inclinometer to measure the hip adduction angle (Reese and Bandy, 2003).

Neural sensitivity evaluation

Examination of the neural system and the treatment techniques involved in managing related issues can often be complex to understand. In recent years, clinicians have

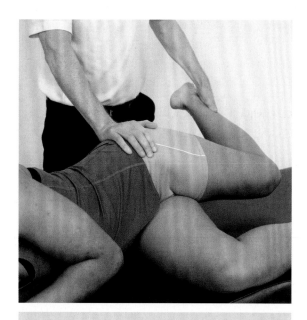

Figure 5.42

been able to familiarize themselves with excellent texts from experts in this field, such as Butler and Shacklock. Neural testing should always be included as part of the clinical evaluation process if symptoms appear to be associated with irritation of the neural components and/ or related structures. I am not going to offer examples of comprehensive clinical tests for evaluating neural deficits because Butler and Shacklock have both published guidelines for clinicians in this particular field. However, I will provide an overview of neural sensitivity testing, especially in regard to the spino-pelvic-hip complex.

Due to the nature of competitive sport, athletes have an increased susceptibility to injury and a greater possibility of developing abnormal functional patterns, which often present with signs and symptoms related to neural sensitivity. Sometimes, the symptoms have never been evaluated. Neural dysfunctions can encompass many pathological issues, but in this section I am discussing only neural dysfunction, affecting neural tissue

responses to sliding and tension. Based on my clinical experience, clinicians should aim primarily to treat the spino-pelvic region for segmental or pelvic restrictions, prior to beginning neural mobilization techniques, to ensure effective treatment of neural-related issues. This will have a direct beneficial impact on the CNS and will also influence muscle and joint relaxation throughout the lower limb, making neural mobilization techniques more comfortable for the patient.

Neural sliding dysfunction can sometimes be observed clinically around the pelvic, hip and groin region in athletes. It may be the result of previous surgery to the area, an intrinsic overload injury or an extrinsic traumatic insult. Essentially, the nerve loses the ability to glide through the tissues and is often tethered, or restricted, by scar tissue. This, in turn, may produce an inflammatory response. Patients generally report an ache or pain at the site of the injury and sometimes describe a burning sensation along the course of the nerve. Increased sensitivity is often apparent on palpation along the nerve, and symptoms are normally correlated with increased tension and discomfort, being provoked by mechanical or sporting activities. Neural sensitivity testing, combined with additional movement modification techniques, may prove useful for reducing symptoms.

Two forms of neural mobilization techniques can be used: sliding and tensioning (Waldhelm et al., 2019). Sliding mobilizations involve gliding the peripheral nerve to increase tension at one end of the nerve bed, followed by increasing the tension of the nerve at the other end of the nerve bed. Neural tensioning, on the other hand, involves lengthening the peripheral nerve from both ends (Coppieters et al., 2009; Beneciuk et al., 2009; Coppieters and Alshami, 2007; Coppieters and Butler, 2008; Shacklock, 1995). It has been proposed that neural mobilization affects the movement of the nerve, the connective tissue around it, axoplasmic flow (that is, fluid flow within nerve tissue extensions) and the vascular circulation of the nerve (Nee et al., 2012).

Case study: Patient K

Let's consider a case relating to neural sliding dysfunction. Patient K is a 28-year-old male professional soccer player, who developed right-sided anterior hip and groin pain as a result of acute tissue overload. He reported groin pain that originated in his iliac fossa and tended to radiate to his groin and scrotum when the action of turning to the right was performed at speed, during on-field training. When analyzing the movements he was likely to perform during this action, I reasoned that this would increase hip joint internal rotation, closing down associated neural structures. Pain was also reported when striking a ball with the inside of his right foot. The mechanism of striking the ball would increase dynamic tension along the length of the nerve and stretch the region during the active hip joint external rotation imposed by this action. Pain was reported on palpation along the course of the inguinal canal and this was similar to his responses to the side-lying obturator nerve test, with an external hip rotation modification. The obturator nerve supplies muscle and skin in the medial thigh. Patient K tested positive for neural sensitivity (Shacklock, 2005).

In this particular case, the hypothesis was that the soccer player had developed a neural dysfunction as a result of acute local tissue overload that had created an inflammatory response, which influenced the sliding motion of the neural structures. Chapter 6 will highlight examples of neural mobilization techniques used to help with this case.

Neural tension dysfunction is normally a result of increased tension and sensitivity and/or a loss of extensibility in nerve tissue. The functional outcome is a lack of active and passive ROM in the muscles and joints of the lower limb when the nerve is "wound up" or placed under tension. However, if the nerve is not placed under tension, then the ROM in the muscles and joints of the lower limb is normal. Symptoms can range from a diffuse, dull ache to pain and paresthesia, with increased sensitivity along the length of the nerve. Neural sensitivity testing highlights a reduction in ROM, as this tends to be the primary functional issue reported by the patient/athlete.

If we consider the issue of neural sensitivity in relation to the posterior thigh, we may ask ourselves: how would we differentiate between neural tension and muscular stiffness in the hamstrings? Consider those athletes who have a reduced SLR test: often, they also report pain and discomfort behind the posterior thigh. If no change in symptoms is evident after introducing sensitizing components to the SLR, it is less likely that the reduced SLR is a result of neural tension; it is more likely to result from muscular tension.

In my experience, I would suggest that clinicians aim to manage neural sensitivity by beginning with effective treatment of the spino-pelvic complex prior to performing neural mobilization techniques. In my opinion, this will assist with reducing lower lumbar segmental restrictions and facilitating muscular relaxation. Furthermore, attention to the possibility that muscle imbalance may be influencing the neural system tension is extremely important: for example, hypertonic quadricep muscles (specifically, rectus femoris) may increase anterior pelvic tilt and tension in the posterior chain.

Techniques for neural sensitivity testing
Straight leg raise (SLR)

- The patient is supine and the clinician takes the leg to be tested into hip flexion with a straight knee, ensuring no accessory frontal or transverse plane motion occurs.

- The clinician can test for proximal symptoms by introducing ankle dorsiflexion (Figure 5.43).

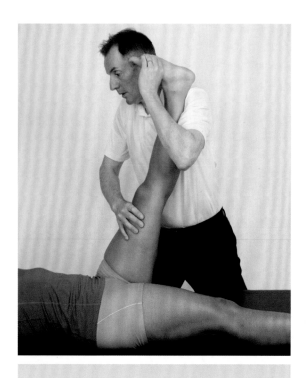

Figure 5.43

- The clinician can test for distal symptoms in the patient's foot or ankle by the degree of hip flexion they have introduced.

- The SLR has been shown to have moderate sensitivity (0.52) but high specificity (0.89) (Majlesi et al., 2008) for detecting neural tension in patients with sciatic pain.

Refining or sensitizing neural testing

- The clinician can combine ankle dorsiflexion and foot eversion with the SLR to bias the tibial nerve.

- The clinician can combine ankle dorsiflexion and foot inversion with the SLR to bias the sural nerve.

- The clinician can combine ankle plantar flexion, foot inversion and hip adduction and internal rotation with the SLR to bias the common peroneal nerve.

Slump sitting

- The patient is seated on the couch and is instructed to perform thoracic and lumbar flexion.

- The clinician applies manual pressure to the lumbar and thoracic spine, between the C7 spinous process and the hip joint, ensuring the vertical distance between these two points is reduced.

- The patient performs cervical flexion and the clinician maintains manual pressure by stabilizing the patient's occiput.

- Knee extension is performed, either actively or passively, and the clinician supports the ankle.

- The clinician applies ankle dorsiflexion; this increases tension through the lumbosacral nerve roots, with particular bias towards tension in the sciatic and tibial nerves (Figure 5.44).

- Refining or sensitizing movements may include contralateral lumbar flexion, hip internal rotation and adduction, and foot movements specific to each peripheral nerve, as highlighted in the previous paragraph.

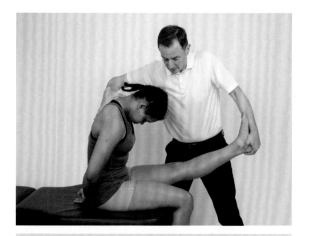

Figure 5.44

- The slump test has been shown to have high sensitivity (0.84) and specificity (0.83) (Majlesi et al., 2008) for detecting neural tension in patients with lumbar disk herniations.

Femoral nerve

- The patient is in a slump position in side lying, holding their knee with their hip flexed, and is instructed to perform cervical flexion.

- The patient extends their upper leg into hip extension and the clinician supports the thigh and encourages knee flexion.

- The clinician increases the hip extension component until tension in the anterior thigh is reported. The patient performs cervical extension and any change in tension in the anterior thigh is noted (Figure 5.45).

- This has been shown to have a high sensitivity (1.00) and specificity (0.83) (Tawa et al., 2017) for detecting tension in the femoral nerve.

- Hip joint lateral and medial rotation can be introduced to test the ilioinguinal and iliohypogastric nerves.

Obturator nerve

- The clinician tests the obturator nerve in the slump, side-lying position, as described for the femoral nerve test (Butler, 2010; Shacklock, 2005).

- Hip abduction is introduced to test the obturator nerve, which is associated with the groin and medial knee (Figure 5.46).

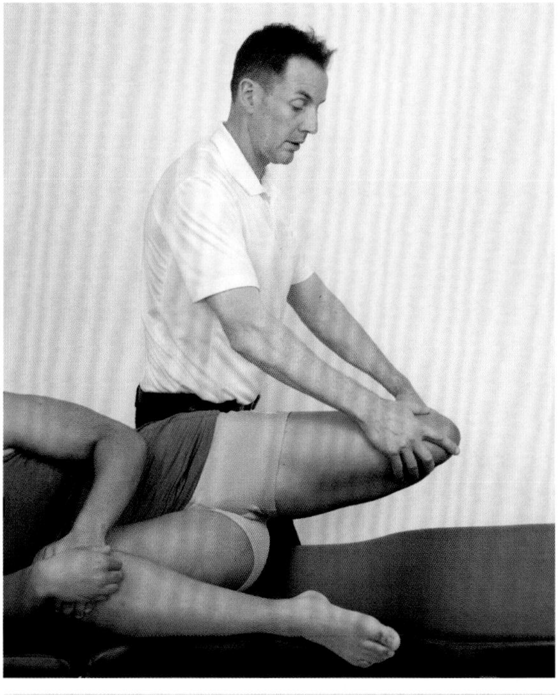

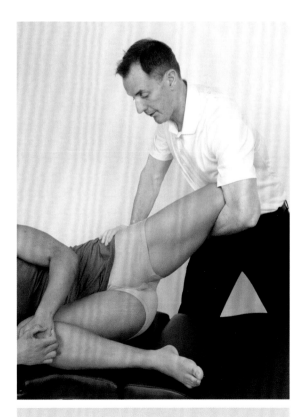

Figure 5.45

Figure 5.46

Muscle strength and capacity evaluation

Strength and capacity evaluations can be used to measure, objectively, the ability of an individual to tolerate variable intensities and durations of load. These may be factors which contribute to their ability to perform a task or action more efficiently (Spencer et al., 2016; Ratamess et al., 2009). The inability of an individual to tolerate mechanical loading demands, due to insufficient tissue capacity, may result in loss of optimal neuromuscular motor control and movement efficiency. If we consider a patient or athlete who has lost the ability to control the motion of spinal flexion as a result of chronic LBP, testing, used appropriately, may help them to focus on addressing posterior chain muscle capacity and restoring function, to enable asymptomatic lumbar flexion.

It is important to stress that testing of strength and muscle capacity should be performed at the correct time and in the correct way: that is, once the reactive phase has reduced and if it is tolerated (refer to Chapter 4 for a discussion of the phases of healing). However, there is no point in testing an individual's capacity if they have a motor control deficit. The deficit obviously needs to be addressed first. Additionally, there is no value in assessing an individual's strength or capacity in the presence of pain because pain inhibits optimal muscle function, and this may result in a reduction in measured force output. As far as possible, the capacity test should aim to reflect the individual's sporting or work-based performance, to provide a relevant measurement of the outcome under consideration.

In a clinical setting, capacity and strength evaluations enable the clinician to document an athlete or patient's progress over time. The handheld dynamometer (HHD) is a useful clinical tool for measuring muscle capacity and has shown a high positive correlation (r=0.91) when compared with a gold standard isokinetic dynamometer (Martin et al., 2006), as well as excellent intra-tester reliability (Thorborg et al., 2016; Le-Ngoc and Janssen, 2011; Thorborg et al., 2010; 2011b). It is a quick, objective, inexpensive tool that may be used to measure function within the clinical setting. This may be useful for insurance purposes, providing an objective evaluation that complements a logical management process, emphasizing strength improvements. It might even help to motivate individuals to help themselves and move away from a passive healthcare model. Patient dependency on passive care is increased when their outcomes and goals are biased towards symptoms, not function. Developing capacity within the tissues, to comply with load through a graded exposure to exercise, can only help to improve the outcome for a patient or athlete, making them "robust" and "bullet-proof."

Case study: Patient L

Consider the case of Patient L, a 32-year-old female runner who had recently developed pubic-related groin pain after returning to running 2 months after the birth of her second child. Initially, her symptoms appeared to start after 3 km but by the time I saw her the distance had reduced to less than 1 km. During the consultation, she reported that she had started Pilates and other core-related exercises post pregnancy and felt frustrated that she had now developed these symptoms. Examination revealed that she had remarkable ranges of mobility, alongside adequate timing and activation of the musculature across her pelvic girdle and hip joints. However, testing of her muscle capacity, with the modified Copenhagen and Sorenson's tests (see below), reproduced her symptoms and showed she had an inability to tolerate load, with reduced compliance in her tissues.

This case highlights how relying purely on mobility and motor control may not be sufficient for athletes to function optimally, reinforcing how essential a graded exposure to load is to developing muscle capacity.

Techniques for muscle strength and capacity testing

HHD testing hip flexors

- The patient is supine, hands holding the side of the couch, with the knee and hip to be tested flexed to 90°.

- The HHD device is positioned over the anterior thigh (Figure 5.47A); the clinician instructs the patient to push against the instrument to the point of discomfort (P1) or as hard as they can (P2).

- This can be modified for HHD testing in an outer range with the patient positioned over the end of the couch (Figure 5.47B).

- Measurements (P1 and P2) are taken from the isometric contraction and compared with the contralateral side.

HHD testing hip extensors

- The patient is prone over the end of the couch, hands holding the side of the couch; the tested leg is taken into hip extension with knee flexion.

- The HHD device is positioned just above the knee and the clinician instructs the patient to push up (Figure 5.48) against the instrument to the point of discomfort (P1) or as hard as they can (P2).

- Measurements (P1 and P2) are taken from the isometric contraction and compared with the contralateral side.

HHD testing hip adductors

- The patient is supine, hands holding the side of the couch, with legs straight.

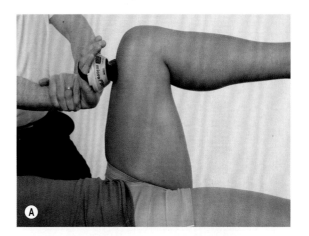

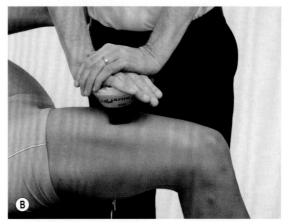

Figure 5.47

- The clinician standardizes the frontal plane range by placing his/her elbow between both malleoli.

- The HHD device is positioned over the medial shin (Figure 5.49) and the clinician instructs the patient to push against the instrument to the point of discomfort (P1) or as hard as they can (P2).

- Measurements (P1 and P2) are taken from the isometric contraction and compared with the contralateral side.

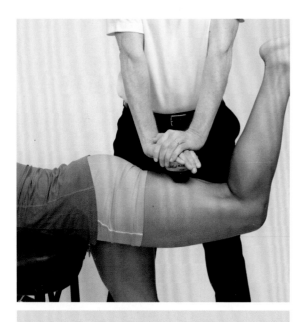

Figure 5.48

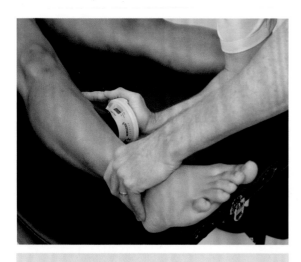

Figure 5.49

HHD testing hip abductors

- The patient is supine, hands holding the side of the couch, with legs straight.

- The clinician standardizes the frontal plane range by placing his/her elbow between both malleoli.

- The HHD device is positioned over the lateral shin (Figure 5.50) and the clinician instructs the patient to push against the instrument to the point of discomfort (P1) or as hard as they can (P2).

- Measurements (P1 and P2) are taken from the isometric contraction and compared with the contralateral side.

Short-lever capacity test: isometric adductor plank (modified Copenhagen)

- The patient is side-lying on a bench, with their upper knee in line with their hip, pelvis and shoulders.

- The clinician instructs the patient to engage their deep abdominals and to bridge (lift pelvis up) and hold the position (Figure 5.51).

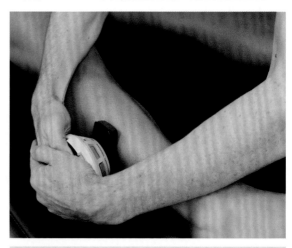

Figure 5.50

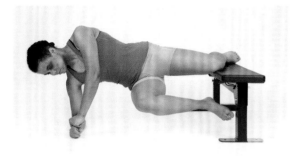

Figure 5.51

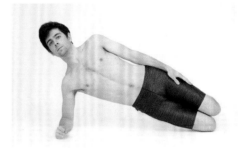

Figure 5.52

- Duration of hold (seconds) is recorded, as a measure of tissue capacity within the adductor complex, and is compared with the contralateral side.

- Load (demand) on the adductor muscles can be increased by performing the test in a longer-lever (straight leg) position.

Modified Sorenson's side-lying short-lever plank

- The patient is side-lying, propped up on their elbow, and knees in line with their hips, pelvis and shoulders.

- The clinician instructs the patient to engage their deep abdominals and to bridge up and hold the position (Figure 5.52).

- Duration of hold (seconds) is recorded, as a measure of tissue capacity of the spinal stabilizers, and is compared with the contralateral side. The test is graded according to McGill (1998) as: normal (5) – able to lift pelvis and hold for 20 seconds; good (4) – able to lift pelvis but difficulty holding for 10 seconds; fair (3) – able to lift pelvis but cannot hold spine for 5 seconds; or poor (2) – unable to lift pelvis.

- Load (demand) on the spinal stabilizers can be increased by performing the test in a longer-lever (straight leg) position.

Sit-to-stand squat

- The patient is seated on a chair or the edge of a couch, with arms folded across their chest, feet positioned with heels on the floor and knees aligned over the second toe. Alternatively, this test may be performed without a chair using a strong Theraband® (TB) Figure 5.53).

- The clinician instructs the patient to drive through their heels and perform a sit-to-stand squat; the test score is represented by how many repetitions of the action the patient performs in 60 seconds.

- This has been shown to have excellent intra-rater reliability (ICC 0.90) (Cliborne et al., 2004) for demonstrating lower limb strength.

- This test can be modified to increase load by performing it on a single-leg.

Conclusion

  This chapter set out to introduce what I would consider to be fundamentals for clinicians, helping them understand the first two components of my "five 'ATEs" framework: *evaluATE* and *educATE*. Remember: this advice is based

Chapter 5

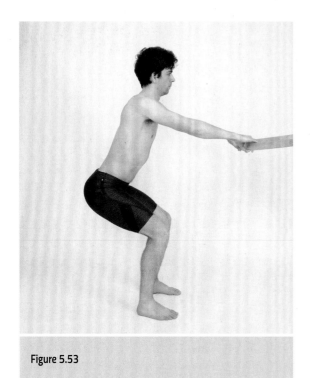

Figure 5.53

on my clinical experience across many years of professional practice. To appreciate these two components of the "five 'ATEs" framework, clinicians should strive to develop a thorough understanding of the five phases of muscular evaluation, which can include all or specific aspects of functional, positional, articular, muscular and neural sensitivity evaluation tests.

In summary, use the *evaluATE* component of the "five 'ATEs" to help *educATE* patients. This can begin during the case history, with the patient being encouraged to tell their story, during which time the beginning of a therapeutic relationship is formulated between patient and clinician. As a clinician, start to develop working hypotheses and test each one accordingly using a battery of tests that can encompass any or all of the five phases of musculoskeletal evaluation. Remember that some tests are statistically stronger than others but that does not mean that you should dismiss the weaker ones entirely. I would encourage you, as clinicians, to try

mini-treatments or symptom modification techniques and to *re-evaluATE* to test your hypotheses and provide a diagnostic outcome for each patient. The information you gain will go a long way towards successfully managing the individual using two further components, *manipulATE and activATE*, which I will discuss in Chapters 6 and 7.

References

Anloague, PA., Chorny, WS., Childs, KE. et al., 2015. The relationship between the femoral nerve tension and hip flexor length. *Journal Novel Physiotherapy*, 5(244). DOI:10.4172/2165-7025.1000244.

Beneciuk, JM., Bishop, MD. and George, SZ., 2009. Effects of upper extremity neural mobilization on thermal pain sensitivity: a sham-controlled study in asymptomatic participants. *Journal Orthopaedic Sports Physical Therapy*, 39, pp. 428–438.

Buckle, J., Spencer, S., Fawcett, L. et al., 2017. Validity of the digital inclinometer and iphone when measuring thoracic spine rotation. *Journal Athletic Training*, 52(9), pp. 820–825.

Butler, D., 2010. *The Neurodynamic Techniques*. Adelaide: Noigroup Publications.

Cibulka, MT., White, DM., Woehrle, J. et al., 2009. Hip pain and mobility deficits – hip osteoarthritis: clinical practice guidelines. *Journal Orthopaedic Sports Physical Therapy*, 39(4), pp. A1–A25.

Cliborne, AV., Waineer, RS., Rhon, DI. et al., 2004. Clinical hip tests and a functional squat test in patients with knee osteoarthritis: reliability, prevalence of positive test findings, and short-term response to hip mobilization. *Journal Orthopaedic Sports Physical Therapy*, 34, pp. 676–685.

Coppieters, MW. and Alshami, AM., 2007. Longitudinal excursion and strain in the median nerve during novel gliding exercises for carpal tunnel syndrome. *Journal Orthopaedic Research*, 25, pp. 972–980.

Coppieters, MW. and Butler, DS., 2008. Do "sliders" slide and "tensioners" tension? An analysis of neurodynamic techniques and considerations regarding their application. *Manual Therapy*, 13, pp. 213–221.

Coppieters, MW., Hough, AD. and Dilley, A., 2009. Different nerve-gliding exercises induce different magnitudes of median nerve longitudinal excursion: an in vivo study using dynamic ultrasound imaging. *Journal Orthopaedic Sports Physical Therapy*, 39(3), pp. 164–171.

Dreyfuss, P., Dreyer, S, Griffin, J. et al., 1994. Positive sacroiliac screening tests in asymptomatic adults. *Spine*, 10, pp. 1138–1143.

Dreyfuss, P., Michaelsen, M., Pauza, K. et al., 1996. The value of medical history and physical examination in diagnosing sacroiliac pain. *Spine*, 21, pp. 2594–2602.

Elkstrom, L., Zhang, Q., Abrahamson, J. et al., 2020. A model for the evaluation of the electric activity and oxygenation in the erector spinae muscle during isometric loading adapted for spine patients. *Journal Orthopaedic Surgery and Research*, 15, p. 155.

Feddock, CA., 2007. The lost art of clinical skills. *American Journal Medicine*, 120, pp. 374–378.

Ferreira, PH., Ferreira, ML., Maher, CG. et al., 2013. The therapeutic alliance between clinicians and patients predicts outcome in chronic low back pain. *Physical Therapy*, 93, pp. 470–478.

Fuentes, J., Armijo-Olivo, S., Funabashi, M. et al., 2014. Enhanced therapeutic alliance modulates pain intensity and muscle pain sensitivity in patients with chronic low back pain: an experimental study. *Physical Therapy*, 94, pp. 477–489.

Gibbons, S., 2007. Assessment and rehabilitation of the stability function of psoas major. *Manuelle Therapie*, 11, pp. 177–187.

Greenman, P., 1996. *Principles of Manual Medicine*. 5th ed. Philadelphia: Lippincott Williams and Wilkins.

Hall, AM., Ferreira, PH., Maher, CG. et al., 2010. The influence of the therapist-patient relationship on treatment outcome in physical rehabilitation: a systematic review. *Physical Therapy*, 90, pp. 1099–1110.

Haneline, MT., Cooperstein, R., Young, M. et al., 2008. Spinal motion palpation: a comparison of studies that assessed intersegmental end feel vs excursion. *Journal Manipulative Physiology Therapy*, 31(8), pp. 616–626.

Hegedus, EJ., Goode, A., Campbell, S. et al., 2008. Physical examination tests of the shoulder: a systematic review with meta-analysis of individual tests. *British Journal Sports Medicine*, 42, pp. 80–92.

Higgins, T., Larson, E. and Schnall, R., 2017. Unravelling the meaning of patient engagement: a concept analysis. *Patient Educational Counseling*, 100, pp. 30–36.

Hill, JC., Dunn, KM., Lewis, M. et al., 2008. A primary care back pain screening tool: identifying patient subgroups for initial treatment. *Arthritis Care and Research*, 59, pp. 632–641.

Hill, JC., Whitehurst, DG., Lewis, M. et al., 2011. Comparison of stratified management for low back pain with current best practice (STarT Back): a randomised controlled trial. *Lancet*, 378, pp. 1560–1571.

Hodges, P., Moseley, G., Gabrielsson, A. et al., 2003. Experimental muscle pain changes feedforward postural responses of the trunk muscles. *Experimental Brain Research*, 151(2), pp. 262–271.

Hölmich, P., Hölmich, LR. and Bjerg, AM., 2004. Clinical examination of athletes with groin pain: an intraobserver and interobserver reliability study. *British Journal of Sports Medicine*, 38(4), pp. 446–451.

Hoyt K., Kneezel T., Castaneda B. et al., 2008. Quantitative sonoelastography for the in vivo assessment of skeletal muscle viscoelasticity. *Physics in Medicine and Biology*, 53(7), pp. 4063–4080.

Hungerford, B., Gilleard, W., Moran, M. et al., 2007. Evaluation of the ability of physical therapists to palpate intrapelvic motion with the stork test on the support side. *Physical Therapy*, 87(7), pp. 879–887.

Hush, JM., Cameron, K. and Mackey, M., 2007. Patient satisfaction with musculoskeletal physical therapy care: a systematic review. *Physical Therapy*, 91, pp. 25–36.

Inscoe, E., Witt, P., Gross, M. et al., 1995. Reliability in evaluating passive intervertebral motion of the lumbar spine. *Journal Manual Manipulative Therapy*, 3(4), pp. 135–143.

Janda, V., 1998. *Muscle Imbalance and Movement Dysfunction*. Course notes, Joint Chiropractic Committee Conference, Anglo-European College of Chiropractors, Bournemouth, UK.

Johansson, H., Sjölander, P. and Sojka, P., 1991. Receptors in the knee joint ligaments and their role in the biomechanics of the joint. *Critical Reviews in Biomedical Engineering*, 18(5), pp. 341–368.

Jones, M., 1992. Clinical reasoning in manual therapy. *Physical Therapy*, 72(12), pp. 875–884.

Lamontagne, M., Kennedy, M. and Beaulé, P., 2009. The effect of cam FAI on hip and pelvic motion during maximum squat. *Clinical Orthopaedics and Related Research*, 467(3), pp. 645–650.

Laslett, M., Aprill, C., McDonald, B. et al., 2005. Diagnosis of sacroiliac joint pain: validity of individual provocation tests and composites of tests. *Manual Therapy*, 10(3), pp. 207–218.

Laslett, M., McDonald, B., Aprill, C. et al., 2006. Clinical predictors of screening lumbar zygapophyseal joint blocks: development of clinical prediction rules. *Spine Journal*, 6(4), pp. 370–379.

Lee, D., 2011. *The Pelvic Girdle. An Integration of Clinical Expertise and Research*. 4th ed. Edinburgh: Churchill Livingstone/Elsevier.

Le-Ngoc, L. and Janssen, J., 2011. Validity and reliability of a hand-held dynamometer for dynamic muscle strength assessment. *Rehabilitation Medicine*, 4, pp. 53–66.

Lequesne, M., Mathieu, P., Vuillemin-Bodaghi, V. et al., 2008. Gluteal tendinopathy in refractory greater trochanter pain syndrome: diagnostic value of two clinical tests. *Arthritis & Rheumatism*, 59(2), pp. 241–246.

Lewit, K., 1999. *Manipulative Therapy in Rehabilitation of the Locomotor System*. 3rd ed. Oxford: Butterworth, pp. 26–29.

MacLeod, R. and McPherson, KM., 2007. Care and compassion: part of the person-centred rehabilitation, inappropriate response or a forgotten art? *Disability Rehabilitation*, 29, pp. 1589–1595.

Majlesi, J., Togay, H., Unalan, H. et al., 2008. The sensitivity and specificity of the slump and the straight leg raising tests in patients with lumbar disc herniation. *Journal Clinical Rheumatology*, 14(2), pp. 87–91.

Martin, HJ., Yule, V., Syddall, HE. et al., 2006. Is hand-held dynamometer useful for the measurement of quadriceps strength in older people? A comparison with the gold standard Biodex dynamometry. *Gerontology*, 52, pp. 154–159.

Martin, HD., Kivlan, BR., Palmer, IJ. et al., 2014. Diagnostic accuracy of clinical tests for sciatic nerve entrapment in the gluteal region. *Knee Surgery, Sports Traumatology, Arthroscopy*, 22(4), pp. 882–888.

McGill, S., 1998. Low back exercises: evidence for improving exercise regimes. *Physical Therapy*, 78, pp. 754–765.

Mead, N. and Power, P., 2000. Patient-centredness: a conceptual framework and review of the empirical literature. *Social Science Medicine*, 51, pp. 1087–1110.

Mens, J., Vleeming, A., Snijders, C. et al., 2002. Reliability and validity of hip adduction strength to measure disease severity in posterior pelvic pain since pregnancy. *Spine*, 27(15), pp. 1674–1679.

Mens, J., Damen, L., Snijders, C. et al., 2006. The mechanical effect of a pelvic belt in patients with pregnancy-related pelvic pain. *Clinical Biomechanics*, 21(2), pp. 122–127.

Meyer, GA., McCulloch, AD. and Lieberman, RL., 2011. A nonlinear model of passive muscle viscosity. *Journal Biomechanical Engineering*, 133(9), pp. 091007-1–091007-9.

Miciak, M., Mayan, M., Brown, C. et al., 2018. The necessary conditions of engagement for the therapeutic relationship in physiotherapy: an interpretive description study. *Archives of Physiotherapy*, 8(3).

Nee, RJ., Vincenzino, B., Jull, GA. et al., 2012. Neural tissue management provides immediate clinically relevant benefits without harmful effects for patients with nerve related neck and arm pain: a randomized trial. *Journal Physiotherapy*, 58(1), pp. 23–31.

O'Sullivan, P., Caneiro, JP., O'Keefe, M. et al., 2018. Cognitive functional therapy: an integrated behavioral approach with articular exercises for the targeted disabling low back pain. *Physical Therapy*, 98, pp. 408–423.

Panzer, D., 1992. The reliability of lumbar motion palpation. *Journal Manipulative and Physiological Therapeutics*, 15(8), pp. 518–524.

Pincus, T., Holt, N., Vogel, S. et al., 2013. Cognitive and affective reassurance and patient outcomes in primary care: a systematic review. *Pain*, 154(11), pp. 2407–2416.

Quack, C., Schenk, P., Laeubli, T. et al., 2007. Do MRI findings correlate with mobility tests? An explorative analysis of the test validity with regard to structure. *European Journal Spine*, 16(6), pp. 803–812.

Ranawat, AS., Guadiana, MA., Slullitel, PA. et al., 2017. Foot progression angle walking test: a dynamic diagnostic assessment for femoroacetabular impingement and hip instability. *Orthopaedic Journal Sports Medicine*, 5(1), p. 2325967116679641.

Ratamess, NA., Alvar, A., Evetoch, TK. et al., 2009. American College of Sports Medicine position stand: progression models in resistance training for healthy adults. *Medicine Science Sports Exercise*, 41(3), pp. 687–708.

Reese, NB. and Bandy, WD., 2003. Use of an inclinometer to measure flexibility of the iliotibial band using the Ober test and the modified Ober test: differences in magnitude and reliability of measurements. *Journal Orthopaedic & Sports Physical Therapy*, 33(6), pp. 326–330.

Reiman, M., Mather, R. and Cook, C., 2015. Physical examination tests for hip dysfunction and injury. *British Journal of Sports Medicine*, 49(6), pp. 357–361.

Riddle, DL. and Freburger, JK., 2002. Evaluation of the presence of sacroiliac joint region dysfunction using a combination of tests: a multicenter intertester reliability study. *Physical Therapy*, 82(8), pp. 772–781.

Roussel, N., Nijs, J., Mottram, S. et al., 2009. Altered lumbopelvic movement control but not generalised joint hypermobility is associated with increased injury in dancers. A prospective study. *Manual Therapy*, 14(6), pp. 630–635.

Rubinstein, SD. and van Tulder, M., 2008. A best-evidence review of diagnostic procedures for neck and low back pain. *Best Practice Research Clinical Rheumatology*, 22, pp. 471–482.

Schönberger, M., Humle, F., Zeeman, P. et al., 2006. Working alliance and patient compliance in brain injury rehabilitation and their relation to social outcome. *Neuropsychological Rehabilitation*, 16, pp. 298–314.

Serner, A., Weir, A., Tol, J. et al., 2016. Can standardised clinical examination of athletes with acute groin injuries predict the presence and location of MRI findings? *British Journal Sports Medicine*, 50(24), pp. 1541–1547.

Shacklock, M., 1995. Neurodynamics. *Physiotherapy*, 81(1), pp. 9–16.

Shacklock, M., 2005. *Clinical Neurodynamics: A New System of Musculoskeletal Treatment*. Edinburgh: Butterworth Heinemann/Elsevier.

Spencer, S., Wolf, A. and Rushton, A., 2016. Spinal-exercise prescription in sport: classifying physical training and rehabilitation by intention outcome. *Journal Athletic Training*, 51(8), pp. 613–628.

Stratford, PW., Binkley, JM. and Riddle, DL., 2000. Development and initial validation of the Back Pain Function Scale. *Spine*, 25, pp. 2095–2102.

Swärd-Aminoff, A., Agnvall, C., Todd, C. et al., 2018. The effect of pelvic tilt and cam on hip range of motion in young elite skiers and nonathletes. *Open Access Journal of Sports Medicine*, 9, pp. 147–156.

Tawa, N., Rhoda, A. and Diener, I., 2017. Accuracy of clinical neurological examination in diagnosing lumbo-sacral radiculopathy: a systemic literature review. *BMC Musculoskeletal Disorders*, 18, p. 93.

Thorborg, K., Peterson, J., Magnusson, SP. et al., 2010. Clinical assessment of hip strength using a hand-held dynamometer is reliable. *Scandinavian Journal Medicine Science in Sports*, 20(3), pp. 493–501.

Thorborg, K., Hölmich, P., Christensen, R. et al., 2011a. The Copenhagen Hip and Groin Outcome Score (HAGOS): development and validation according to the COSMIN checklist. *British Journal Sports Medicine*, 45(6), pp. 478–491.

Thorborg, K., Serner, A., Peterson, J. et al., 2011b. Hip adduction and abduction strength profiles in elite soccer players: implications for clinical evaluation of hip adductor muscle recovery after injury. *American Journal Sports Medicine*, 39(1), pp. 121–126.

Thorborg, K., Bandholm, T., Zebis, M. et al., 2016. Large strengthening effect of a hip-flexor training programme:

a randomized controlled trial. *Knee Surgery Sports Traumatology Arthroscopy*, 24, pp. 2346–2352.

Van Dillen, L., Maluf, K. and Sahrmann, S., 2009. Further examination of modifying patient-preferred movement and alignment strategies in patients with low back pain during symptomatic tests. *Manual Therapy*, 14(1), pp. 52–60.

Verrall, G., Slavotinek, J., Barnes, P. et al., 2005. Description of pain provocation tests used for the diagnosis of sports-related chronic groin pain: relationship of tests to defined clinical (pain and tenderness) and MRI (pubic bone marrow oedema) criteria. *Scandinavian Journal of Medicine and Science in Sports*, 15(1), pp. 36–42.

Vleeming, A., Stoeckart, R., , A. et al., 1990a. Relation between form and function in the sacroiliac joint. *Spine*, 15(2), pp. 130–132.

Vleeming, A., Volkers, A., Snijders, C. et al., 1990b. Relation between form and function in the sacroiliac joint. *Spine*, 15(2), pp. 133–136.

Waldhelm, A., Gacek, M., Davis, H. et al., 2019. Acute effects of neural gliding on athletic performance. *Internal Journal Sports Physical Therapy*, 14(4), pp. 603–612.

Yong, P., Alias, N. and Shuaib, I., 2003. Correlation of clinical presentation, radiography and magnetic resonance imaging for low back pain. A preliminary survey. *Journal Hong Kong College Radiology*, 6, pp. 144–151.

Youdas, J., Mraz, S., Norstad, B. et al., 2007. Determining meaningful changes in pelvic-on-femoral position during the Trendelenburg test. *Journal of Sport Rehabilitation*, 16(4), pp. 326–335.

Chapter 6 structure

Introduction	169
Joint manipulation	170
Soft tissue manipulation	170
Muscle activation techniques	170
Neurophysiology of joint manipulation	171
Neurophysiology of soft tissue manipulation	173
Neurophysiology of muscle activation techniques	173
Effects of joint manipulation	174
Effects of soft tissue manipulation	175
Effects of muscle activation techniques	175
Combined effects of joint, soft tissue manipulation and muscle activation	175
Manipulative therapy and patient safety	176
Pre-manipulation provocative testing	178
Techniques for pre-manipulation provocative testing	180
Thoracic spine and rib techniques	181
Lumbar spine techniques	188
Pelvic girdle techniques	191
Hip joint techniques	196
Neural dynamic techniques	203
Common mistakes with manual therapy	205
Conclusion	205

Introduction

Manipulation is often synonymous with treatment from a musculoskeletal practitioner, yet there is also a range of ways in which "touch" and "effective hands on" can be used to help reassure patients and develop a therapeutic relationship between clinician and patient. The use of manual therapy has attracted considerable criticism over the last few years (Oostendorp, 2018). In fact, many clinicians have questioned the value of using a manipulative hands-on approach to treatment (Collins et al., 2017) and have turned instead to an alternative, patient-centered, active approach to deliver healthcare (Kolb et al., 2020). It is highly likely that this change is a reflection of the recent recommendations for more consistent, scientific, evidence-based approaches to managing musculoskeletal pain (Lin et al., 2020). Getting patients better by making them stronger, and empowering and motivating them to help themselves, may appear to have much greater value than using manual therapy and a tissue-based diagnostic approach (Gifford, 1998).

While I completely agree that encouraging active care, as quickly as possible, will lead to more satisfactory outcomes, clinicians should be mindful and take care with embracing the latest approach too eagerly, as the pendulum can swing and treatments change, much like the proverbial hemlines in fashion. I think it makes logical sense to consider incorporating manual therapy into an active approach. For example, manual therapy can be used as a symptom modification technique (Lewis, 2009) and also for evaluation of the local mobility and stability components of movement control within the framework of regional interdependence (Alrwaily et al., 2016; Sueki et al., 2013). Furthermore, in my opinion, effective hands-on "touch" may make a significant contribution to patient reassurance and this may help to develop a therapeutic relationship between the two

parties. Therefore, early use of appropriate manipulation (2–4 treatment sessions) for pain modulation (Cook, 2021) may be indicated to help patients progress towards a more active lifestyle.

With that in mind, let's consider the case of Patient M.

Case study: Patient M

Patient M is a 24-year-old female professional track athlete. On race day morning, she presented reporting right-sided low back pain (LBP). She had been reviewed the evening before and was moving appropriately. At that time, the conclusion was that there was no need to perform any manipulative techniques. However, when she reported LBP on race day, the clinician had to start to consider the previous day's other activities: she had made a 4-hour journey, involving travel by car and plane, and may have slept awkwardly in an unfamiliar bed. These factors, combined with the mental pressure of the race, should lead the clinician to ask: "Did I miss something last night?" Whether or not something was missed, one thing is absolutely clear: the need to *evaluATE*.

Active evaluation highlights a right-sided restriction into extension in her lower lumbar spine; passive evaluation highlights reduced range of movement (ROM) at the level of L4–5. Gluteal tone has increased on the right, with reduced active and passive hip joint ROM, and palpation reveals tight myofascial bands within the gluteus maximus and medius muscles. The clinician hypothesizes that this may be a reactive L4–5 facet joint irritation, which may have increased neural tone in the gluteal muscles as they are innervated at that level. Explaining to the athlete that, more than likely, her symptoms are due to the long day of traveling and sleeping in a different bed helps to reassure her somewhat. But now the clinician has a decision to make! This athlete needs to be pain-free to race, so with that in mind there is a dilemma. Should she be treated with exercises to improve her neuromuscular control of movement or manipulated to resolve the symptoms efficiently and effectively? If the clinician manipulates, are either articular or soft tissue components addressed – or both of these?

This athlete is presenting with a movement restriction; therefore, appropriate manual therapy could help to reduce symptoms, modulate pain and quickly restore function.

The point that I am making in relating this case history is that manual therapy, used in the correct context, can be an extremely powerful tool. In my opinion, manipulation is a skillful art, and therefore not one easily attained by attending a weekend training course, for example, when practitioners want to add manipulation to their toolbox of skills. Those clinicians who practice manipulation proficiently have developed and refined their skills over years of training and experience. However, defining manipulation is extremely difficult. It appears that every discipline in physical therapy has a slightly different interpretation. In addition, does manipulation relate only to joints or should it include soft tissues? In this chapter, I use the term "manipulation" to describe any technique (joint, soft tissue or muscle activation) that is used to affect the articular, myofascial and nervous systems.

Joint manipulation

According to Evans and Lucas (2010), manipulation should involve two joint surfaces that have been moved apart. These authors proposed two categories of empirically derived features to characterize manipulation: the action and the mechanical response.

In the action:

- a force is applied to the recipient

- the line of action of this force is perpendicular to the articular surface of the affected joint.

In the mechanical response:

- application of a force creates joint motion

- joint motion includes separation of the articular surfaces

- joint cavitation occurs within the affected joint.

Soft tissue manipulation

Loghmani and Whitted (2016) defined soft tissue manipulation (STM) as "a powerful form of mechanotherapy that involves applying a non-invasive mechanical stimulus to the soft tissues of the body, to influence molecular, cellular and tissue structure and function through the process of mechanotransduction." Mechanotherapy is defined as any intervention that uses a mechanical stimulus to affect a biological change, and mechanotransduction is the process of converting mechanical stimuli into cellular, molecular and tissue responses.

STM may encompass many forms of treatment and involve either a direct or an indirect approach. An example of a direct approach is when the barrier to resistance is challenged, such as during a specific myofascial release; an example of an indirect approach is when the clinician works away from the barrier, such as during a strain–counterstrain or positional release technique. Table 6.1 summarizes examples of approaches to STM.

Muscle activation techniques

The rationale for applying muscle activation techniques originates from the use of proprioceptive neuromuscular facilitation (PNF) and muscle energy techniques (METs). These rely on the patient contracting against manually applied resistance, resulting in an isometric or isotonic contraction. Although there is limited evidence available concerning the efficacy of using muscle activation techniques, their clinical effectiveness makes them invaluable for retraining the motor system. This may

Table 6.1 Examples of soft tissue manipulation techniques

Technique	Aim
Deep transverse friction	Specifically devised to work on muscles, tendons and ligaments by cross-fiber manipulation
Instrument-assisted soft tissue manipulation	Specifically designed handheld devices for mobilization and manipulation of soft tissue
Inhibition techniques	Direct pressure to specific trigger points or tender points
Myofascial release techniques	Specific techniques to release restrictions in the myofascial tissue that have not responded to other forms of soft tissue manipulation
Strain–counterstrain	An indirect technique, such as positional release, that involves working away from the barrier of resistance

involve either activating and retraining of inhibited muscles, or increasing the extensibility of a shortened muscle (contracture), or helping to mobilize a restricted joint (Fryer, 2006; 2011).

Neurophysiology of joint manipulation

Joint manipulation refers to the "thrust" applied during a high-velocity, low-amplitude thrust (HVLA) technique. Under normal physiological conditions, this results in an audible "pop" or "crack" heard within the joint. While joint manipulation is widely used by clinicians to modulate acute and chronic pain, there is limited scientific evidence concerning the neurophysiology behind this process. It is believed that pain modulation may occur through one, or a combination of, the following three possible mechanisms.

Pain gate mechanism

Description of the pain gate mechanism (Figure 6.1) dates back to the 1960s and is based on research by Melzack and Wall (1965). They theorized that pain was modulated by a gate mechanism, located in the lamina of the dorsal horn in the spinal cord. They proposed the theory that pain was a balance between opposing stimuli (Kandel et al., 2000). It was speculated that the nociceptive, smaller-diameter fibers could open the gate, while non-nociceptive, larger-diameter fibers from the joint capsule mechanoreceptors, muscle spindles and cutaneous mechanoreceptors could

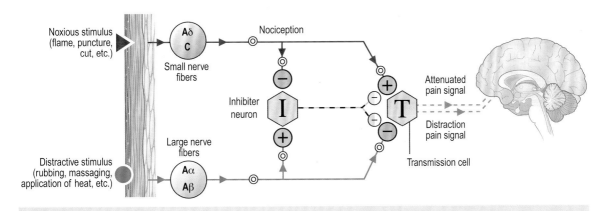

Figure 6.1
Pain gate mechanism.

close the gate. If joint manipulation provides a mechanical impulse applied at speed with sufficient force to move a joint, this may modulate the pain gate mechanism by creating an afferent barrage of non-nociceptive input from the larger-diameter fibers (muscle spindles and the facet joint mechanoreceptors) (Potter et al., 2005; Lederman, 1997), leading to a reduction in symptoms.

Descending pain mechanism

In the field of manipulative therapy, there is a large body of evidence to support the theory that hypoalgesia (pain reduction), after manipulation, is the result of a descending pain mechanism (Figure 6.2) controlled by the brain (Potter et al., 2005; Sterling et al., 2001; Vincenzino et al., 1998). The periaqueductal gray (PAG), an area of gray matter in the brain, surrounds the third ventricle and, when stimulated, produces analgesia via the descending PAG pathways (Reynolds, 1969). The dorsal PAG, when stimulated, modulates pain through a fast-acting, non-opioid analgesia response, whereas the ventral PAG modulates pain through a longer-acting, opioid analgesia response (Satpute et al., 2013). Sympathetic excitation occurs as a result of stimulating the dorsal PAG, as opposed to sympathetic inhibition, which occurs as a result of stimulating the ventral PAG (Sterling, 2001). The mechanical stimulus of actual joint manipulation, when compared with sham

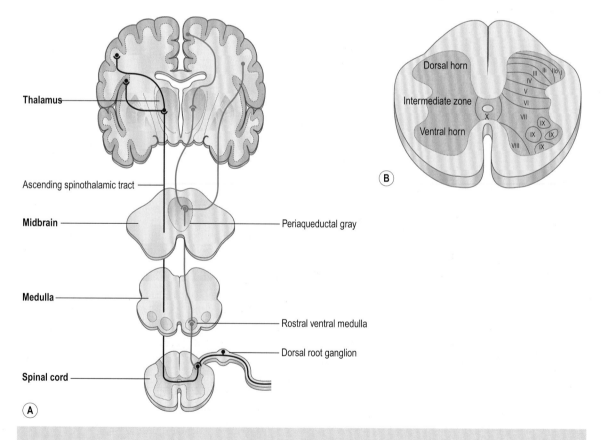

Figure 6.2
Descending pain mechanism.

manipulation, has been shown to influence hypoalgesia and sympathetic excitation, which in turn may modulate pain through the endogenous activation of the descending pathways, mediated through the dorsal PAG (Sterling et al., 2001; Vincenzino et al., 1998).

Neurotransmitters

Neurotransmitters have been shown to play an important role in pain modulation (Kandel et al., 2000). Substance P is a neurotransmitter that has been shown to modulate pain. It is produced in the dorsal root ganglion and released into the peripheral tissues and the dorsal horn of the spinal cord by C fibers, which influence nociceptive input (Kandel et al., 2000). Pain modulation may also result from an increase in beta-endorphins, released by the endogenous anti-nociceptive system (Potter et al., 2005; Kandel et al., 2000). Secreted by the pituitary gland, beta-endorphins assert an anti-nociceptive influence by decreasing the effectiveness of substance P in the dorsal horn of the spinal cord, reducing input to the higher centers. Joint manipulation, in some studies, has shown a hypoalgesic effect due to the anti-nociceptive influence of plasma beta-endorphin levels following HVLA (Thomson et al., 2009; Vernon et al., 1986).

Neurophysiology of soft tissue manipulation

STM can be viewed as a form of mechanotherapy. This is defined as any intervention that uses a mechanical stimulus to effect a biological change (Huang et al., 2013; Khan and Scott, 2009). All cells within the body will respond to mechanical stimuli, and STM, used appropriately, may directly influence cellular responses, molecular pathways, and tissue structure, function, healing, repair and regeneration (Best et al., 2013). It is critical for health, survival and function for cells to have the ability to sense changes within their environment and translate these changes into biochemical signals (mechanotransduction) (Thompson et al., 2016).

STM, delivered through application of a controlled physical force, will create localized changes in tissues.

When tissue change is detected, it is converted into signals that may have profound biological effects, mediated by intra-cellular and extra-cellular signaling responses. The extra-cellular matrix (ECM) is primarily composed of water and fibrous proteins, such as collagen; it provides a structure for cells and has a role within cell function, growth, healing and repair. The ECM creates an environment which maintains the reciprocal structural and functional relationships that lead to connective tissue organization. It is hypothesized that STM, through mechanical stimuli, creates a cascade effect, initiated by "stress" to the so-called "cytoskeleton" of the cell. This is sensed by small molecules that cross the membrane (ECM integrins) and connect the ECM to the environment within the cell (Martino et al., 2018). This concept is not new. Wolff's law states that the remodeling of bone occurs in response to physical stress. Davis's law can be viewed as the soft tissue equivalent, describing how soft tissue will remodel itself in line with imposed demands.

Neurophysiology of muscle activation techniques

The underlying neurophysiological effect of any form of muscle activation technique is likely to involve a number of mechanisms. For example, the effect of METs may include pain modulation, increased tissue extensibility, changes in proprioception, motor programming and motor control, and fluid dynamics (Fryer, 2011).

Pain modulation

Hypoalgesia may develop as a result of an increased tolerance to stretching, which may involve central and peripheral mechanisms (Fryer and Fossum, 2010; Fryer, 2006). These include activation of muscle and joint mechanoreceptors and centrally mediated pathways, such as the PAG in the midbrain, or non-opioid serotonergic and noradrenergic descending inhibitory pathways. Sympathoexcitation has been shown to occur by activation of the lateral and dorsolateral PAG in response to muscle contraction (Seseke et al., 2006; Li and Mitchell, 2003). Similarly, activation of descending, non-opioid inhibitory pathways has been shown to occur after joint mobilization (Paungmali et al., 2004; Skyba et al., 2003). Improved fluid dynamics as a consequence of brief muscle contractions may assist with hypoalgesia (Havas et al., 1997), and mechanical forces have an impact on fibroblast activity because of changes in interstitial pressure (Langevin et al., 2005). It is also speculated that pain modulation may reduce inflammatory cytokines and desensitize peripheral receptors (Fryer, 2011).

Increased muscle extensibility

Increased muscle extensibility may occur as a result of changes in viscoelastic and plastic tissue properties (Taylor et al., 1997; Lederman, 2005) and this may influence extra-cellular fluid dynamics (Fryer, 2011; Fryer and Fossum, 2010; Schleip, 2003) and fibroblast mechanotransduction (Langevin et al., 2004; Schleip, 2003). Previously, reflex relaxation was cited in many texts as a mechanism for improving ROM, muscle length and tissue changes following the application of a given soft tissue technique (Fryer and Fossum, 2010; Fryer, 2006). However, no study to date has shown a reduction in the electromyographic (EMG) activity following MET, although increases in low-level EMG activity have been reported after MET (Ferber et al., 2002; Osternig et al., 1987).

Altered motor control

There is persuasive evidence that altered proprioception, motor programming and motor control may occur as a result of muscle activation techniques. Evidence has shown that spinal pain disrupts proprioception and inhibits motor control, decreasing the awareness of spinal motion and position (Lee et al., 2008; Grip et al., 2007; Taimela et al., 1999). This is observed regularly in elite sport, when athletes develop LBP as a result of muscle fatigue from soft tissue overload. Therefore, if muscle activation promotes movement around joints through low-threshold muscle recruitment, it may be reasoned that it also has an impact on proprioceptive feedback, motor control and motor learning.

Effects of joint manipulation

Facet joints

Most clinicians will equate joint manipulation with the "thrust" technique applied during an HVLA thrust. To understand how this may work, we need to be aware that facet joints have a limit, or threshold, for withstanding external force, depending on their location in the spine. For example, the thoracic spine has been shown to have a threshold of up to 500 N, whereas the lumbar spine has a lower threshold of 400 N (Brennan, 1995). When an external force, such as an HVLA exceeding the threshold of the facet joint, is applied, joint cavitation occurs within the synovial fluid of the joint, resulting in an audible "pop" or "crack" (Evans and Lucas, 2010).

Intervertebral disks

Joint manipulation may also have an effect on the intervertebral disk. Pressure changes within the intervertebral disk have been shown to correlate with intervertebral movement. Maigne and Guillon (2000) demonstrated that a small increase in intradiskal pressure occurred when an HVLA was performed, and this was followed by a small decrease in intradiskal pressure at the end of the HVLA. It is suggested that joint repositioning occurs following manipulation to separate the articular surfaces and reduce the intradiskal pressure (Oliphant, 2004), and that manipulation of a protruding disk may help to return it to its optimal position (Maigne and Nieves, 2005). Unfortunately, current scientific evidence to support the manipulation of the intervertebral disk for LBP is lacking.

Muscle tissue

A reduction in muscle activity following HVLA is often observed clinically. This may result from stretching the spinal paravertebral muscles when applying an HVLA technique. The style of technique may also be important. For example, a long-lever manipulation will stretch the paravertebral muscles further than a short-lever technique (Gyer et al., 2017). A reduction in muscle tone may occur following an HVLA technique through a combination of intervertebral disk movement, facet joint separation and paraspinal muscle stretch. It is possible that these factors may all help to modulate the gamma and alpha motor neuron reflex activity (Maigne and Vautravers, 2003) and result in a reduction in muscle tone.

Case study: more on Patient M

Thinking back to the case of Patient M, the athlete with LBP on race day, joint manipulation may well be indicated to improve her movement dysfunction, but I have seen some clinicians shy away from this approach. Among possible reasons for such reluctance is the unwillingness of the clinician or practitioner to perform a maneuver that may make the athlete's/patient's symptoms worse, either if the manipulative technique is not adequate to treat the issue, or if irritation arises as a side effect of input to the neural and musculoskeletal systems, which can occur after manipulation. Their skill level may not be adequate to perform such a subtle manipulation. This is not a problem in itself, as there are many other approaches. However, if it is used appropriately with an athlete or patient, manipulation can provide a very powerful treatment. In the case of Patient M, using joint manipulation is a quick and effective way to modulate her pain, allowing her to carry on with her normal warm-up routine, which will help to encourage joint mobility and up-regulate (that is, restore homeostatic mechanisms to) the nervous system.

Effects of soft tissue manipulation

Muscle and connective tissue

Connective tissue surrounds, and is continuous with, muscle tissue; consequently, STM will affect both structures. Increased ROM and improved muscle function have both been shown to occur following STM (Kivlan

et al., 2015; Iwatsuki et al., 2001). STM delivered with instruments has been shown to increase the number of fibroblasts, the cells responsible for collagen deposition. It may therefore be reasoned that an increase in fibroblast activity will positively influence soft tissue healing (Gehlsen et al., 1999). STM may also benefit recovery after sport participation, reducing recovery time (Schillinger et al., 2006). For example, a more rapid decrease in the enzymes implicated in muscle cell damage has been shown to occur following exercise (Schillinger et al., 2006), suggesting that STM could decrease recovery time after exercise and increase muscle strength after application.

Effects of muscle activation techniques

The therapeutic effects of muscle activation techniques, such as MET, are proposed to occur through a number of pathways:

- beneficial changes in motor control following spinal pain or fatigue, resulting in increased muscle activation or restored function at a joint

- increased muscle tolerance to stretching because of greater tissue elasticity and/or extensibility, reducing contractures ("shortened muscles")

- enhanced viscoelastic and plastic tissue properties of myofascial structures

- pain modulation, through an analgesic response mediated by muscle and joint mechanoreceptors and involving central pathways, such as the PAG or non-opioid, serotonergic and noradrenergic descending inhibitory pathways.

Combined effects of joint, soft tissue manipulation and muscle activation

Blood and lymphatic flow

It has been proposed that joint and soft tissue manipulation enhances blood flow to damaged tissues, increasing the removal of toxic substances and decreasing edema (Maigne and Vautravers, 2003; Vario et al., 2009). STM has been shown to have a positive effect on fluid dynamics via the formation of new vessels, which facilitates the healing process and ensures an adequate blood supply to the tissues. In addition, joint and soft tissue manipulation lead to a higher skin temperature, increases in blood flow and the potential for more rapid removal of waste products from the area (Portillo-Soto et al., 2014; Okamoto et al., 2014).

Placebo

Patients report experiencing a significant psychological benefit from having both joint and soft tissue manipulation. Unfortunately, this had led many critics of manipulative therapy to claim that the effect of manipulation is purely placebo in nature. Of course, a placebo effect may occur when a clinician places their hands on a patient or when the patient feels the immediate effect of pain relief following a joint manipulation and this should not be under-estimated: in itself it may be a useful tool with which to modulate pain and it should be seen as a positive and integral aspect of treatment (Potter et al., 2005).

Case study: more on Patient M

So, what if the decision had been taken to use STM with Patient M, prior to her race, to benefit her symptoms? Most clinicians would probably use a combination of joint and STM techniques. However, if a clinician is not competent or may not have been trained in joint manipulation, they will choose the treatment they feel comfortable with. STM has its benefits but sometimes, with an underlying articular issue, it can simply irritate the presenting condition. Another mistake a clinician may make is to spend too much time treating a patient with soft tissue techniques. What is being achieved with excessive soft tissue treatment? Any athlete that spends too much time on the treatment couch, prior to a race or competition, may become lethargic and end up with desensitized tissues from an afferent barrage (that

is, excessive "input") to the nervous system (Maigne and Vautravers, 2003). It may be hypothesized that, in this instance, STM could ultimately impair performance, as evidence suggests (Moran et al., 2018; Fletcher, 2010; Goodwin et al., 2007). This is precisely one of the reasons why manual therapy has attracted criticism. Who does the treatment benefit? Does it feed the ego of the athlete or does it make the clinician feel important? My concern is the athlete becomes a couch-dependent patient, and if the practitioner is not scrupulous in avoiding this type of dependency, it could have a detrimental effect and play into negatively reinforcing the athlete's ego or the concept of the clinician as guru.

Manipulative therapy and patient safety

It is extremely difficult to assess and determine protocols and establish guidelines for the risk assessment of manipulative therapy. The most significant reasons for this are inconsistency and evidence that suggests accuracy and high levels of reliability are lacking to evaluate patients prior to manipulation (Puentedura et al., 2012; Refshauge, 2002). Historically, the majority of the research around this subject has been predominantly focused on the spine: in particular, the cervical spine. Although they are touched on in this chapter, there will not be any cervical spinal manipulative techniques presented in this book because my preference is to concentrate on the thoracic, lumbar and pelvic regions; in my experience, treating these regions produces consistently good patient outcomes for spino-pelvic-hip musculoskeletal issues.

The suitability of manipulative therapy techniques, such as HVLA, needs to be considered during the process of patient evaluation. An in-depth case history should provide the clinician with information about the present patient and will also include information about past history and medical history, as well as an insight into the patient as an individual. The evaluation should be thorough enough to take into consideration the patient's functional ability, and to determine the safety and efficacy of performing manipulative therapy techniques by screening the patient during clinical examination. This process may include a request for laboratory tests to investigate inflammatory markers, and diagnostic imaging to investigate potential pathology; it will also include neurological evaluations.

Pre-manipulation tests

Prior to any manipulative HVLA thrust technique being administered, it is important to discuss the risks and benefits with the patient. If I feel the technique is indicated and the patient has verbally consented, it is a legal requirement to obtain the patient's written consent prior to performing any evaluation and treatment. In most cases, where an adverse reaction to HVLA techniques has been reported, a poor level of communication and a lack of interaction between the clinician and patient are likely to have been at the heart of the issue, in my opinion. Table 6.2 provides examples of factors that could give rise to adverse reactions from manipulative techniques such as HVLA (Refshauge et al., 2002).

Common side effects of manipulative therapy

Most side effects experienced after manipulative therapy are not serious, the majority generally resolving within 24–48 hours of treatment (Cagnie et al., 2004). It has

Table 6.3 Adverse complications of manipulative therapy

Level of severity	Complication	Frequency (%)
Mild to moderate	Localized discomfort, stiffness, fatigue Increased or radiating pain Weakness Paresthesia Visual disturbances Vertigo Loss of consciousness	33–61
Serious	Stroke Vertebral/carotid artery dissection Myelopathy Dural tear Pathological fractures Rib fracture Disk herniation Cauda equina syndrome Death	Extremely rare

been shown that approximately 55 percent of patients may experience minor side effects, such as localized discomfort, fatigue and headaches, especially after cervical or thoracic manipulation (Senstad et al., 1997). Serious adverse complications from manipulative therapy are extremely rare; these are listed in Table 6.3 (Gouveia et al., 2009; Ernst, 2007; World Health Organization, 2005).

Contra-indications to manipulative therapy

A number of contra-indications to manipulative therapy exist and are generally classified as relative or absolute (Table 6.4) (World Health Organization, 2005: Gibbons and Tehan, 2004; Liem and Dobler, 2014). Clinicians may use these contra-indications to inform clinical decisions. This ensures that the risks and benefits of performing manipulative therapy are considered prior to performing treatment, and judgments are made based on whether or not to expose patients to potential risks or complications. In the case of a relative contra-indication, the manipulative technique should be modified and applied with the appropriate level of care and consideration, to minimize

Table 6.2 Possible reasons for adverse reactions to manipulative therapy

- Poor communication between clinician and patient, leading to lack of patient understanding
- Poor diagnostic skills due to inadequate evaluation
- Inappropriate technique
- Excessive use of manipulative technique
- Underlying herniated disk
- Underlying arterial disease or disorders, such as coronary artery disease

Table 6.4 Contra-indications to manipulative therapy	
Relative	**Absolute**
• Acute disk herniation • Spondylolisthesis • Vascular pathology • Bleeding disorders or taking anticoagulants • Hypermobility • Osteopenia • Psychological issues	• Inflammatory conditions (rheumatoid arthritis and seronegative spondyloarthropathies) • Atlantoaxial instability • Fractures and dislocations • Avascular necrosis • Acute infections (osteomyelitis) • Metabolic conditions (osteomalacia, osteopenia, osteoporosis) • Spinal anomalies (spina bifida, deformations) • Iatrogenic from long-term steroid medication • Tumor (spinal cord, malignant bone, meningeal, giant cell, osteoblastoma, osteoid osteoma) • Progressive neurological deficits (cervical myelopathy, meningitis, spinal cord compression, nerve compression, intracranial hypertension, cauda equina syndrome, hydrocephalus) • Vascular pathology (vertebrobasilar insufficiency, aortic aneurysm, vascular calcification, bleeding disorders)

Table 6.5 Red flags for manipulative therapy
• Previous diagnosis of vertebrobasilar insufficiency • Signs and symptoms of spondylitis and spondylolisthesis • Previous history of joint surgery • Facial/intra-oral anesthesia or paresthesia • History of long-term steroid use • History of traumatic event • Women at menopause • Psychogenic issues • Nystagmus • Osteopenia • Scoliosis • Diplopia or visual disturbances • Ataxia and coordination issues • Dizziness, vertigo, light-headedness • Blurred vision • Nausea • Sudden fall without loss of consciousness or drop attack • Dysarthria • Sensation of ringing or buzzing in ears • Dysphagia • Aggravation of any of the above symptoms from manipulation • No improvement or worsening of symptoms following manipulation

exposure to adverse side effects. Compare this with an absolute contra-indication, when the manipulative technique should not be delivered, as it may result in life-threatening complications. However, the presence of a contra-indication in one region of the body does not necessarily exclude the use of manipulative techniques in other regions.

Red flags

Symptoms considered to be red flags are highlighted in Table 6.5. These may indicate the presence of a serious underlying medical condition. It is recommended that

clinicians should be aware of known contra-indications so that they can determine whether manipulative techniques, such as HVLA, are to be used appropriately (Refshauge et al., 2002; Childs et al., 2005).

Pre-manipulation provocative testing

Pre-manipulation provocative evaluations may help to reduce potential complications arising from using manipulative techniques to treat the thoracic and/or lumbar spine (Thiel and Rix, 2005). Although often criticized for its lack of reliability, validity and accuracy, especially with regard to the cervical spine (Rivett et al., 2005; Magarey et al., 2004), pre-manipulation provocative testing is still employed regularly in clinical practice and in sports medicine. It must be stressed that it is not my intention, in this book, to discuss the safety aspects of cervical spine manipulation. I will focus specifically on the thoracolumbar spine and pelvis. I think it is important to emphasize again that a thorough subjective case history, in combination with objective evaluations, helps to inform good clinical reasoning processes.

A final point I would like to emphasize is that pre-manipulation provocative testing can be used right up to the moment before the manipulation is delivered. This involves setting up the patient in the position of manipulation and placing them at the barrier of restriction (the pre-thrust position known as the barrier or zone elasticity located between the physiological and anatomical barriers incorporating the "neutral zone", Figure 6.3; Gibbons and Tehan, 2001; Evans and Breen, 2006) by removing the slack in the tissues, without necessarily delivering an HVLA technique. I always ask if a patient is comfortable with this position and use it as a means to evaluate the patient's tolerance, to observe any possibility of an increase in pain, and to familiarize the patient with the position in which the manipulative technique may be delivered. If the patient is not comfortable, I adapt my technique accordingly, using an alternative approach such as articular mobilization or a MET. I have often performed the "set-up" prior to delivering an HVLA technique and found that the patient tenses, fails to relax or attempts to resist my pressure. This is particularly common with athletes who have played in a number of different countries. They have often been exposed to different variations or styles of manipulative therapy techniques and may have had bad experiences from being too frequently or forcefully manipulated. If the patient has no issues with being placed in the pre-provocative testing position, then an HVLA technique may be safely delivered.

Clinical implications

The contra-indications to muscle activation techniques and joint and soft tissue manipulation may overlap on many occasions. Vascular conditions are an example of when not to treat a patient with either technique. Nevertheless, the technique may be modified, or a different style or approach may be used, with the same result achieved. For example, an athlete with a suspected rib contusion who is waiting for an MRI examination may still be treated to reduce biomechanical strain to the area of concern. HVLA techniques may be a local contra-indication, but using specific soft tissue manipulation, such as strain–counterstrain techniques, or muscle activation techniques may prove to be beneficial in reducing localized pain.

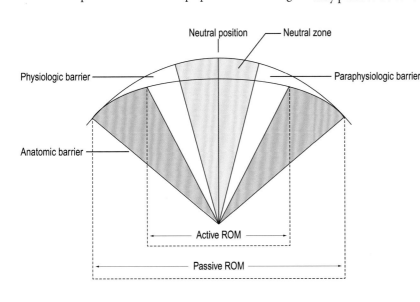

Figure 6.3
The barrier concept.
ROM: range of movement.

Below is a summary of the pre-manipulation provocative evaluations I often use to assist in my decision-making processes, prior to employing manipulative techniques for the thoracic and lumbar spine. Please refer to Chapter 5 for more information.

Techniques for pre-manipulation provocative testing

Anterior/posterior rib compression

There are many occasions when athletes involved in contact sports have suffered possible rib fractures, contusions or avulsions of the oblique muscles from their attachments. Although there is no validity for using the anterior/posterior compression test, it can be performed prior to other diagnostic evaluations, such as a magnetic resonance imaging (MRI) scan; a positive test would rule out any HVLA manipulative techniques. The anterior/posterior compression test can be performed in sitting or standing.

- The clinician places one hand on the anterior ribs and the other hand on the posterior ribcage, applying compression by squeezing the hands together and then releasing the pressure (Magee, 2014).

- Pain or specific point tenderness on compression of the ribcage, or respiratory restriction with both inhalation and exhalation, may be indicative of a possible rib fracture or a possible contusion of the soft tissues and/or bony structures.

Straight leg raise (SLR; Butler, 2010; Shacklock, 2005)

Clinically, this test is extremely useful if there is any suspicion of nerve root irritation to the lumbar spine. The SLR test has been shown to have 52 percent sensitivity and 89 percent specificity in diagnosing or assessing sciatica (Majlesi et al., 2008). I often use it alongside other neurological examinations, such as dermatome and myotome testing, to evaluate muscle power, reflexes and two-point discrimination in the lower limbs. A positive test, combined with reduced power

and reflexes, would rule out specific HVLA manipulative techniques to the area involved.

- The patient is supine and the clinician takes the leg to be tested into hip flexion with a straight knee, ensuring no accessory frontal or transverse plane motion occurs.

- The clinician can test for proximal symptoms by introducing ankle dorsiflexion.

- The clinician can test for distal symptoms in the patient's foot or ankle by varying the degree of hip flexion introduced.

- The same procedure is repeated on the contralateral leg (Magee, 2014; Majlesi et al., 2008).

Sensitizing the evaluation

- The clinician can combine ankle dorsiflexion and foot eversion with the SLR to bias the tibial nerve.

- The clinician can combine ankle dorsiflexion and foot inversion with the SLR to bias the sural nerve.

- The clinician can combine ankle plantar flexion, foot inversion and hip adduction and internal rotation with the SLR to bias the common peroneal nerve.

Slump sitting

This has been shown to be a more sensitive test for lumbar disk herniation. The slump sitting evaluation has been shown to have 84 percent sensitivity and 83 percent specificity (Majlesi et al., 2008) in identifying this condition.

- The patient sits on the couch and is instructed to perform thoracic and lumbar flexion.

- The clinician applies manual pressure to the lumbar and thoracic spine between the C7 spinous process and the hip joint, ensuring the vertical distance between these two points is reduced.

- The patient performs cervical flexion and the clinician maintains the manual pressure by stabilizing the patient's occiput.

- Knee extension is performed either actively or passively and the clinician supports the ankle.

- The clinician applies ankle dorsiflexion; this increases tension through the lumbosacral nerve roots and the sciatic and tibial nerves.

- Sensitizing movements may include contralateral lumbar flexion, hip internal rotation and adduction, and foot movements specific to each peripheral nerve (Magee, 2014; Majlesi et al., 2008).

Femoral nerve

- The patient is slump side-lying, holding their leg in hip and knee flexion, and is instructed to perform cervical flexion.

- The patient extends their upper leg into hip extension and the clinician supports the thigh and encourages knee flexion.

- The clinician increases the hip extension component until tension in the anterior thigh is reported. The patient performs cervical extension and any change in tension in the anterior thigh is noted.

- This has been shown to have a high sensitivity (1.00) and specificity (0.83) (Tawa et al., 2017) for detecting femoral nerve root irritation.

- Hip joint lateral and medial rotation can be introduced to test the ilioinguinal and iliohypogastric nerves.

Obturator nerve

- The clinician tests the obturator nerve in the slump side-lying position, similar to the femoral nerve test (Butler, 2010; Shacklock, 2005).

- Hip abduction is introduced to test the neurogenic components of the groin and medial knee.

Lumbar quadrant

The lumbar quadrant test is used to evaluate the possibility of facet joint pathology or the cause of the pain; if pain radiating into the legs is experienced, it may also be an indication that nerve root irritation is present, requiring the inclusion of neurological tests (SLR, slump, power/reflexes, two-point discrimination) in combination with this evaluation. The lumbar quadrant test is similar to the extension/rotation test, with the latter demonstrating 100 percent sensitivity but only 22 percent specificity (Laslett et al., 2006) for lumbar facet joint pathology.

- The patient stands with the clinician behind them; the clinician stabilizes the ilium with one hand and applies pressure to the shoulder with their other hand.

- The clinician takes the patient into extension, lateral flexion and rotation towards the side of pain.

- This position is held for 3 seconds (Stuber et al., 2014).

 ## Thoracic spine and rib techniques
Thoracic manipulation seated
HVLA T7–12 (Figure 6.4)

- The patient is seated as far back on the couch as possible and instructed to fold their arms across their chest.

- The clinician can place a rolled-up towel below the contact point of the segment that is to be manipulated and places both arms around the patient's lower elbow. Both clinician and patient interlock their fingers.

- The patient is instructed to inhale and exhale. As they exhale, the clinician engages the barrier and applies compression; manipulation may be performed.

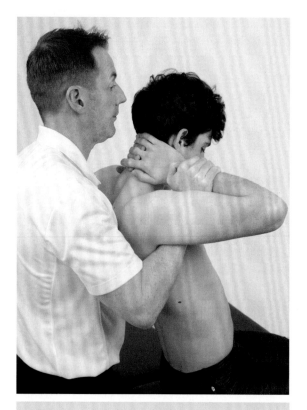

Figure 6.4

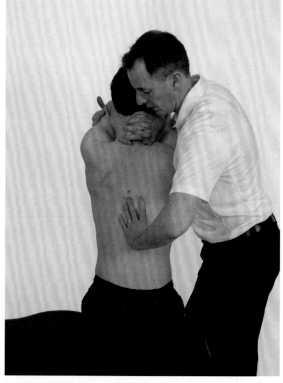

Figure 6.5

MET – extension (Figure 6.5)

- The patient is seated with hands interlocked behind the head.

- The clinician takes the patient's weight on their forearms.

- Segmental thoracic spine ROM can be evaluated and the level of restriction noted.

- This technique can be used as either an articulatory, a myofascial or a MET treatment, or as a combination involving all three in this position.

MET – rotation (Figure 6.6)

- The patient is seated with their arms folded across their chest.

- The clinician stabilizes the patient's opposite shoulder.

- Segmental motion is palpated through side bending and rotation.

- This technique can be used as either an articulatory, a myofascial or a MET technique/treatment, or as a combination involving all three.

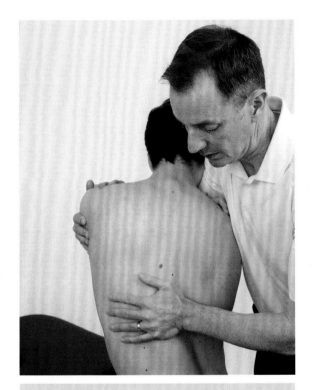

Figure 6.6

STM active release – flexion/extension (Figure 6.7)

- This technique is similar to the MET but the patient is instructed to perform an active flexion/extension motion, while the clinician actively releases the soft tissues.

Thoracic manipulation prone
HVLA (butterfly) T2–10 (Figure 6.8)

- The patient is prone and the clinician locates the segment that requires manipulation.

- The clinician contacts the transverse process with the ipsilateral pisiform bone of the dominant hand.

- The clinician contacts the transverse process of the contralateral side with pisiform bone of the other hand. This creates the butterfly.

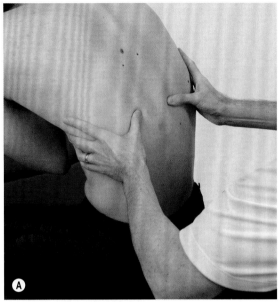

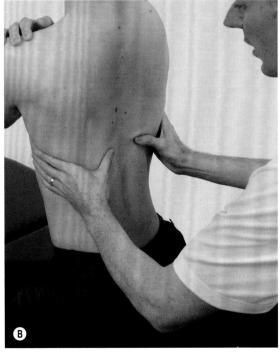

Figure 6.7

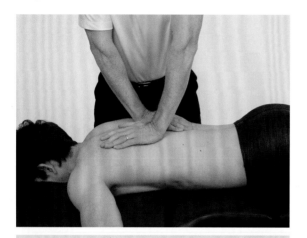

Figure 6.8

- The patient is instructed to inhale and exhale. As they exhale, the clinician introduces equal compression through both arms, which are almost locked at the elbows.

- Manipulation can be delivered in a downward direction, as if pushing through the couch, at the end of exhalation.

Thoracic manipulation supine
HVLA T2–12 (Figure 6.9)

- The patient is supine and instructed to cross their arms over their chest; the opposite arm to where the clinician is standing should be the lower arm.

- The clinician rolls the patient towards them to identify the segment that requires manipulation.

- The clinician adapts their hand position so as to make contact with the spinous process below the segment that requires manipulation, while their other hand stabilizes the patient's elbows.

- The patient is instructed to inhale and exhale. As they start to exhale, the clinician rolls the patient over their

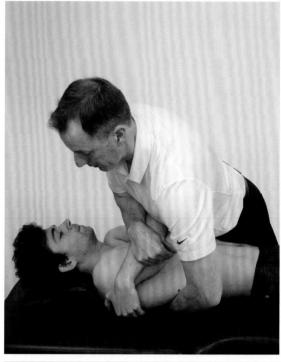

Figure 6.9

applicating hand (the hand delivering the maneuver) and at the same time starts to introduce compression through applying pressure to the patient's elbows.

- At the end of exhalation, maximum compression is achieved and manipulation is delivered in a superior oblique direction, through the patient's shoulders, in line with the angle of the facet joints.

Rib manipulation prone
HVLA ribs 6–10 (Figure 6.10)

- The patient is prone while the clinician is standing. Contact is made at the specific rib angle that requires manipulation.

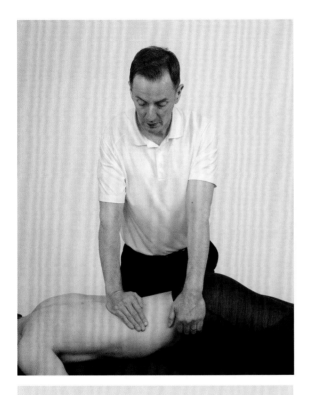

Figure 6.10

- The clinician stabilizes the anterior superior iliac spine (ASIS) with the other hand and instructs the patient to inhale and exhale.

- As the patient exhales, the clinician lifts and rotates the pelvis until the barrier is met.

- The clinician lifts and rotates the ASIS towards them, while simultaneously applying pressure through the specific rib angle.

- Manipulation is delivered by thrusting simultaneously in the direction of the couch, by applying pressure on the rib angle and lifting and rotating the pelvis.

- The set-up position for this technique can be used to perform a MET to treat restrictions in ribs 6–12.

- The clinician stabilizes the ASIS with the other hand and lifts and rotates the pelvis until the barrier is met.

- The patient inhales and pulls their pelvis towards the couch, activating the quadratus lumborum muscle for 2–3 seconds as the clinician applies lateral pressure to the involved rib. This sequence can be repeated 3–5 times.

Rib manipulation supine
HVLA ribs 2–10 (Figure 6.11)

- The patient is supine and instructed to cross their arms over one another.

- The clinician reaches across the patient, contacts the medial border of the scapula and rotates the patient towards them.

- The rib that requires manipulation is identified and contact is made through the thenar eminence of the clinician's hand (in some cases, the fist can be used) (Figure 6.11A).

- The patient is instructed to inhale and exhale; as they exhale, the clinician rolls them over the contact hand (the one delivering manipulation), while simultaneously moving the patient's elbows over the hand that is in contact with the specific rib.

- As compression is built up around the contact hand, the manipulation can be delivered (Figure 6.11B).

MET ribs 6–9 (Figure 6.12)

- The clinician contacts the posterosuperior surface of ribs 6–9.

- The patient inhales, holds their breath and extends the shoulder for 2–3 seconds, activating the serratus anterior muscle.

- The patient relaxes and the clinician stretches caudally on the posterosuperior surface of ribs 6–9. This can be repeated 3–5 times and the patient re-evaluated.

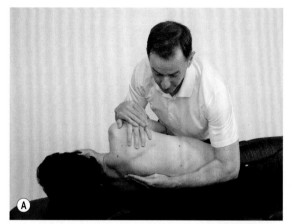

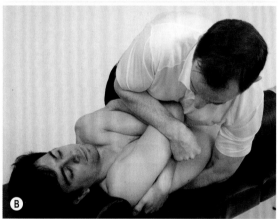

Figure 6.11

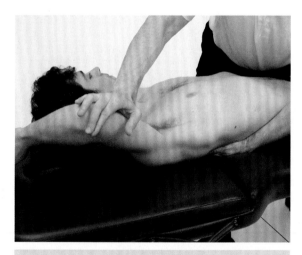

Figure 6.12

STM abdominals, particularly oblique muscles (Figure 6.13AB)

- The patient is supine and the clinician palpates and tests for altered respiratory mechanics, loss of translation and spring through the lower ribcage.

- If one side is identified as having lost ROM, the clinician palpates for trigger points (TrPs) and tender points (TnPs) along the oblique and rectus abdominis muscles.

- Inhibition techniques are used to address restrictions in the abdominal tissues, and the clinician may encourage positional release techniques.

- The clinician crowds (draws together) the tissues into a position where they are most relaxed for the patient's comfort and this position is held for 90 seconds.

- Once the tissue has relaxed, this can be followed with gentle stretching and breathing techniques to normalize rib mechanics and the length–tension relationship within the rectus abdominis/oblique musculature.

STM diaphragm (Figure 6.14)

- The patient is supine and the clinician palpates and tests for altered respiratory mechanics and loss of translation and spring through the lower ribcage.

- If one side is identified as having lost ROM, the clinician palpates for TrPs and TnPs along the diaphragm muscle; this may be more comfortable if the patient has their knees and hips flexed.

- Inhibition techniques are used to address restrictions or dysfunction in the diaphragm; the clinician encourages active inhalation and exhalation to facilitate retraining of the thoracic canister.

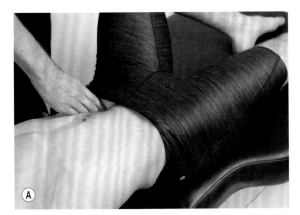

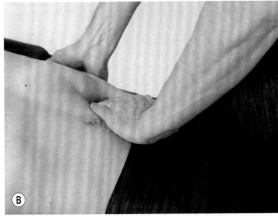

Figure 6.13

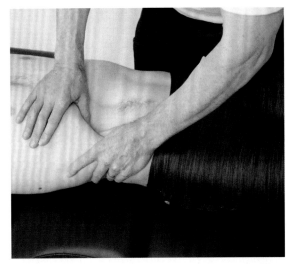

Figure 6.14

Rib manipulation seated
HVLA ribs 3–10 (Figure 6.15)

- The patient is seated and instructed to cross their arms, one on top of the other.

- The clinician makes contact with the inferior elbow and introduces rotation, so the clinician's shoulder is supporting the patient.

- The specific rib angle is located and pisiform contact made, reducing any slack in the soft tissues.

- The elbow is lowered to ensure an inferior to superior angle of drive is achieved.

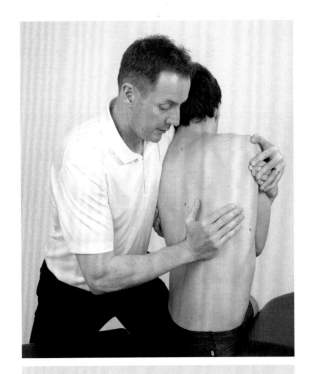

Figure 6.15

- The patient is instructed to inhale and exhale. As they exhale, rotation is introduced away from the side of the rib that is to be manipulated.

- When the barrier has built up, a thrust is delivered obliquely through the rib angle, to manipulate away from the specific segment.

MET ribs 3–10 (Figure 6.16)

- The patient is seated with one hand placed behind their neck.

- The clinician identifies the specific rib angle that requires manipulation and contact is made through application of the thumb or fingers as the clinician controls the patient's elbow simultaneously with their other hand.

- The clinician maintains posterolateral pressure on the rib angle and, depending on the restriction,

instructs the patient to pull their elbow laterally, medially, superiorly or inferiorly.

- Three to five repetitions of 3–5 muscle contractions are made to restore function and then the patient is re-evaluated.

Lumbar spine techniques
HVLA side-lying (thoracolumbar junction) (Figure 6.17)

- The patient is side-lying with their symptomatic side up; the bottom leg is straight and the top leg is bent at the knee, with the foot placed behind the popliteal fossa.

- The clinician places their upper arm between the patient's upper arm and body to make contact with the T12 spinous process.

- The clinician's other hand contacts the spinous process of L1, with the forearm placed in the gluteal crease of the pelvis.

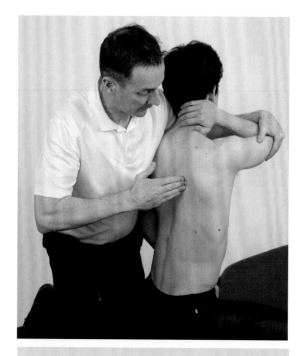

Figure 6.16

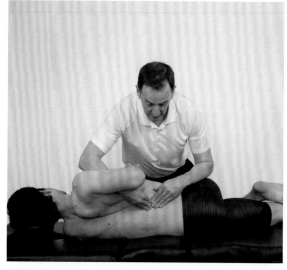

Figure 6.17

- The patient is instructed to inhale and exhale. At the end of exhalation, the clinician engages the barrier by introducing compression and rotation forces through the ribs and pelvic girdle.

- When the barrier is met, a thrust is delivered to manipulate the segment.

HVLA side-lying (L2 to L5–S1) (Figure 6.18)

- The patient is side-lying with their symptomatic side up; the bottom leg is straight and the top leg is bent at the knee, with the foot placed behind or below the popliteal fossa.

- The clinician places their upper arm between the patient's upper arm and body, while the clinician's forearm is placed in the gluteal crease of the pelvis, introducing a rotational component.

- The specific segment to be manipulated is identified.

- The patient is instructed to inhale and exhale. At the end of exhalation, the clinician engages the barrier and a thrust is delivered to manipulate the segment.

HVLA side-lying (leg-off-table modification) (Figure 6.19)

- The set-up and manipulation are delivered similarly to those described above, but instead of placing the patient's top leg behind the popliteal fossa, the leg is encouraged to drop off the couch.

- The clinician can further modify this technique by placing the patient's leg between their own legs and introducing traction by dropping their body weight to deliver the thrust; this is particularly useful for restricted segments.

- This technique can be modified and used for lumbar mobilization; it may also be combined with a neural dynamic technique.

- Some patients may not be able to flex their upper knee, due to hip or knee joint osteoarthritis, hip or knee joint replacements, flaccid or spastic paralysis in the lower extremity, or amputation.

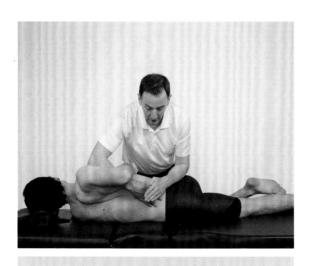

Figure 6.18

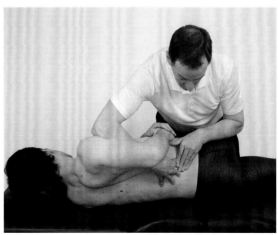

Figure 6.19

STM quadratus lumborum and lateral sling (Figure 6.20)

- The patient is side-lying; the upper leg is off the couch and the upper arm is holding onto the head of the couch. A pillow may be placed under the trunk to facilitate lateral flexion.

- Through palpation, the clinician evaluates the lateral line to determine the region of greatest myofascial tension.

- Once the region of tension has been identified, STM can be performed, while the patient is encouraged to breathe and stretch their upper arm and leg in opposite directions as the clinician releases the soft tissue tension.

- This technique can be adapted into a MET and used to address dysfunction and restrictions in the following muscles: tensor fasciae latae (TFL), lateral gluteals, quadratus lumborum, lumbar erector spinae, thoracolumbar fascia and latissimus dorsi.

MET quadratus lumborum (Figure 6.21)

- The patient is side-lying, with the lower leg held at the knee to stabilize the pelvis and the upper leg off the couch.

- The clinician straddles the patient's upper leg and grasps the iliac crest until a barrier is introduced by the clinician applying pressure to the ilium.

- Contraction occurs in quadratus lumborum as the patient pushes against the clinician's resistance for 3–5 seconds.

- Stretch is induced as the patient relaxes and the clinician stretches into the new barrier; this action can be repeated a further 3–5 times. A greater stretch may be achieved if the patient stretches the upper arm above the head.

MET erector spinae – flexion (Figure 6.22)

- The patient is seated with their back to the clinician, legs hanging over the couch and arms hanging down between their legs.

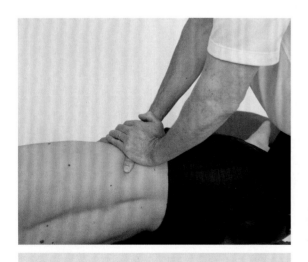

Figure 6.20

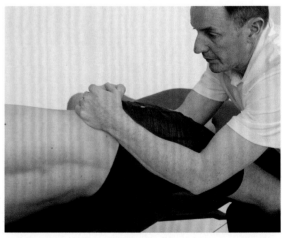

Figure 6.21

- The clinician places one hand on the patient's shoulder girdle and the other hand stabilizes the patient's lumbosacral spine.

- Contraction occurs when the patient actively extends towards an upright position, against resistance from the clinician.

- Inhalation and holding the breath for 7–10 seconds may be encouraged during the contraction phase.

- The patient relaxes and exhales, and the new barrier is met. After the final barrier is achieved, the patient may contract further, against the clinician and towards the restriction barrier, while inhaling and holding the breath for 7–10 seconds, to encourage antagonist muscular contraction.

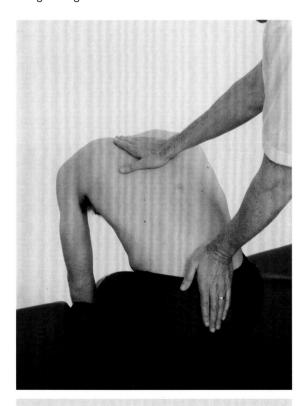

Figure 6.22

- This technique can be adapted to become an active release technique.

Pelvic girdle techniques
HVLA innominate prone (Figure 6.23)

- The patient is prone on the couch with the clinician standing at their right side.

- The clinician supports the patient's left knee and places the other hand on the left iliac crest, just above the posterior superior iliac spine (PSIS).

- The clinician raises the patient's leg and introduces adduction to build up the barrier, while simultaneously applying pressure on the iliac crest.

- The patient is instructed to inhale and exhale. As they exhale, a manipulation is delivered to the innominate by applying a thrust through the PSIS.

HVLA innominate supine (Chicago) (Figure 6.24)

- The patient is supine and the clinician places the patient's upper and lower body in a right side-lying position, to loose-pack the ilia.

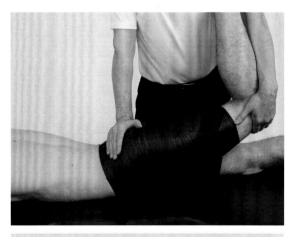

Figure 6.23

- The clinician places their right hand between the patient's arm and chest and introduces rotation, until the barrier is engaged, while stabilizing the patient's right ilium with their left hand.

- The patient is instructed to inhale and exhale. As they exhale, pressure is applied simultaneously through the ASIS and by rotation of the patient's upper body.

- As pressure is increased, a manipulation is delivered through the ASIS.

HVLA innominate side-lying (Figure 6.25)

- This technique is used to manipulate the innominate in a *posterior* direction.

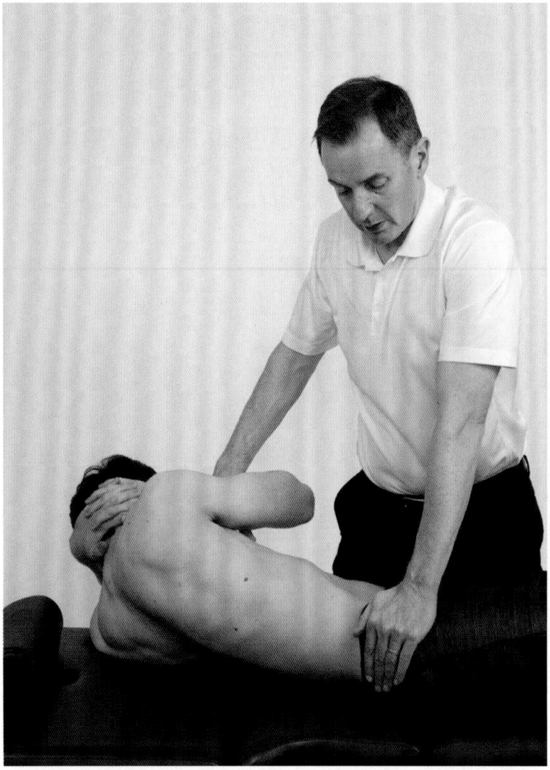

- The patient is side-lying, symptomatic side facing upwards, and instructed to straighten the bottom leg; the top leg is bent at the knee, with the foot placed in the popliteal fossa.

- The clinician places their hand through the patient's elbow or upper arm and increases pressure to stabilize the patient's upper body.

- The clinician's other hand contacts the ischial tuberosity and the patient is instructed to inhale and exhale, while the barrier is engaged by the clinician and rotation and compression are introduced.

- A thrust is delivered through the heel of the clinician's hand, to manipulate the innominate in a *posterior* direction.

HVLA innominate side-lying (Figure 6.26)

- This technique is used to manipulate the innominate in an *anterior* direction.

- The patient is side-lying, symptomatic side facing upwards, and instructed to straighten the bottom leg; the top leg is bent at the knee with the foot placed in the popliteal fossa.

Figure 6.24

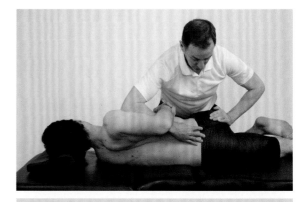

Figure 6.25

- The clinician places their hand through the patient's elbow or upper arm and increases pressure to stabilize the patient's upper body.

- The clinician's other hand contacts the PSIS, and the patient is instructed to inhale and exhale, while the barrier is engaged by the clinician and rotation and compression are introduced.

- A thrust is delivered through the heel of the clinician's hand, to manipulate the innominate in an *anterior* direction.

HVLA sacroiliac joint (SIJ) supine (Figure 6.27)

- The patient is supine and the clinician interlocks their hands around the patient's ankle on the symptomatic side.

- The clinician introduces flexion, adduction and internal rotation motion to close-pack the SIJ.

- The patient is instructed to inhale and exhale. On exhalation, a thrust is delivered caudally to manipulate the innominate.

- This technique can also be used for manipulation of the lumbosacral joint.

MET SIJ prone (Figure 6.28)

- The patient is prone on the couch with the clinician standing at their right side.

- The clinician supports the patient's left knee and places the other hand on the left iliac crest, just above the PSIS.

- The clinician raises the patient's leg to build up the barrier and simultaneously applies pressure on the iliac crest. Contraction occurs as the patient pulls the leg towards the couch, against the clinician's resistance, for 3–5 seconds.

- The patient relaxes and the clinician takes up tension to the new barrier. This can be repeated 3–5 times and the patient re-evaluated.

MET SIJ supine (Figure 6.29)

- The patient is supine and the clinician places the patient's upper and lower body in a right side-lying position, to loose-pack the ilia.

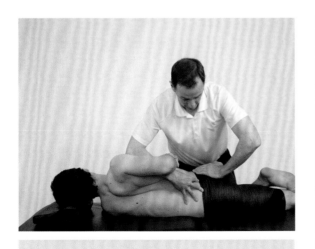

Figure 6.26

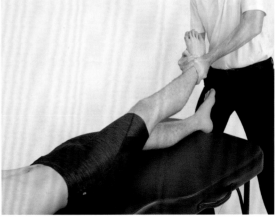

Figure 6.27

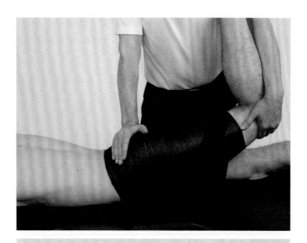

Figure 6.28

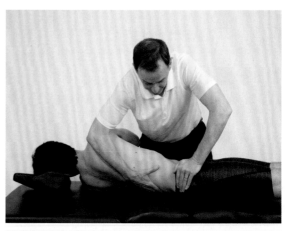

Figure 6.29

- The clinician places their right hand behind patient's torso and introduces rotation until the barrier is engaged, while stabilizing the patient's right ilium with their left hand.

- Contraction occurs as the patient rotates the upper body into right rotation, against the resistance of the clinician.

- As the patient relaxes, the clinician takes up the new position of bind (until the new barrier is reached), by rotating the right innominate posteriorly.

MET innominate posterior in side lying (Figure 6.30)

- The patient is in side-lying position on the couch, with the dysfunctional side up. The clinician is standing, facing the patient.

- The patient's bottom leg is straightened and the top leg is flexed to 90° and stabilized against the clinician's hip.

- The clinician's left hand palpates the right SIJ and controls the patient's right knee; adduction,

abduction and internal and external rotation are introduced, with flexion, to the barrier point.

- Contraction of the target muscle is achieved by the patient flexing their right leg against the clinician's resistance for 3–5 seconds.

- The patient relaxes and the clinician takes up the new barrier. This can be repeated 3–5 times and the patient re-evaluated.

MET innominate anterior in side-lying (Figure 6.31)

- The patient is in a side-lying position on the couch with the dysfunctional side up. The clinician is standing, facing the patient.

- The patient's bottom leg is straightened and the top leg is flexed to 90° and stabilized against the clinician's hip.

- The clinician's right hand palpates the right SIJ and controls the patient's right knee; adduction, abduction and internal and external rotation are introduced, with flexion, until the barrier is met.

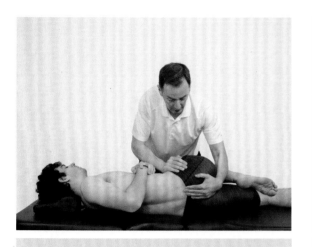

Figure 6.30

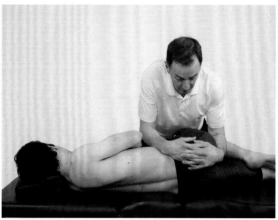

Figure 6.31

- Contraction of the target muscle is achieved by the patient straightening the right leg against the clinician's resistance for 3–5 seconds.

- The patient relaxes and the clinician takes up the new barrier. This can be repeated 3–5 times and the patient re-evaluated.

MET symphysis pubis (Figure 6.32)

- The patient is supine with the knees bent and the feet placed flat on the couch.

- The clinician places their hands around the patient's knees, offers resistance, and instructs the patient to push their knees apart for 3–5 seconds, to create an isometric contraction of the hip abductors.

- The clinician then changes hand position and resists the patient squeezing their knees together for 3–5 seconds, creating an isometric contraction of the adductor muscles.

- This process is repeated 3–5 times and the patient re-evaluated.

- Using this technique, a joint cavitation may occur in the symphysis pubis without having to use any unnecessary force.

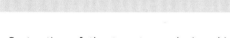 **Hip joint techniques**
HVLA hip joint supine (Figure 6.33)

- The patient is supine and the clinician interlocks their fingers around the ankle of the patient's symptomatic hip.

- The clinician introduces flexion, adduction and internal rotation to close-pack the hip joint.

- The patient is instructed to inhale and exhale. On exhalation, a caudal thrust is applied to manipulate the hip joint.

HVLA hip joint prone (Figure 6.34)

- The patient is prone as the clinician contacts the posterior aspect of the distal femur with one hand and takes hold of the anterior thigh with the other hand.

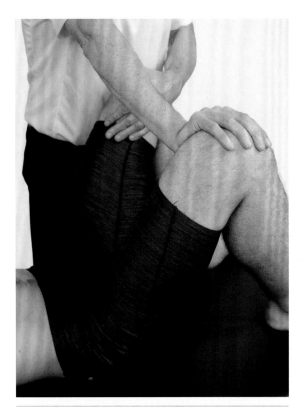

Figure 6.32

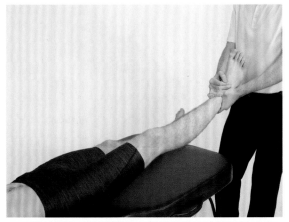

Figure 6.33

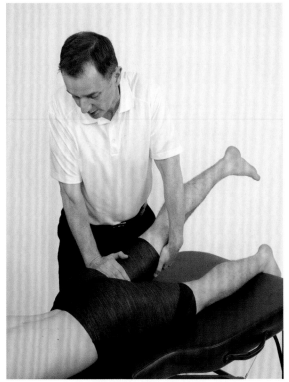

Figure 6.34

- The hip is taken passively into extension, with internal and external rotation, and adduction and abduction, being introduced to find the barrier.

- The patient is instructed to inhale and exhale. On exhalation, the clinician introduces a thrust to perform an anterior manipulation of the hip joint.

- This technique can be extremely useful for reducing tension in the anterior hip capsule.

Anterior hip capsule stretch (Figure 6.35)

- The patient is prone and the clinician takes control of the leg, increasing knee flexion and hip abduction.

- The clinician stabilizes the greater trochanter with one hand and the other hand is placed on the ankle.

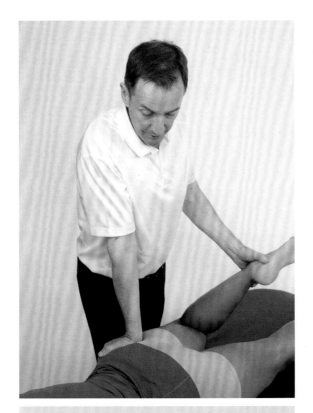

Figure 6.35

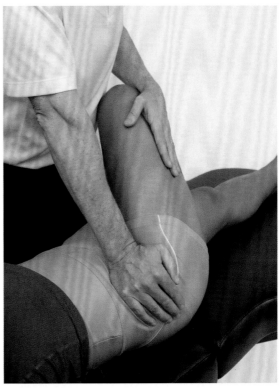

Figure 6.36

- Passive external hip rotation motion is encouraged to the barrier, in an attempt to help stretch or mobilize the anterior hip capsule.

Posterior hip capsule stretch (Figure 6.36)

- The patient is supine; the clinician reaches across the patient and takes control of the leg, increasing the patient's degree of knee joint flexion by placing one leg over the other.

- The clinician stabilizes the pelvic girdle and passive hip internal rotation and adduction are encouraged to the barrier, in an attempt to stretch or mobilize the posterior hip capsule.

STM tensor fasciae latae (TFL)/iliotibial band (ITB) (Figure 6.37)

- The patient is side-lying, problematic leg uppermost, with the knee resting on a prop.

- The clinician uses SMT to release the myofascial tension in the TFL/ITB; this can be adapted to encourage an active release technique, to facilitate active hip extension and abduction.

- Similarly, this technique may be adapted as a MET or neural dynamic technique.

197

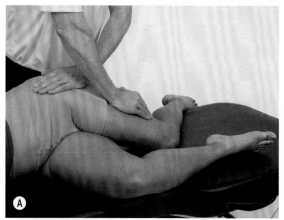

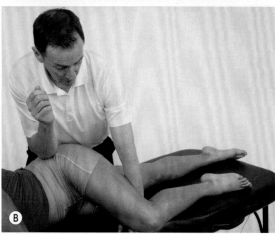

Figure 6.37

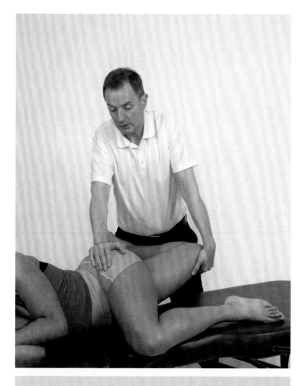

Figure 6.38

MET TFL/ITB (Figure 6.38)

- The patient is side-lying, upper leg flexed to 90° and lower leg straight.

- The clinician supports the lower leg and engages the barrier.

- Contraction occurs when the patient abducts their hip against the clinician's resistance.

- The clinician passively adducts the leg by moving it upwards while stabilizing the pelvis, introducing a stretch to the adductors.

STM deep hip external rotators (Figure 6.39)

- The patient is side-lying, problematic leg uppermost, resting the knee on the couch.

- The clinician uses palpation to identify the restriction within the myofascial tissue and uses SMT to restore appropriate length–tension within this structure.

- This can be adapted to become an active release or MET technique.

MET deep hip external rotators (Figure 6.40)

- The patient lies supine, leg flexed at the knee and crossed over the other leg.

- The clinician engages the barrier by stabilizing the opposite hip.

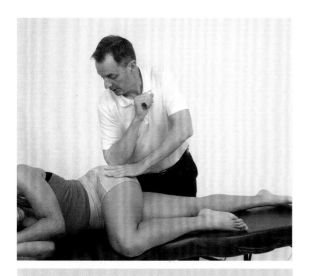

Figure 6.39

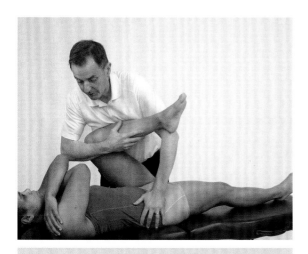

Figure 6.40

- Contraction is brought about by the patient pushing the flexed knee against the clinician's resistance.

- Stretch is introduced to the deep posterior hip region as the clinician pushes the flexed knee across the patient's body.

STM obturator membrane (Figure 6.41)

- This technique is extremely useful for helping to facilitate hip joint internal rotation, and to help relax the adductor tissues prior to applying STM or MET techniques in this region.

- The patient is supine with the knee and hip flexed; the clinician palpates inside the obturator membrane for TrPs or TnPs, and an inhibition technique (direct pressure) is held for approximately 90 seconds, or until relaxation is palpated in the obturator membrane.

- As the tissues relax, the patient is encouraged to actively relax their leg, allowing it to slide down the bed until straight.

- This technique can be combined simultaneously with STM to release the iliacus muscle.

STM adductors in supine (Figure 6.42)

- This technique can be performed in supine or side-lying.

- In supine the patient is relaxed, with the problematic leg resting on the clinician's thigh or on a prop.

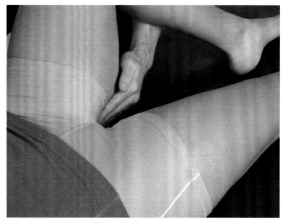

Figure 6.41

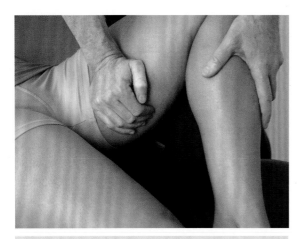

Figure 6.42

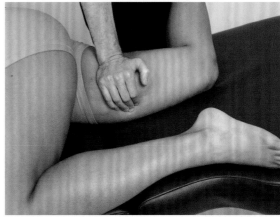

Figure 6.43

- In side lying (Figure 6.43) the lower (problematic) leg is positioned straight and the upper leg is crossed over it, exposing the adductors.

- The adductor muscles are palpated and the clinician pays specific attention to any myofascial tension identified within the adductor musculature.

- STM may include inhibition or combined active release techniques, to restore the length–tension relationships within the adductor musculature.

MET adductors (Figure 6.44)

- The patient lies supine and the clinician passively abducts the leg to be treated until the barrier is met.

- Contraction is brought about by the patient adducting against the clinician's resistance. Stretch is introduced to the adductors as the clinician passively moves the patient's leg further into abduction.

- If the abducted leg is flexed at the knee, the short adductors (pectineus and adductors brevis, longus and magnus) are targeted.

STM iliacus (Figure 6.45)

- The patient is supine, knee and hip joint flexed on the problematic side.

- The clinician begins to palpate from the iliac crest, moving medially and easing the ascending/descending colon out of the way, until a TrP or TnP is palpated.

- Inhibition techniques are applied for approximately 90 seconds or until relaxation occurs within the tissues.

- If this is too uncomfortable, a positional release technique may be used to dampen down the symptoms and relax the tissue further.

- Once relaxation has occurred within the tissue, the patient is instructed to slide the leg straight, encouraging lengthening and relaxation of the muscle tissue.

MET iliacus (Figure 6.46)

- The patient is in an adapted Thomas test position over the end of a couch.

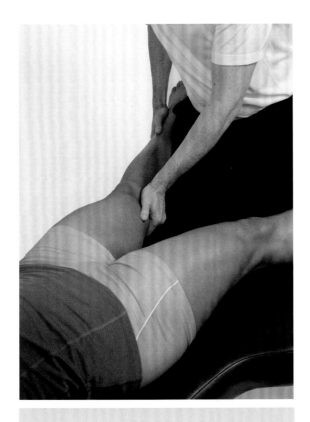

Figure 6.44

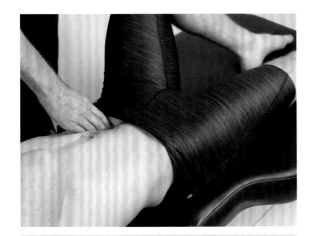

Figure 6.45

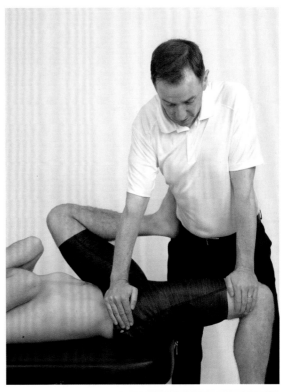

Figure 6.46

- The clinician stabilizes the patient's innominate on the side to be treated. Contraction is brought about by the patient actively flexing their hip against the clinician's resistance.

- The clinician moves the thigh further into passive hip extension while stabilizing the patient's innominate, to introduce stretch to the iliacus.

MET psoas and rectus femoris (Figure 6.47)

- The patient is in an adapted Thomas test position over the end of a couch.

- Contraction is introduced (brought about) by the patient actively flexing the hip against the clinician's resistance.

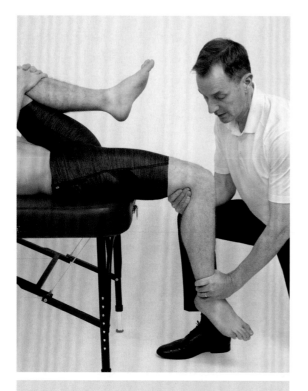

Figure 6.47

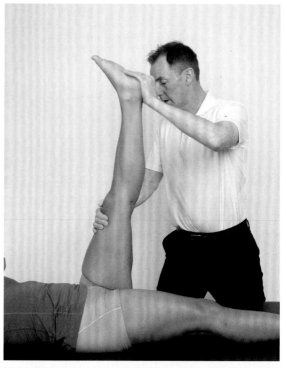

Figure 6.48

- The clinician moves the thigh further into passive hip extension while stabilizing the patient's pelvis, to introduce a stretch to the psoas.

- Rectus femoris contraction is introduced by the patient actively extending their knee against the clinician's resistance.

- The clinician moves the knee further into passive flexion, to induce a stretch in rectus femoris.

MET hamstrings (Figure 6.48)

- The patient lies supine, with the leg to be treated flexed at the hip and supported by the clinician.

- The barrier is engaged and contraction is introduced by the patient extending their leg against the clinician's resistance.

- Resistance can be performed either in a straight leg or in a laterally/medially rotated leg, according to which hamstring fibers are to be treated.

- Taking the leg further into hip flexion induces a greater stretch in the hamstrings.

- Introducing hip joint internal or external rotation will put more emphasis on the biceps femoris and medial hamstrings, respectively.

- This technique can be combined with a neural mobilization.

Neural dynamic techniques
Sciatic nerve straight leg raise (SLR) *(Figure 6.49)*

- The patient is supine and the clinician introduces ankle dorsiflexion and SLR with one hand, while stabilizing and monitoring knee extension with the other hand.

- Sensitizing movements of the ankle (inversion/eversion/plantar flexion) may be introduced. Similarly, the sensitizing movements of hip adduction/internal rotation may be introduced.

- To perform a sliding technique, the SLR is slowly taken to the barrier and the patient is instructed to perform

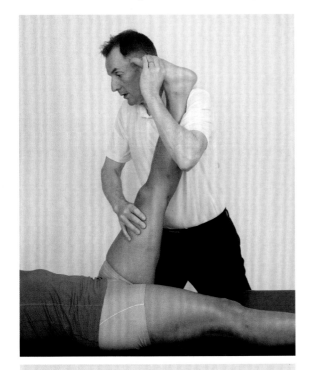

Figure 6.49

neck flexion; at this point, the SLR is released from the barrier. The clinician observes for any change in symptoms.

- A neural dynamic slider is performed, combining neck flexion/extension with hip flexion/extension, as 2–3 sets of 10–15 repetitions, and then the patient is re-evaluated.

- Common problems experienced in applying this technique may be caused by allowing the knee joint to flex and/or failing to control frontal and transverse plane hip motion, which can all affect the sensitizing components.

Femoral nerve (Figure 6.50)

- The patient is in slump side-lying, holding the lower leg just below the knee in hip flexion, and is instructed to perform cervical flexion.

- The patient extends the upper leg into hip extension, and the clinician supports the thigh and encourages knee flexion.

- The clinician increases the hip extension and knee flexion components, until tension in the anterior thigh is reported. The patient performs cervical extension and any change in tension in the anterior thigh is noted. At this point, the thigh is taken off tension by introducing knee extension and any change in symptoms is observed.

- A neural slider technique is performed, combining neck flexion/extension alternately with knee flexion/extension, for 2–3 sets of 10–15 repetitions, and then the patient is re-evaluated.

- Hip joint lateral and medial rotation can be introduced with this neural dynamic technique to bias the ilioinguinal and iliohypogastric nerves.

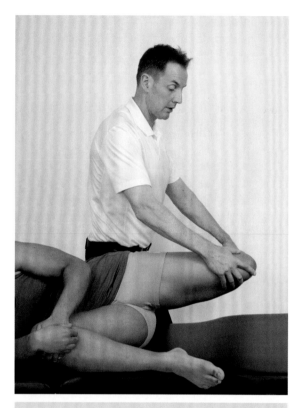

Figure 6.50

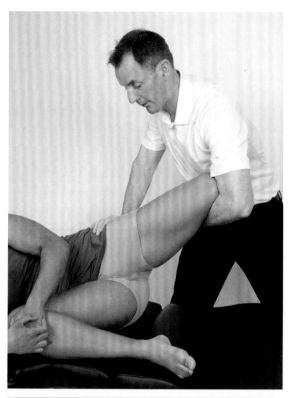

Figure 6.51

Obturator nerve (Figure 6.51)

- The clinician tests the obturator nerve in the slump side-lying position, as described previously for the femoral nerve test.

- Hip abduction is introduced to test the neurogenic components which affect (innervate) the groin and medial knee.

- The clinician increases the hip extension, knee flexion and hip abduction components until tension in the anterior thigh and groin is reported. The patient performs cervical extension and any change in tension in the anterior thigh and groin is noted. At this point, the thigh is taken off tension by introducing hip adduction and any change in symptoms observed.

- A neural dynamic slider technique is performed, combining neck flexion/extension alternately with hip abduction/adduction for 2–3 sets of 10–15 repetitions, and then the patient is re-evaluated.

Common mistakes with manual therapy

- Too much manual therapy may encourage patients to become dependent on passive care. This is not a fault with manual therapy but more an issue of perception or expectation.

- Too much deep soft tissue manipulation offers nothing more than desensitization of the area from an afferent barrage (Maigne and Vautravers, 2003), leaving patients sore, tender and bruised after treatment (Cambron et al., 2007).

- Too much stretching may have an adverse impact on the quality of tissue tone; it may reduce muscle stiffness and impair motor control, producing aberrant movement patterns (McHugh and Cosgrave, 2010).

Conclusion

As previously described, manipulation is often synonymous with musculoskeletal treatment. There are many ways in which "touch" and "hands on" can be used to deliver treatment. It was the intention in this chapter to highlight examples of manipulation (joint and soft tissue) for the spino-pelvic-hip complex that can be administered safely to ensure successful treatment outcomes. There are no "silver bullets" for managing patients with musculoskeletal pain or injuries, and manipulation may be used effectively to provide short-term pain relief (2–4 treatments), to allow patients to progress to a more active recovery.

In my opinion, manipulation, assuming good technique (*manipulATE*) and sound assessment (*evaluATE*), positions itself well within my "five 'ATEs" framework. Furthermore, having the knowledge and an understanding of this framework will help clinicians to become more flexible and to integrate the principles of biomedical and bio-psychosocial healthcare models into an elite sporting environment. For patients, having a clearer understanding of the benefits of manipulation and where it sits within my "five 'ATEs" framework will help to reassure and *educATE*, which can only serve to offer a more successful multi-modal approach to patient care.

References

Alwaily, M., Timko, M., Schneider, M. et al., 2016. Treatment-based classification system for low back pain: revision and update. *Physical Therapy*, 96(7), pp. 1057–1066.

Best, T., Gharaibeh, B. and Huard, J., 2013. Stem cells angiogenesis and muscle healing: a potential role in massage therapies? *British Journal Sports Medicine*, 47, pp. 556–560.

Brennan, PC., 1995. Review of the systemic effects of spinal manipulation. In: Gatterman, MI. (ed.), *Foundations of Chiropractic Subluxation*. St Louis: Mosby/Elsevier.

Butler, D., 2010. *The Neurodynamic Techniques*. Melbourne: Noigroup Publications.

Cagnie, B., Vinck, E., Beernaert, A. et al., 2004. How common are side effects of spinal manipulation and can these be predicted? *Manual Therapy*, 9 (3), pp. 151–156.

Cambron, JA., Dexheimer, J., Coe, P. et al., 2007. Side effects of massage therapy: a cross-sectional study of 100 clients. *Journal Alternative Complementary Medicine*, 13(8), pp. 793–796.

Childs, J., Flynn, T., Fritz, J. et al., 2005. Screening for vertebrobasilar insufficiency in patients with neck pain: manual therapy decision-making in the presence of uncertainty. *Journal Orthopaedic Sports Physical Therapy*, 35(5), pp. 300–306.

Collins, CK., Masaracchio, M., Brismee, J-M. and 2017. The future of orthopaedic manual therapy: what are we missing? *Journal Manual Manipulative Therapy*, 25(4), pp. 169–171.

Cook, C., 2021. The demonization of manual therapy. *MSK – Muskuloskelettale Physiotherapie*, 25, pp. 125–132.

Ernst, E., 2007. Adverse effects of spinal manipulation: a systemic review. *Journal Royal Society Medicine*, 100(7), pp. 330–338.

Evans, D. and Breen, A., 2006. A biomechanical model for mechanically efficient cavitation production during spinal manipulation: prethrust position and the neutral zone. *Journal Manipulative and Physiological Therapeutics*, 29(1), pp. 71–82.

Evans, D., and Lucas, N., 2010. What is "manipulation"? A reappraisal. *Manual Therapy*, 15(3), pp. 286–291.

Ferber, R., Osternig, LR., Gravelle, DC., 2002. Effect of PNF stretch techniques on knee flexor muscle EMG activity in older adults. *Journal Electromyography Kinesiology*, 12, pp. 391–397.

Fletcher, IM., 2010. The effects of precompetition massage on the kinematic parameters of 20-m sprint performance. *Journal Strength Conditioning Research*, 24(5), pp. 1179–1183.

Fryer, G., 2006. Chapter 4: Muscle energy technique: research and efficacy. In: Chaitow, L. (ed.), *Muscle Energy Techniques*. 3rd ed. Edinburgh: Churchill Livingstone/Elsevier, pp. 109–132.

Fryer, G., 2011. Muscle energy technique: an evidence-informed approach. *International Journal Osteopathic Medicine*, 14(1), pp. 3–9.

Fryer, G. and Fossum, C., 2010. Therapeutic mechanisms underlying muscle energy approaches. In: Fernández-de-las-Peñas, C., Arendt-Nielsen, L. and Gerwin, RD. (eds),

Tension-type and Cervicogenic Headache: Pathophysiology, Diagnosis, and Management. Sudbury, MA: Jones and Bartlett, pp. 221–229.

Gehlsen, GM., Ganion, LR., Helfst, R. 1999. Fibroblast responses to variation in soft tissue mobilization pressure. *Medicine Science Sports Exercise*, 31, pp. 531–535.

Gibbons, P. and Tehan, P., 2001. Patient positioning and spinal locking for lumbar spine rotation manipulation. *Manual Therapy*, 6(3), pp. 130–138.

Gibbons, P. and Tehan, P., 2004. *Manipulation von Wirbelsäule, Thorax and Becken.* Munich: Urban & Fischer/Elsevier.

Gifford, L., 1998. Pain, the tissues and the nervous system: a conceptual model. *Physiotherapy*, 84(1), pp. 27–36.

Goodwin, JE., Glaister, M., Howatson, G. et al., 2007. Effect or pre-performance lower-limb massage on thirty-meter sprint running. *Journal Strength Conditioning Research*, 21(4), pp. 1028–1031.

Gouveia, L., Castonho, P. and Ferreira, J., 2009. Safety of chiropractic interventions: a systemic review. *Spine*, 34(11), pp. E405–E413.

Grip, H., Sundelin, G., Gerdle, B. et al., 2007. Variations in the axis of motion during head repositioning – a comparison of subjects with whiplash-associated disorders or non-specific neck pain and healthy controls. *Clinical Biomechanics*, 22(8), pp. 865–873.

Gyer, G., Michael, J. and Davis, R., 2017. *Osteopathic and Chiropractic Techniques for Manual Therapists: A Comprehensive Guide to Spinal and Peripheral Manipulations.* London: Singing Dragon.

Havas, E., Parviainen, T., Vuorela, J. et al., 1997. Lymph flow dynamics in exercising human skeletal muscle as detected by scintigraphy. *Journal Physiology*, 504, pp. 233–239.

Huang, C., Holfeld, J., Schaden, W. et al., 2013. Mechanotherapy: revisiting physical therapy and recruiting mechanobiology for a new era in medicine. *Trends Molecular Medicine*, 10, pp. 555–564.

Iwatsuki, H., Ikuta, Y. and Shinoda, K., 2001. Deep friction massage on the masticatory muscles in stroke patients increases biting force. *Journal Physical Therapy Science*, 13, pp. 17–20.

Kandel, ER., Schwartz, JH. and Jessell, TM., 2000. *Principles of Neural Science.* 4th ed. London: McGraw-Hill.

Khan, KM. and Scott, A., 2009. Mechanotherapy: how physical therapists' prescription of exercise promotes tissue repair. *British Journal Sports Medicine*, 43, pp. 247–252.

Kivlan, BR., Carcia, CR., Clemente, FR. et al., 2015. The effect of Astym(R) therapy on muscle strength: a blinded, randomized, clinically controlled trial. *BMC Musculoskeletal Disorders*, 16, p. 325.

Kolb, WH., McDevitt, AW., Young, J. et al., 2020. The evolution of manual therapy education, what are we waiting for? *Journal Manual Manipulative Therapy*, 28(1), pp. 1–3.

Langevin, HM., Cornbrooks, CJ. and Taatjes, DJ., 2004. Fibroblasts form a body-wide cellular network. *Histochemistry Cell Biology*, 122(1), pp. 7–15.

Langevin, HM., Bouffard, NA., Badger, GJ. et al., 2005. Dynamic fibroblast cytoskeletal response to subcutaneous tissue stretch ex vivo and in vivo. *American Journal Physiology-Cell Physiology*, 288(3), pp. C747–756.

Laslett, M., McDonald, B., Aprill, C. et al., 2006. Clinical predictors of screening zygapophyseal joint blocks: development of clinical prediction rules. *Spine Journal*, 6, pp. 370–379.

Lederman, E. 1997. Overview and clinical application. In: *Fundamentals of Manual Therapy.* London: Churchill Livingstone, pp. 213–20.

Lederman, E., 2005. *The Science and Practice of Manual Therapy.* 2nd ed. Edinburgh: Churchill Livingstone/Elsevier.

Lee, HY., Wang, JD., Yao, G. et al., 2008. Association between cervicocephalic kinesthetic sensibility and frequency of subclinical neck pain. *Manual Therapy*, 13(5), pp. 419–425.

Lewis, J., 2009. Rotator cuff tendinopathy/subacromial impingement syndrome: is it time for a new method of assessment? *British Journal Sports Medicine*, 43, pp. 259–264.

Li, J. and Mitchell, JH., 2003. Glutamate release in midbrain periaqueductal gray by activation of skeletal muscle receptors and arterial baroreceptors. *Am J Physiol Heart Circ Physiol*, 285(1), pp. H.137–144.

Liem, T. and Dobler, T., 2014. *Leitfaden Osteopathic: Parietale Techniken.* Jena: Urban & Fischer/Elsevier.

Lin, I., Wiles, L., Waller, R. et al., 2020. What does best practice for musculoskeletal pain look like? Eleven consistent recommendations from high-quality clinical guidelines: systematic review. *British Journal Sports Medicine*, 54, pp. 79–86.

Loghmani, MT. and Whitted, M., 2016. Soft tissue manipulation: a powerful form of mechanotherapy. *Physiotherapy Rehabilitation*, 1: 122. DOI:10.4172/2573-0312.1000122.

Magarey, M., Rebbeck, T., Coughlan, B. et al., 2004. Pre-manipulative testing of the cervical spine review, revision and new clinical guidelines. *Manual Therapy*, 9(2), pp. 95–108.

Magee, D., 2014. *Orthopaedic Physical Assessment.* 5th ed. Philadelphia: W.B. Saunders.

Maigne, J. and Guillon, F., 2000. Highlighting of intervertebral movements and variations of intradiskal pressure during lumbar manipulation: a feasibility study. *Journal of Manipulative and Physiological Therapeutics*, 23(8), pp. 531–535.

Maigne, R. and Nieves, W., 2005. *Diagnosis and Treatment of Pain of Vertebral origin.* Vol. 1. Boca Raton, FL: Taylor & Francis.

Maigne, J. and Vautravers, P., 2003. Mechanism of action of spinal manipulative therapy. *Joint Bone Spine*, 70(5), pp. 336–341.

Majlesi, J., Togay, H., Ünalan, H. et al., 2008. The sensitivity and specificity of the slump and straight leg raise tests in patients with lumbar disc herniation. *Journal Clinical Rheumatology*, 14(2), pp. 87–91.

Martino, F., Perestrelo, AR., Vinarský, V. et al., 2018. Cellular mechanotransduction: from tension to function. *Frontiers in Physiology,* 9, p. 824. Available at: <https://doi.org/10.3389/fphys.2018.00824> [accessed February 17, 2022].

McHugh, MP. and Cosgrave, CH., 2010. To stretch or not to stretch: the role of stretching in injury prevention and performance. *Scandinavian Journal Medicine Science Sports*, 20(2), pp. 169–181.

Melzack, R. and Wall, P., 1965. Pain mechanisms: a new theory. *Science*, 150(3699), pp. 971–979.

Moran, RN., Hauth, JM. and Rabena, R., 2018. The effect of massage on acceleration and sprint performance in track and field athletes. *Complementary Therapy Clinical Practice*, 30, pp. 1–5.

Okamato, T., Masuhara, M. and Ikuta, K., 2014. Acute effects of self-myofascial release using a foam roller on arterial function. *Journal Strength and Conditioning*, 28, pp. 69–73.

Oliphant, D., 2004. Safety of spinal manipulation in the treatment of lumbar disk herniations: a systematic review and risk assessment. *Journal Manipulative Physiological Therapeutics,* 27(3), pp. 197–210.

Oostendorp, R., 2018. Credibility of manual therapy is at stake. "Where do we go from here?" *Journal Manual Manipulative Therapy*, 26(4), pp. 189–192.

Osternig, LR., Robertson, R., Troxel, RK. et al., 1987. Muscle activation during proprioceptive neuromuscular facilitation (PNF) stretching techniques. *American Journal Physical Medicine*, 66(5), pp. 298–307.

Paungmali, A., O'Leary, S., Souvlis, T. et al., 2004. Naloxone fails to antagonize initial hypoalgesic effect of a manual therapy treatment for lateral epicondylalgia. *Journal Manipulative Physiological Therapy*, 27(3), pp. 180–185.

Portillo-Soto, A., Eberman, L., Demchak, T. et al., 2014. Comparison of blood flow changes with soft tissue mobilization and massage therapy. *Alternative Complementary Medicine*, 20, pp. 932–936.

Potter, L., McCarthy, C. and Oldham, J., 2005. Physiological effects of spinal manipulation: a review of proposed theories. *Physical Therapy Reviews*, 3, pp. 163–170.

Puentedura, E., March, J., Anders, J. et al., 2012. Safety of cervical spine manipulation: are adverse events preventable and are manipulations being performed appropriately? A review of 134 case reports. *Journal of Manual Manipulative Therapy*, 20(2), pp. 66–74.

Refshauge, K., Parry, S., Shirley, D. et al., 2002. Professional responsibility in relation to cervical manipulation. *Australian Journal Physiotherapy*, 48(3), pp. 171–179.

Reynolds, DV., 1969. Surgery in the rat during electrical analgesia induced by focal brain stimulation. *Science*, 25, 164(3878), pp. 444–445.

Rivett, D., Thomas, L. and Bolton, B., 2005. Pre-manipulative testing: where do we go from here? *New Zealand Journal Physiotherapy*, 33(23), pp. 78–84.

Satpute, A., Wager, T., Cohen-Adad, J. et al., 2013. Identification of discrete functional subregions of the human periaqueductal gray. *Proceedings National Academy Sciences*, 110(42), pp. 17101–17106.

Schillinger, A., Koenig, D., Haefele, C. et al., 2006. Effect of manual lymph drainage on the course of serum levels of muscle enzymes after treadmill exercise. *American Journal Physical Medicine Rehabilitation*, 85, pp. 516–520.

Schleip, R., 2003. Fascial plasticity – a new neurobiological explanation. Part 1. *Journal of Bodywork & Movement Therapies*, 7(1), pp. 11–19.

Senstad, O., Leboeuf-Yde, C. and Borchgrevink, C., 1997. Frequency and characteristics of side effects of manipulative therapy. *Spine*, 22(4), pp. 435–440.

Seseke, S., Baudewig, J., Kallenberg, K. et al., 2006. Voluntary pelvic floor muscle control – an fMRI study. *Neuroimage*, 31(4), pp. 1399–1407.

Shacklock, M., 2005. *Clinical Neurodynamics: A New System of Musculoskeletal Treatment.* Edinburgh: Butterworth Heinemann/Elsevier.

Skyba, DA., Radhakrishnan, R., Rohlwing, JJ. et al., 2003. Joint manipulation reduces hyperalgesia by activation of monoamine receptors but not opioid or GABA receptors in the spinal cord. *Pain*, 106, pp. 159–168.

Sterling, M., Jull, G. and Wright, A., 2001. Cervical mobilisation: concurrent effects on pain, sympathetic nervous system activity and motor activity. *Manual Therapy*, 6, pp. 72–81.

Stuber, K., Lerede, C., Kristmanson, K. et al., 2014. The diagnostic accuracy of the Kemp's test: a systematic review. *Journal Canadian Chiropractic Association*, 58(3), pp. 258–267.

Sueki, DG., Cleland, JA. and Wainner, RS., 2013. A regional interdependence model of musculoskeletal dysfunction: research, mechanisms and clinical implications. *Journal Manual Manipulative Therapy*, 21(2), pp. 90–102.

Taimela, S., Kankaanpaa, M. and Luoto, S. 1999. The effect of lumbar fatigue on the ability to sense a change in lumbar position. *Spine*, 24(13), pp. 1322–1327.

Tawa, N., Rhoda, A. and Diener, I., 2017. Accuracy of clinical neurological examination in diagnosing lumbosacral radiculopathy: a systemic literature review. *BMC Musculoskeletal Disorders*, 18, p. 93.

Taylor, DC., Brooks, DE. and Ryan, JB., 1997. Visco-elastic characteristics of muscle: passive stretching versus muscular contractions. *Medicine & Science Sport Exercise*, 29(12), pp. 1619–1624.

Thiel, H. and Rix, G., 2005. Is it time to stop functional pre-manipulation testing of the cervical spine? *Manual Therapy*, 10(2), pp. 105–110.

Thompson, WR., Scott, A., Loghmani, MT. et al., 2016. Understanding mechanobiology: physical therapists as a force in mechanotherapy and musculoskeletal regenerative rehabilitation. *Physical Therapy*, 96, pp. 560–569.

Thomson, O., Haig, L. and Mansfield, H., 2009. The effects of high-velocity low-amplitude thrust manipulation and mobilisation techniques on pressure pain threshold in the lumbar spine. *International Journal Osteopathic Medicine*, 12(2), pp. 56–62.

Vario, G., Miller, S., McBrier, N. et al., 2009. Systematic review of efficacy for manual lymphatic drainage techniques in sports medicine and rehabilitation: an evidence-based practice approach. *Journal Manipulative Therapy*, 17, pp. e80–89.

Vernon, HT., Dhami, MS., Howley, TP. et al., 1986. Spinal manipulation and beta-endorphin: a controlled study of the effect of a spinal manipulation on plasma beta-endorphin levels in normal males. *Journal Manipulative Physiology Therapeutics*, 9, pp. 115–123.

Vincenzino, B., Collins, D. and Wright, A. 1988. An investigation of the interrelationship between manipulative therapy-induced hypoalgesia and sympathoexcitation. *Journal Manipulative Physiology Therapeutics*, 21, pp. 448–453.

World Health Organization, 2005. *WHO Guidelines on Basic Training and Safety in Chiropractic*. Geneva: World Health Organization.

Chapter 7 structure

Introduction   211

Mobility   216

Examples of activation techniques for mobility   217

Motor control   224

Examples of activation techniques for motor control   226

Muscle capacity and strength   234

Examples of activation techniques for muscle

capacity and strength   236

Conclusion   247

Introduction

In my opinion, activation incorporates the training principles necessary for an athlete to make a sustainable change or adaptation in their body. This will occur through graded exposure to appropriate mobility, motor control, muscle capacity and strengthening exercises. Such an approach helps *educATE* the athlete or patient, allowing them to take ownership of their condition. The aim is to restore the balance between progressive tissue load and muscle capacity. When this is achieved, a clinical progression for successfully managing patients is created, as highlighted in Figure 7.1.

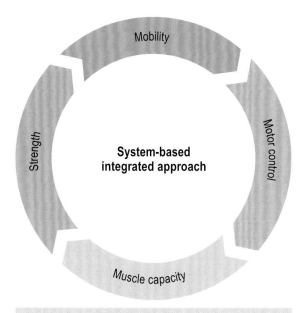

Figure 7.1
Clinical progression for activation.

Muscle inhibition is a major cause of non-functional movement patterns in athletes and in the general public (Oscar, 2012). As a consequence of muscle inhibition, substitution strategies are developed, which lead to the over-recruitment of muscle synergists to assist the inhibited muscle (Sahrmann, 2002). The result may have huge ramifications for the motor control, muscle capacity and strength of any individual.

Clinical gem

A good example of this occurs across the hip joint, in relation to the frequently observed over-recruitment of the tensor fasciae latae (TFL) muscle to assist frontal plane hip abduction during single-leg stance. The TFL is also a flexor and internal rotator of the hip, and so when it becomes the dominant prime mover, this only serves to increase its inhibitory effect on the gluteus medius muscle. Why? Due to the increased internal rotation of the hip joint, gluteus medius is put under greater levels of physiological demand, resulting in a loss of joint centration; this reduces optimum function in the frontal plane, resulting in the loss of *lateral hip control* (that is, efficient maintenance of frontal plane alignment). This can be confirmed with the side-lying hip abduction test. When the leg is taken into hip abduction and extension, it will test weak if gluteus medius is inhibited. However, if you take the leg into hip abduction and flexion, it will test stronger, due to the increased activity of the TFL. Remember, the TFL is also a hip joint flexor.

Program design

Specific rehabilitation principles should guide the training or rehabilitation requirements for the athlete or patient. Table 7.1 shows what I consider to be the key "fundamental principles" for designing a rehabilitation training program. At a minimum, this should include the demands and requirements of any task or sport,

Table 7.1 Highlighting the principles and definition of program design

Principle	Definition
Individual	Design the rehabilitation program for the individual. Consider age, gender, health, goals, motivation and any restraints relating to the injury or surgery
Overload	Progressive overload allows the body to make gains from training and exercise, according to the manner in which it trains
Specificity	Muscle action specificity (isometric, concentric, eccentric) Muscle group specificity (training the muscles involved in the activity or sport) Velocity specificity (training gains, specific to the velocities in which exercises are performed, including through ranges: inner, mid and outer)
Volume/ intensity	Volume relates to the amount of activity in a session (such as repetitions and sets) Intensity relates to how hard the body is working during physical activity. Load increases physiological demand; therefore, the intensity of performance in response to higher loads is elevated
Frequency	The number of training sessions per specific timeframe (weekly)
Rest	The length of time for recovery (e.g., between repetitions and sets)
Types of resistance	Body weight, Theraband®, free weights, kettle bells, machines, eccentric/flywheel and aquatic resistance
Periodization	Manipulation of training variables (load, sets, repetitions) to maximize adaptation; this may be determined according to micro (e.g., weekly) or macro (e.g., 8–12-week) cycles

appropriate for the specific individual, to assist in a return to their desired level of activities (Reiman and Lorenz, 2011). For example, an athlete who has just undergone hip surgery may want to develop hip flexion mobility and motor control through the range of hip flexion, so they can lift their hip comfortably when seated. This would require low-threshold hip flexion exercises at 30 percent maximum voluntary contraction (MVC), which could be repeated regularly throughout the day and performed 5–7 times weekly. The *Medical Dictionary for Health Professions and Nursing* (2012) defines MVC as the greatest amount of tension a muscle can generate, which is usually the instantaneous highest measured force during a test, depending on the parameters of the testing protocol. This differs significantly, however, depending on where the athlete is in their rehabilitation. An athlete at a later stage of their rehabilitation program would need to start replicating the demands of their sport, perhaps introducing activities such as high-speed running and actions requiring explosive power, with longer bouts of rest and recovery prescribed between sets and training sessions (Reiman and Lorenz, 2011; Iosia and Bishop, 2008; Rhea et al., 2006).

The program should be designed to take into consideration, and address, any specific muscle impairments or imbalances that may have contributed to the injury or that could be implicated in re-injury, alongside encouraging appropriate recovery strategies (Mihata et al., 2009; Croisier et al., 2008). Order of exercise during a training session is an important consideration when prescribing volume- and load-specific rehabilitation outcome. Generally speaking, multi-joint functional exercises require greater levels of coordination, skill and energy, and would normally be prescribed first in any training session, to limit fatigue (Powers, 2003). However, rehabilitation programs can vary considerably. For example, isolation exercises or non-functional exercises may be prescribed first, to begin targeting the weak link within the kinetic chain, before putting all the links together during functional exercise.

Specific consideration should be directed to the load and volume of these exercises; if a motor control deficit is present, neuromuscular fatigue may occur quite quickly. Similarly, careful consideration should be given to rehabilitating an athlete according to sport and body type. Muscles of the spinal column are predominantly slow-twitch, type 1 fibers (MacDonald et al., 2006; Thorstensson and Carlson, 1987) requiring high-repetition, low-load training (see Chapter 1). This contrasts with other more explosive muscles, such as quadriceps and gastrocnemius, which contain predominantly type 2 fibers and act as prime movers, which would require a greater emphasis on strength-based programs (Reiman and Lorenz, 2011).

Clinical gem

 I have found that introducing super-sets is a way to limit the exposure of an inhibited muscle group to neuromuscular fatigue in patients with motor control deficits. Super-setting involves alternating agonist and antagonist muscle groups (Powers, 2003). Working the antagonist muscle group directly after the agonist provides a short period of rest for the agonist group of muscles, which limits fatigue.

Progression

Exercises that incorporate motor control, control through range (mobility), muscle capacity and strength should all aim to challenge patients and athletes. While knowledge and understanding of corrective exercise may be limited in some cases, the role of the clinician, in this instance, is to *educATE* and help develop confidence in the safety and efficacy of movement-based exercises, and to actively encourage their undertaking. However, exercises that increase pain or develop it to unacceptable levels, either during or after a rehabilitation session, should be avoided. Similarly, too many low-threshold exercises should not be

prescribed, as these will slow down the recovery process and will not lead to strength adaptation, which may be a requirement for return to sport or functional demands. Increasing the length of recovery time and inhibiting the rehabilitation progress are likely to result in the patient or athlete seeking another opinion or approach.

There are two general rules of thumb for progressing exercises:

- Perform the exercise through a range of movement (ROM), then progress by increasing or extending the ROM, increasing the load, increasing the number of repetitions or reducing the recovery.

- Perform the exercise for the prescribed repetitions. For example, while ×10–15 repetitions ×2–3 sets may be one prescription, with a higher load a lower volume would be prescribed, depending on the desired outcome; that is, if the intensity were increased, the prescription would look different.

There are two particular categories of patients that clinicians should be aware of when prescribing rehabilitation exercises: those who can push themselves to the boundary of pain, perhaps to a 4/10 limit or higher on the Visual Analogue Scale (VAS), and those who need to be pain-free. The issue with patients in the former category (pain) is that they may feel they should work into pain, thinking that it is helping them, when in most cases it is just irritating their tissues. The problem with patients in the latter category (pain-free) is their perception of pain. Sometimes, chronic musculoskeletal patients report that their exercises are reproducing their pain when, in fact, all that is happening is that they are experiencing discomfort from using a weakened muscle or from post-exercise delayed-onset muscle soreness (DOMS) (Cheung et al., 2003). This is an educational issue for both parties. For example, if the clinician prescribes a program that lacks the appropriate level of loading or if the patient does not work hard enough, they will not progress. Similarly, if the program is too intense or the patient works too hard, it can hinder progress. A systematic review comparing painful and non-painful exercises for musculoskeletal conditions concluded that exercise approaches that worked into a pain threshold demonstrated superior short-term outcomes, compared with pain-free exercises (Smith et al., 2017).

Activation theory

Activation techniques play a significant role in managing patients back to performing at normal levels of their valued activities. Prior to beginning an activation program, it is useful to evaluate the mobility of tight, restricted muscles and to administer treatment to manipulate these tissues, which may be extremely beneficial. Starting strength training without addressing this issue may lead to reinforcement of faulty movement patterns.

Clinical gem

To take an example, if a loss of active hip extension is noted, treatment could begin by using reciprocal inhibition techniques (Iles, 1986) for the restricted anterior hip structures, such as the TFL and the rectus femoris muscles, to improve mobility prior to undertaking an active hip extension training program. This can then be incorporated into the athlete's or patient's training, by introducing exercises such as a single-leg high bridge and progressing over time to a reverse lunge to "open up" their anterior chain, while still maintaining a hip extension bias.

Although it may appear logical that activation techniques follow the stage of manipulation, it is not necessarily always the case. For example, if the deep hip flexor muscle (psoas major) is tested and found to be inhibited, then activation techniques for this muscle may begin straight away. However, a position must be found to train this muscle in isolation, without increasing activity in the superficial musculature. For example, supine lying might be more appropriate than a sitting position, as over-recruitment of the TFL in sitting may negatively influence joint centration, and only serve to reinforce the faulty hip flexion movement pattern.

Case study: Patient N

Consider the case of Patient N, who presents reporting a history of long-term back pain. Advice and help have previously been sought from just about every type of manipulative therapist in existence! Unfortunately, Patient N is still in pain.

Clinical gem

It is important to realize here that manipulation will not work. If you *evaluATE* the case carefully, you must conclude that therapists have already tried and failed with manipulation as an option. It is always tempting to think that if a patient has not tried your own individual style of manipulation, it might just work. However, I think this patient needs to be educated. I frequently tell a patient that the only person who will make them better is themself.

Case study: more on Patient N

In this context, for this patient, neuromuscular low-threshold motor control exercises are much more appropriate. Giving ownership, providing an active healthcare approach and educating through movement control exercises will go much further than any passive intervention.

Skeletal muscle tissue physiology plays a significant role in the performance of any particular muscle group. However, performing high-intensity exercise bouts may also lead to decreased levels in performance as a direct result of skeletal muscle fatigue (Kilduff et al., 2007; Jessen and Ebben, 2003; Jones and Lees, 2003). I believe most intrinsic musculoskeletal issues arise due to neuromuscular fatigue. Keeping this in mind and remembering that the body possesses an inherent ability to adapt, I do not find it surprising that the evidence suggests that substitution strategies develop through over-recruitment of muscle synergists as a result of fatigue (Sahrmann, 2002). It may be reasonable to assume that fatigue and muscle inhibition are correlated with a reduction in athletic performance, as has been demonstrated (Suter and Lindsay, 2001; Garland and McComas, 1990).

 Many strategies have been suggested for assisting with the activation of inhibited muscles; these include techniques that incorporate visualization, palpation, isometric contractions and breathing strategies. I use all of them, at some stage or another, on a daily basis in the clinical environment.

Visualization

 Visualization and mental imagery have been used to help improve alignment and movement patterns for many years (McGill, 2004). Thinking about a particular body part has been shown to activate the somatosensory portion of the cortex. In recent years, this has been demonstrated through increased brain activity on magnetic resonance imaging (MRI) while visualization techniques have been performed (Umphred, 2007). Athletes often use this approach to help enhance performance outcomes prior to races or competitions. Similarly, verbal cues such as "imagine," "feel," "activate" and "lengthen" have all been proposed as powerful cues for activation of the deep muscular system (Lee, 2011).

Palpation

 Soft tissue manipulation has often been cited as a treatment option for muscle inhibition (Frost, 2002; Walther, 2000). This approach involves cross-friction mobilization over the origin and insertion of a weak, inhibited muscle, which results in an immediate increase in strength of that muscle. This may be due to mechanical pressure affecting muscle spindle and Golgi tendon organ activity within the target muscles, or to mechanoreceptor activity facilitating the alpha motor neurons (Frost, 2002) (see Chapter 1). Deep, slow and lateral stimulation, administered through palpation techniques, has also been shown to affect the mechanoreceptors within the fascial system, increasing blood flow, improving flexibility and resetting muscle tone (Lindsay, 2008). In addition, other palpation techniques, including rapid tapping and brushing, have been shown to stimulate muscle spindle activity (Page et al., 2010). Similarly, electrostimulation, through the use of a Compex® device, may also promote the activation of inhibited muscles (Gondin et al., 2011; Billot et al., 2010).

Isometric contractions

 The rationale for application of muscle activation techniques may be based in the theory of post-activation potentiation (PAP), which states that muscular force output is enhanced with resistance activities (Robbins, 2005). For example, it has been shown that activation after a set of heavy squats, prior to performing vertical and horizontal jumps, enhances the jumping performance in athletes. A proposed explanation is that performance may be enhanced as a result of pre-loading the neuromuscular system, which elicits an excited or sensitive neural state (Robbins, 2005).

Clinically, this knowledge may be applied through isometric resistance exercises, to improve strength and joint stability. One benefit is that the technique can still be used, even when full ROM may not be available (Bandy and Sanders, 2001). This may be progressed to isotonic (contraction) mode, as soon as range is restored; however, under isometric conditions, muscle response to increased resistance has been shown to be greater, compared with isotonic conditions (Umphred, 2007).

The patient is instructed to perform a contraction at 10–25 percent MVC for 5–10 seconds' duration, against the clinician's resistance. This may be continued for 3–5 repetitions and resistance gradually increased to 50 percent MVC.

Breathing strategies

 Normalizing and restoring optimal diaphragmatic breathing techniques may influence the overall stabilization and strength of the entire locomotor system (Hodges et al., 2005). Thus, inefficient breathing could result in muscle imbalance, motor control alterations and physiological adaptations (Bradley and Esformes, 2014). Decreased abdominal motion, relative to upper thoracic motion, can be taken as confirmation of poor diaphragm function (Vickery, 2007). The diaphragm is capable of performing both a postural and a respiratory function, and disruption in one function may affect the capability of the other (Hodges et al., 2007). As we have seen, "if breathing is not normalized, no other movement pattern can be" (Lewit, 1994). Bradley and Esformes (2014) have shown that greater levels of movement dysfunction are exhibited in patients with breathing pattern disorders. As a result, incorporating breathing evaluation into clinical practice could be useful for clinicians, as disorders may contribute to poor or altered motor control and movement deficits.

Clinical gem

 In my clinical experience, once a breathing pattern dysfunction has been identified, manipulation may help to normalize tissue tension across this region. Greenman (1996) suggested that dysfunction within the thoracic region, although often pain-free, can heavily influence breathing mechanics. Joint or soft tissue manipulation may encourage optimal muscle activation patterns, improving oxygenation to the tissues, and leading to a reduction in sympathetic activity and an up-regulation in parasympathetic activity. Examples of treatment approaches used in clinical practice include:

- inhibition techniques, to address trigger points (TrPs) and tender points (TnPs) in the oblique/rectus abdominis muscles

- spinal manipulation to the thoracolumbar region

- neuromuscular motor control activation exercises to encourage optimum function of the diaphragm.

Mobility

 Mobility is defined as the freedom of movement that is readily available around a specific joint (Spencer et al., 2016). Efficient movement represents a balance between soft tissue extensibility and articular mobility (Figure 7.2). For example, restrictions in spinal mobility have been identified in athletes with low back pain (LBP) (Campbell et al., 2014; Vad et al., 2004; Lindsay and Horton, 2002), and a loss of mobility in the cocking leg

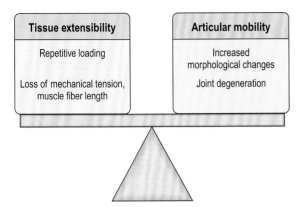

Figure 7.2
Influence of soft tissue and articular systems on mobility.

of soccer players has been shown to increase vulnerability to musculoskeletal injury (Tak and Langhout, 2014).

Tissue extensibility may be influenced by repetitive directional loading, which may lead to a loss of mechanical tension associated with tissue remodeling and the subsequent loss of fiber length (Langevin and Sherman, 2007; Sahrmann, 2002). Repetitive loading (that is, exercise, training or repeated daily tasks) can alter the potential balance, tipping the scale towards greater stiffness in muscle tissues. However, loss of mechanical tension and muscle fiber length changes are not the only physiological explanations for increased stiffness or reduction in extensibility; hypertrophy increases the intrinsic stiffness of muscle tissue due to an increase in non-elastic tissue components associated with adaptation to a hypertrophic stimulus.

Articular mobility may be influenced by increased morphological changes within a joint, such as hip joint cam femoroacetabular impingement (FAI) syndrome (Griffin et al., 2016). It has been proposed that such an increase in morphological changes may eventually result in increased joint degenerative changes such as osteoarthritis (OA) (Griffin et al., 2016).

Optimal mobility may provide the basis for the development of motor control (Boyle, 2010). Loss of mobility may give rise to adaptive or maladaptive strategies, through which an individual attempts to recreate active stability and maintain function. However, in the presence of pain and increased levels of psychological stress (that is, cognitively mediated), as opposed to stress on tissue (biomechanical), it may lead to the development of inefficient motor control patterns (Cook et al., 2010).

Examples of activation techniques for mobility
Psoas stretch (Figure 7.3)

- Indications: (1) Extension-related LBP and or sacroiliac joint (SIJ) pain, (2) Loss of active sagittal plane hip ROM, (3) Flexed forward standing posture, (4) Loss of active posterior pelvic tilt.

- Specific attention should be paid to engaging abdominals to limit excessive lumbar lordosis.

- The patient should glide forward on the hip that is being stretched until tension is developed across the anterior hip, although the tension may be felt in the lateral hip due to an over-active TFL.

- Stretch may be increased by encouraging (1) Lateral flexion away from the side being stretched and taking the arm overhead (Figure 7.4), (2) Rotation towards the side being stretched (Figure 7.5).

- Stretch should be felt only in the anterior thigh and hip, not the lower back.

Rectus femoris stretch (Figure 7.6)

- Indications: (1) Extension-related LBP and or SIJ pain, (2) Loss of active sagittal plane hip ROM.

- Specific attention should be paid to engaging abdominals to limit excessive lumbar lordosis.

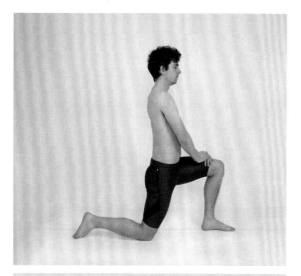

Figure 7.3

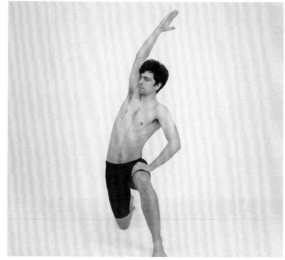

Figure 7.5

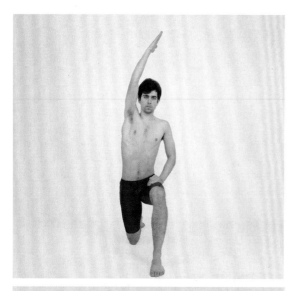

Figure 7.4

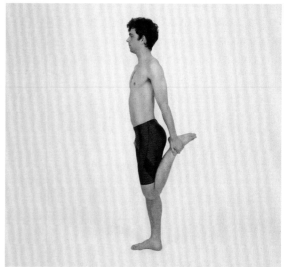

Figure 7.6

- The patient should focus on extending the thigh, rather than knee flexion.

- This stretch may be combined with the psoas stretch.

- Stretch should be felt only in the anterior thigh and hip, not the lower back.

Adductor stretch (Figure 7.7)

- Indications: (1) Hip joint/SIJ dysfunction or medial knee pain, (2) Adductor-related groin pain with loss of frontal plane ROM, (3) Loss of lateral hip control in single-leg (SL) stance.

- Specific attention should be paid to stretching muscle, rather than aggravating the hip joint.

- The patient can rotate the knee internally/externally to bias different fibers of the adductor muscles.

Hamstring stretch (Figure 7.8)

- Indications: (1) Posterior chain-related impairments due to hypomobility, (2) Loss of lumbar flexion ROM, (3) Recurrent hamstring issues.

- Specific attention should be paid to stretching the muscle rather than the sciatic nerve.

- The patient can rotate the knee internally/externally to bias different hamstring muscles, or flex

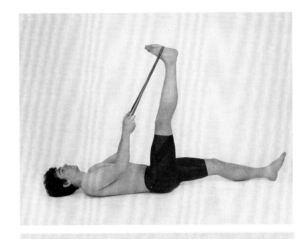

Figure 7.8

the hip and knee to bias different portions of the muscles.

Gluteus maximus stretch (GMx; Figure 7.9)

- Indications: (1) Posterior chain-related impairments due to hypomobility, (2) LBP, SIJ and buttock pain, (3) Loss of hip flexion ROM.

- Specific attention should be paid to avoiding aggravating or irritating the hip: e.g., in FAI syndrome or hip OA, reproducing groin pain, the patient should be shown how to maintain alignment and limit range during the stretch.

Piriformis stretch (Figure 7.10)

- Indications: (1) SIJ dysfunction, posterior thigh and buttock pain, (2) Pseudo-sciatica pain, (3) Over-activity, compensating for inhibited gluteus medius (GMed).

- Specific attention should be paid to not reproducing anterior hip and groin pain.

- Stretch should be felt specifically in the deep buttock.

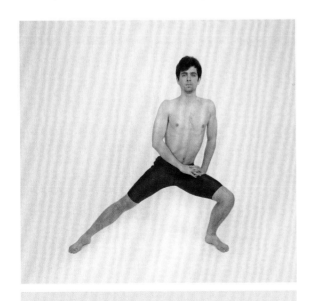

Figure 7.7

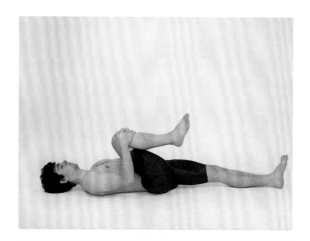

Figure 7.9

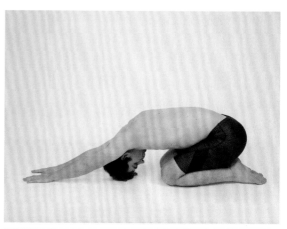

Figure 7.11

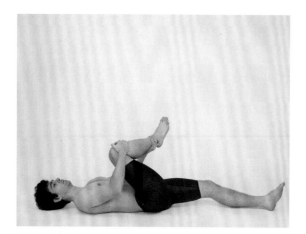

Figure 7.10

Erector spinae flexion stretch (Figure 7.11)

- Indications: (1) Loss of sagittal plane lumbar flexion due to myofascial stiffness, (2) LBP and/or SIJ pain.

- Specific attention should be paid to prevent over-stretching the lower lumbar spine and SIJ joints beyond normal physiological ROM.

Erector spinae supine rotation stretch (Figure 7.12)

- Indications: (1) Hip- and groin-related pain, (2) Loss of thoracolumbar rotation ROM, (3) Quadratus lumborum stiffness or spasm.

- Encourage a stable base by stretching the arms out and maintain control by keeping the shoulder girdle on the floor, while rotating through the hips and keeping the knees bent and feet on the floor.

- Use the oblique muscles rather than rotating through the lower lumbar spine.

- Encourage breathing to facilitate a better stretch: e.g., inhale during the held phase and exhale during the relaxation phase.

- Intensity of stretch can be increased by crossing one leg over the other or by raising the legs to 90°.

Erector spinae extension self-mobilization (Figure 7.13)

- Indications: (1) Lower lumbar intervertebral disk lesions, (2) Postural re-education to assist with loss of thoracic spine extension ROM, (3) Hypertonic rectus abdominis muscles.

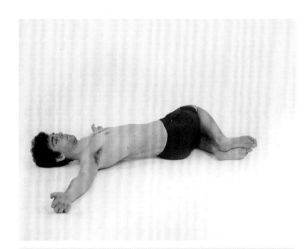

Figure 7.12

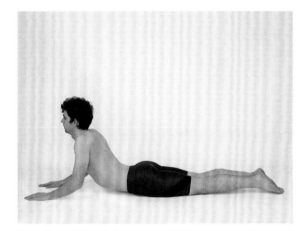

Figure 7.13

- Specific attention should be paid to not hyper-extending and irritating the lower lumbar facet joints.

Thoracolumbar spine: side-lying self-mobilization - archer rotation (Figure 7.14AB)

- Indications: (1) Improving thoracolumbar rotation ROM.

- Specific attention should be paid to activating the adductor muscles of the top leg, to maintain lumbar stability.

- Specific attention should be paid to not over-rotating the lower lumbar segments.

- Encourage breathing to facilitate relaxation and increased ROM, e.g., inhale as the shoulder and thoracic spine ROM increases.

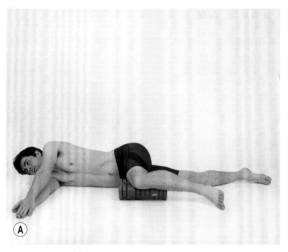

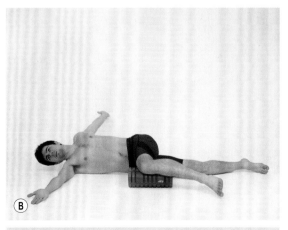

Figure 7.14

- Specific shoulder retraction and extension, to encourage upper and mid-thoracic rotation ROM.

Thoracic extension: supine self-mobilization with towel (Figure 7.15)

- Indications: (1) Loss of upper thoracic ROM, (2) Anterior shoulder restriction ROM, (3) Cervical spine pain due to hypomobility in upper thoracic spine.

- A small pillow may help to avoid hyper-extending the cervical spine.

- Ensure the knees are flexed and the feet on the floor.

Thoracic extension: self-mobilization – modified dead bug (Figure 7.16)

- Indications: (1) Loss of thoracic spine extension ROM, (2) LBP extension "hinging," (3) Shoulder joint stiffness or myofascial insufficiency/loss of extensibility affecting spinal mechanics.

- Specific attention should be paid to maintaining a neutral lumbar spine.

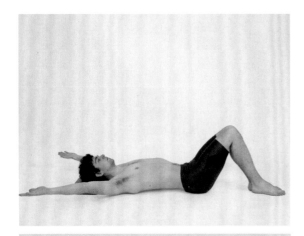

Figure 7.15

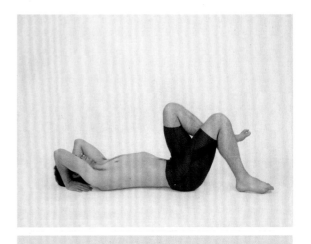

Figure 7.16

- Avoid flaring of the lower ribcage.

- The cervical spine can be supported with a pillow or cushion if the patient demonstrates excessive upper thoracic kyphosis.

Thoracic self-mobilization: seated (Figure 7.17)

- Indications: (1) Loss of thoracic spine extension, (2) Lower lumbar extension "hinging."

- In sitting, the lumbar spine is relatively stable, hands are placed behind the head and fingers interlocked to stabilize the cervical spine, and thoracic mobility is encouraged in sagittal, frontal and transverse planes.

Thoracic extension standing self-mobilization: against wall (Figure 7.18AB)

- Indications: (1) Loss of thoracic extension to neutral ROM, (2) Lower lumbar extension "hinging" LBP.

- Ensure that the head, shoulders and lower back are placed against a wall.

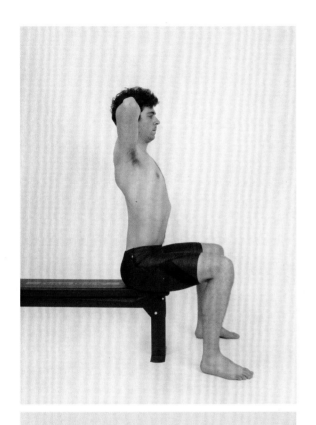

Figure 7.17

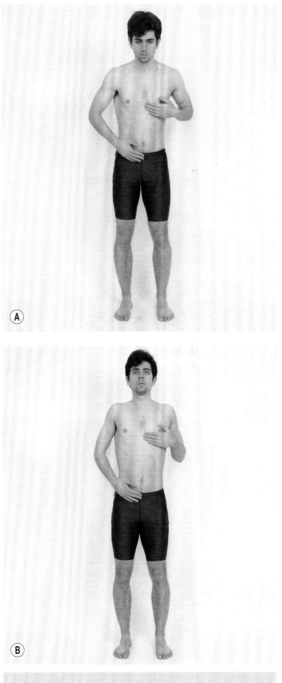

Figure 7.18

- Relax the knees and engage the abdominals, particularly the obliques, to prevent flaring of the lower ribcage.

- The patient should place one hand on the sternum and one hand on the pubic bone.

- The upper thoracic spine should be encouraged to relax and flex, while maintaining a neutral lumbar spine by engaging the abdominals; active thoracic extension should be encouraged (Figure 7.18B).

Thoracic segmental rotation self-mobilization: heel to pelvis (Figure 7.19)

- Indications: (1) Loss of thoracic rotation ROM, (2) Loss of hip joint rotation.

- Encourage sitting back on to the sitting bones (ischial tuberosities), if hip and knee joints allow, to minimize lumbar motion.

- One hand is placed behind the head to encourage glenohumeral joint (GHJ) external rotation (alternatively, the hand can be placed behind the back to encourage internal rotation).

- Active thoracic rotation should be encouraged in an axial plane, to increase length throughout the spine.

- In addition, a Theraband® (TB) may be used, to offer light resistance and control through the range.

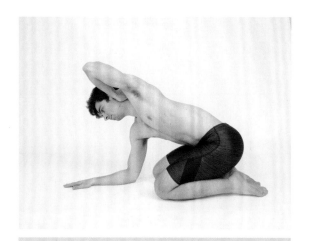

Figure 7.19

Motor control

Motor control is described as the process that maintains optimal alignment and initiates, directs and grades purposeful movement for performing a skillful task (Spencer et al., 2016). It is dependent on a person having the capacity of muscle to perform the task, on processing of sensory input, on interpretation of stability and dynamic activity, and on established motor strategies in response to unpredictable and unexpected movement challenges (Figure 7.20) (Hodges and Mosley, 2003). According to Panjabi's control system, the central nervous system determines motor control requirements through contraction of the deep and superficial muscles, in order to provide stability and coordinated dynamic mobility, which are regulated via feed-back and feed-forward control mechanisms (Diedrichsen et al., 2010). If an athlete is to perform efficiently, the level of stability and the degree of dynamic mobility will become task-specific, and will be determined by the demands of the intended movement, the load demands required to perform it, and the perception of the risks that may be associated with that activity (van Dieën and de Looze, 1999).

Motor control adaptation to pain can be influenced by corrective exercise. For example, it has previously been shown that prescribing specific motor control exercises to restore delayed or reduced activation of the transversus abdominis (Tsao and Hodges, 2007)

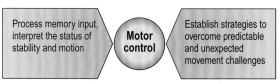

Figure 7.20
Strategies for developing motor control.

and multifidus (Tsao et al., 2010) produces a positive effect, even after training has ceased (Tsao and Hodges, 2008). Athletes who participate in sports that produce high-level loads on their spine, hips and groin need to be able to distribute these forces evenly, to minimize the risk of overloading tissues (Adams and Nolan, 2007; Cholewicki and McGill, 1992). Failure to maintain alignment when performing low-threshold, as well as high-threshold, activities may increase the potential risk of tissue damage, especially during repetitive loading (Monnier et al., 2012).

Failure to manage load transfer during low-threshold exercises may result from motor control incompetence or from behavior that may be associated with pain or injury (Hodges, 2011). However, other variables may also be implicated, such as fatigue from over-training, failure to understand instructions given by a trainer, or the athlete's mood. Failure to manage load transfer during higher-threshold exercises may be due to insufficient muscle capacity. This is the ability of an athlete to produce and tolerate varying degrees or levels of intensity at durations required to perform a particular sport (Ratamess et al., 2009; Siff, 2003). Optimal function requires coordinated neuromuscular control, combined with intersegmental kinetic chain mobility (Panjabi, 2003). For example, performing skills at maximum speed requires proximal-to-distal sequencing, to ensure that the distal segment in the kinetic chain can maximally perform a specific task, such as kicking a ball (Shan and Westerhoff, 2005). Failure to achieve load transfer during intersegmental motion tasks may result in altered motor patterns and potential tissue damage through uneven load distribution (Hides et al., 2010; Van Dillen et al., 1998).

Motor control exercises should provide a challenge to the neuromuscular system, through progressive difficulty and variability, and encourage intersegmental tasks, with the aim of retraining appropriate muscle recruitment and facilitating coordinated movement and proprioceptive awareness around the spine, hip and groin (Naito et al., 2012; Brumagne et al., 1999).

Case study: Patient O

 Patient O is a 17-year-old male track and field athlete, who has recently been training abroad. He intends to seek a scholarship, based on his athletic ability. After 7 weeks of increased loading, he sustained a traumatic incident to his right anterior hip. A sports medicine clinician diagnosed psoas tendinitis and injected his psoas tendon, recommending that he should have regular soft tissue manipulation to this region. Patient O followed the clinician's advice but unfortunately remained symptomatic. He sought advice from a second clinician, who told him he needed complete rest. Unfortunately, this did not help either. On returning to the UK, he was reviewed by a third clinician, who, after organizing MRI of the hip and pelvis, made a different diagnosis of pubic-related groin pain. At this point, Patient O received a protein-rich plasma (PRP) injection into the pubic region. When Patient O presented, he reported feeling better but was still unable to train. Evaluation highlighted the following:

1. SL stance test demonstrated to be positive on the right, highlighting an inability to maintain force closure through the pelvis and hip joint

2. anterior groin pain at end-of-range lumbar extension

3. an inability to perform a squat

4. positive resisted abdominals test, which reproduced pain over his right lower abdominals

5. positive active straight leg raise (ASLR) on the right

6. loss of hip flexion and internal rotation ROM

7. pain on resisted SL adductor testing that was symptomatically modified by hip joint internal rotation

8. loss of hip abduction inner range in side lying.

 In my opinion, Patient O had developed a non-functional issue. As you can see from points 1–8 above, his evaluation highlighted many painful entities (Falvey et al., 2016). It is extremely difficult in cases like this to use a classification of pathology relating to anatomical structures (Hölmich, 2007) to make a definitive diagnosis (Falvey et al., 2016). Some of Patient O's symptoms also appeared to be driven by nervousness, fear and anxiety around re-injuring himself. I explained that if I could modify his symptoms, it would enable me to provide a prognostic outcome for his condition; he agreed to me trying this approach.

 I started educating Patient O on how to perform intersegmental motor control exercises, as this approach has previously shown high rates of return to sporting participation (King et al., 2018). We began with inner-range activation of gluteus medius in side lying. The purpose was to open up his anteromedial hip by facilitating external rotation and to provide increased frontal plane ROM. Within 2–3 sets of exercises, Patient O could perform a side-lying hip abduction test, pain-free. On retesting hip joint ROM, flexion and internal rotation were seen to have improved. We progressed to supersetting his adductor muscles, using low-threshold, pain-free manual resistance exercises through ROM. After 3 sets of 6–8 repetitions, on retesting his SL resisted adductor test Patient O had no discomfort; his ASLR and abdominal testing were also pain-free. On functional re-evaluation, he could perform an SL stance and an appropriate squat.

 This case highlights the benefit of implementing techniques for low-threshold neuromuscular activation, rather than joint or soft tissue manipulation. In addition, Patient O could now perform functional movements, and by modifying his symptoms quickly and following an appropriate exercise rehabilitation plan, he could begin to incorporate range and control, and start to move through range, using motor control exercises. He progressed quickly over the following weeks to late-stage

rehabilitation, which included muscle capacity and strength; these aspects will be discussed later in this chapter.

Clinical gem

Dosage for motor control exercises should reflect the classification of a low-threshold activity – 30 percent MVC – and should be performed as 3–5 sets of 20 repetitions, or for 30–60 seconds, 5–7 times weekly.

Examples of activation techniques for motor control

Psoas neuromuscular: supine activation (Figure 7.21)

- Indications: (1) Loss of strength with resisted psoas testing, (2) Thoracolumbar translation with ASLR, (3) Flexion, adduction, internal rotation (FADIR) positive testing, (3) Long psoas identified on Thomas test, (4) Snapping hip syndrome.

- The patient is encouraged to visualize drawing or sucking their femur/thigh bone into its socket.

- The patient may palpate medially and inferiorly to the anterior superior iliac spine (ASIS) to assist with this process.

- Avoid over-recruitment of the lower abdominal muscles.

- Avoid "hitching" the lower lumbar spine with excessive ipsilateral abdominal and quadratus lumborum contraction.

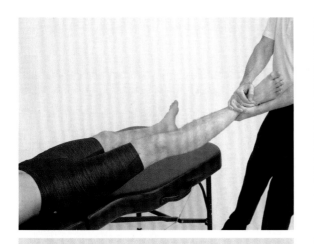

Figure 7.21

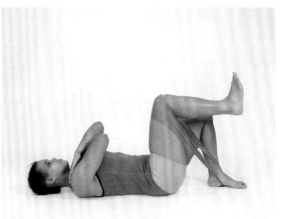

Figure 7.22

- The clinician may offer resistance by applying gentle long-lever traction of the hip.

- Encourage hip joint external rotation and abduction to reduce activity in the TFL.

Psoas neuromuscular: supine activation with TB (Figure 7.22)

- Increase intensity by using a TB around the knee, stabilized under the opposite foot.

- Ensure sagittal plane motion and avoid allowing the patient to drop into frontal plane adduction.

- Encourage minimal activity in the TFL by reminding the patient of psoas suction ("drawing their thigh bone into its socket") activation prior to exercise.

Psoas neuromuscular: sitting activation with TB (Figure 7.23)

- Progression of intensity to sitting.

- A neutral spine should be maintained by instructing the patient to place one hand on the sternum and the

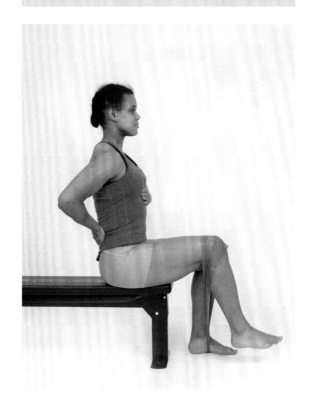

Figure 7.23

other on the lumbar spine, ensuring the hands remain parallel.

- Avoid working into excessive ranges of hip flexion, as this may aggravate symptoms.

Psoas neuromuscular: standing activation with TB (Figure 7.24)

- Ensure lateral control is maintained with the contralateral leg.

- Ensure sagittal plane motion in the hip that is flexed and avoid allowing the patient to drop into frontal plane adduction.

- Arm movements may be exaggerated, as in the "running man" drill, to maintain stability and control.

Psoas neuromuscular: functional step-up activation (Figure 7.25)

- This is a natural progression but ensure adequate ankle dorsiflexion and knee stability are maintained, avoiding excessive subtalar pronation and/or knee joint valgus/varus.

GMed neuromuscular: side-lying activation (Figure 7.26)

- Indications: (1) LBP and or SIJ pain, (2) Loss of lateral control such as positive SL stance or positive Trendelenburg sign (see Chapter 3), (3) Anterior hip and groin pain resulting from an overactive TFL, (4) Iliotibial band (ITB) syndrome.

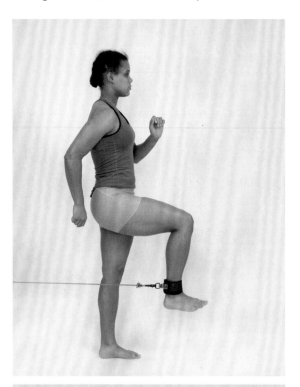

Figure 7.24

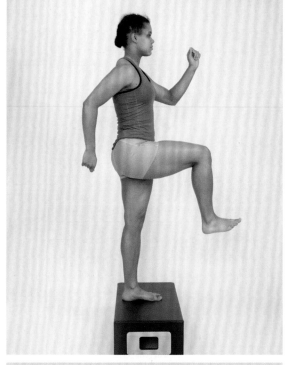

Figure 7.25

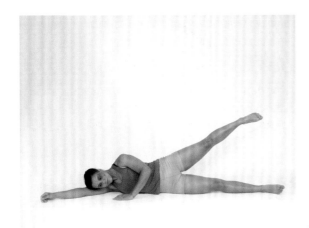

Figure 7.26

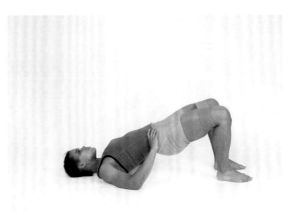

Figure 7.27

- The patient is side-lying and instructed to engage their abdominals, lengthen their upper hip, abduct and, in the position of maximum abduction, actively extend their heel, increasing activity in the posterior GMed.

- This may be modified to a shorter-lever approach by positioning the patient's foot against a wall and instructing the patient to actively extend, while producing hip abduction.

- Avoid excessive abduction as this may encourage lateral flexion of the lumbar spine.

- Specific attention should be paid to avoid the upper leg moving into flexion while performing abduction, as this only encourages increased activity in the TFL.

GMed neuromuscular: double-leg (DL) bridge with hip abduction activation, with TB or Pilates ring (Figure 7.27)

- The patient is instructed how to perform a hip extension pattern in a DL bridge, to ensure segmental lumbar control.

- The hip extension position is held and the patient instructed to avoid flaring of the lower ribcage by engaging the abdominals, particularly the oblique muscles.

- The hip joints are taken into abduction using the TB as resistance.

- Ensure a similar frontal plane range is maintained in both hips.

- The patient may move the feet closer or rock onto their heels to bias GMx; alternatively, move the feet further away to bias hamstring recruitment.

GMed neuromuscular: side-lying activation with TB (short lever), progression 1 (Figure 7.28)

- Progression of DL bridge into SL short lever against gravity.

- Specific attention should be paid to ensuring an appropriate starting position, the top leg abducted into extension to increase activity in the posterior GMed.

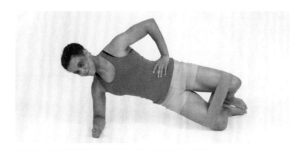

Figure 7.28

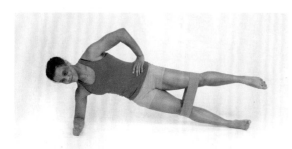

Figure 7.29

GMed neuromuscular: side-lying activation with TB (long lever), progression 2 (Figure 7.29)

- Progression of SL short lever against gravity into long lever.

- Specific attention should be paid to ensuring an appropriate starting position, the top leg abducted into extension to increase activity in the posterior GMed.

Adductor neuromuscular: side-lying activation for short adductors (pectineus, adductor brevis and longus) (Figure 7.30)

- Indications: (1) Recurrent adductor or groin strains, (2) SIJ or symphysis pubis dysfunction, (3) Loss of strength on testing the adductor musculature.

- The patient is side lying, with the leg to be trained resting underneath their body on the couch.

- The leg is lifted by the clinician and placed into internal rotation; the patient is instructed to hold the leg against gravity for 3–5 seconds.

- Manual resistance may be encouraged by the clinician to increase activation of the short adductors; similarly, soft tissue manipulation techniques may be used prior to beginning the exercise, to increase neuromuscular activation patterns.

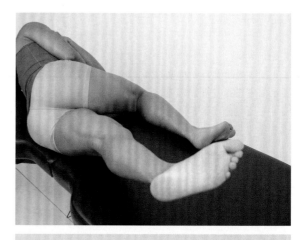

Figure 7.30

Adductor neuromuscular: side-lying activation adductor magnus (Figure 7.31)

- The patient is side lying, with the leg to be trained resting underneath their body on the couch.

- The leg is lifted by the clinician and placed into external rotation; the patient is instructed to hold the leg against gravity for 3–5 seconds.

- Manual resistance may be encouraged by the clinician to increase activation of the short adductors; similarly, soft tissue manipulation techniques may be used prior to beginning the exercise, to increase neuromuscular activation patterns.

Adductor neuromuscular: supine activation with Pilates ring (Figure 7.32)

- The patient is supine, with a Pilates ring placed between the legs, and is instructed to engage the abdominals and gently squeeze the sides of the ring together, holding for 5 seconds.

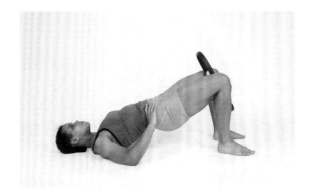

Figure 7.32

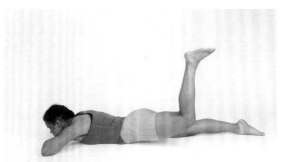

Figure 7.33

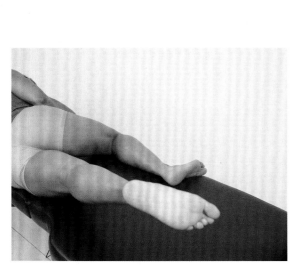

Figure 7.31

- This can be progressed into a DL bridge with hip adduction, similar to the GMed exercise, and positioning of the feet can be modified to ensure more activity in either the GMx or hamstring muscles.

GMx neuromuscular: prone activation (Figure 7.33)

- Indications: (1) LBP and or SIJ pain, (2) Recurrent hamstring strains.

- The patient is prone lying; flexes the knee on the tested leg and takes the hip into passive extension.

231

- Abduction and external rotation may be encouraged, to help increase activity of the GMx.

- The patient is instructed to hold the leg in position as the clinician lets go for 5–10 seconds.

- Manual resistance may be encouraged to increase activity of GMx.

- Avoid excessive lumbar lordosis occurring, by increasing activation of the abdominal muscles.

GMx neuromuscular: supine activation in SL (Figure 7.34)

- Natural progression from above: the patient is in DL bridge position and instructed to lift one foot off the floor.

- Manual resistance may be applied to the knee of the raised leg, while the patient maintains frontal and transverse plane alignment (Figure 7.35).

- Avoid this exercise if excessive cramping of the hamstring muscles is reported.

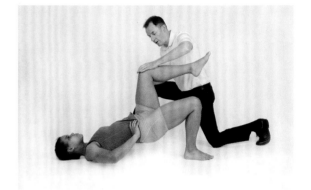

Figure 7.35

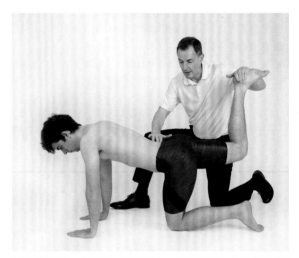

Figure 7.36

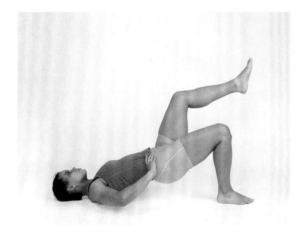

Figure 7.34

GMx neuromuscular: four-point kneeling activation (Figure 7.36)

- The patient is positioned in four-point kneeling and instructed to activate the abdominal muscles.

- One leg is taken into hip extension, with the knee bent at 90° to target the GMx, and the contraction is held for 5–10 seconds.

- The clinician should observe for excessive lumbar lordosis as the patient begins to fatigue.

- This can be modified to increase the load by performing a similar exercise off the end of the bed (e.g., by performing hip extension in standing, with one hip propped against the end of the treatment couch).

GMx neuromuscular: hip hinge activation (Figure 7.37AB)

- Indications: (1) Preparatory exercise that should be used prior to performing a squat, (2) Useful to actively lengthen a hypertonic shortened anterior chain, (3) The first 30° of flexion should come from the hip joint; as a result, this exercise helps to retrain that movement pattern.

- Avoid letting the lumbar spine creep into excessive lordosis or sway back; the emphasis should be placed on sitting through the hips.

Lumbar spine neuromuscular: standing flexion (waiter's bow) (Figure 7.38)

- Indications: (1) Retraining movement pattern for lumbar flexion control, (2) Developing capacity for lumbar flexion, (3) Improving posterior chain myofascial and neural mobility.

- The patient stands with the feet shoulder width apart and knees slightly bent; ask them to squeeze gently with fingers and thumb of one hand and "pinch" the lumbar erector spinae muscles.

- Instruct the patient to slowly bend forward, pushing through the hips and keeping a neutral spine; as soon as the "pinch" is lost, stop and return to neutral, reset and repeat.

- A progression of this exercise is good mornings, for lumbar spine flexion control.

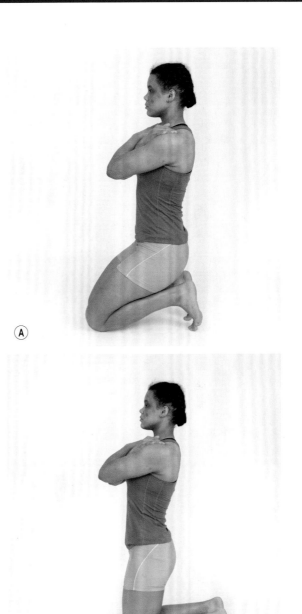

(A)

(B)

Figure 7.37

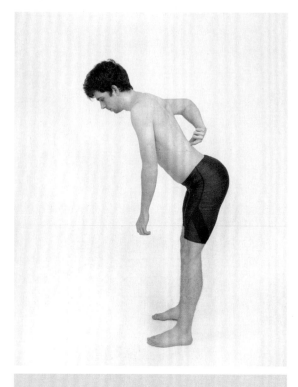

Figure 7.38

Muscle capacity and strength

 While activation focuses on tissue mobility and motor control deficits, the purpose of integration techniques is to encourage progressive loading to help build muscle capacity within the tissues. This allows individuals to become more robust and essentially "bullet-proofs" them, prior to returning to their normal sporting activities. As muscle capacity improves, the athlete may be progressed through strength- and eventually sports-specific phases. Special consideration should be given to the effect on athletes of increasing training load, intensity and duration. Adequate recovery must be included in these stages to allow the athlete time to recover, reset and then push on again.

Clinical gem

 Muscle capacity training should involve 2–3 sessions per week at 60–80 percent MVC. Training exposure should be prescribed at 3–5 sets of 12–15 repetitions or 3–6 times 10 second isometric holds, with 1–2 minutes' recovery between sets.

Muscle capacity

Muscle capacity (Figure 7.39) is defined as an individual's ability to produce and tolerate varying degrees or levels of intensity at durations required to perform a particular sport (Ratamess et al., 2009; Siff, 2003). It should be viewed as a training outcome, rather than a performance outcome, resulting in muscle, tendon and metabolic biogenetic adaptation (Langberg et al., 2000; Van Cutsem et al., 1998). Adaptations in muscle capacity allow for the development of load tolerance, robustness and resilience within the musculoskeletal system, and enable the capacity of the tissues to mirror the volume, intensity and duration required for performance sport (Siff, 2003).

Motor control deficits and biomechanical insufficiency may result in a loss of neuromuscular capacity and an inability to meet the demands of increased mechanical loading (Borghuis et al., 2008). For example, optimal muscle capacity across the pelvic girdle should take into consideration an athlete's ability to transfer and absorb repeated submaximal forces through the pelvis, to help develop a platform for strength training and high-performance sport. Inefficiency within the abdominal musculature, resulting in loss of muscular endurance, may be a risk factor for recurrence of injury (Jones et al., 2005). Similarly, structural changes within the musculature, such as fatty deposits, muscular atrophy and fiber-type modification, have also been shown

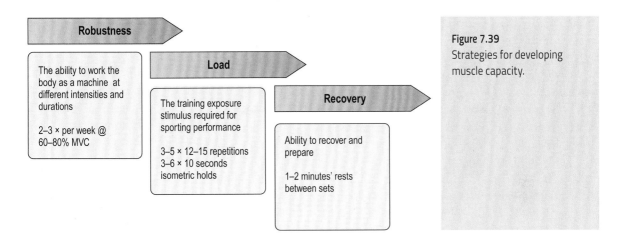

Figure 7.39
Strategies for developing muscle capacity.

Robustness

The ability to work the body as a machine at different intensities and durations

2–3 × per week @ 60–80% MVC

Load

The training exposure stimulus required for sporting performance

3–5 × 12–15 repetitions
3–6 × 10 seconds isometric holds

Recovery

Ability to recover and prepare

1–2 minutes' rests between sets

to occur in patients with chronic LBP (D'hooge et al., 2012; Danneels et al., 2000); if an athlete is exposed to this, it could contribute to suboptimal responses to the training stimulus and, therefore, an increase in potential injury.

Muscle strength

Muscular strength is defined as the ability of an individual to produce force, with maximal strength being the largest amount of force that can be produced (Stone et al., 2004). Rate of force development (RFD) is defined as the rate of rise of contractile force at the beginning of a muscle action and is time-dependent (Aagaard et al., 2002). RFD can be viewed as dynamic, resulting from global external production of power, or static, from stiffening or producing force to offer protection. The production of force and/or stiffness is dependent on morphological and neurological factors. Morphological factors include the cross-sectional area of the muscle, muscle-pennation angle, fascicle length and fiber type (Cormie et al., 2011). Neurological factors that influence strength include motor-recruitment, firing frequency and intermuscular coordination (Cormie et al., 2009).

It is beyond the scope of this book to discuss strength and conditioning training in great detail. There are many published texts in this field and I encourage readers to refer to those included in the reference list at the end of this chapter. For our purposes here, it is worth considering that the peak values for dynamic RFD and power are closely related, and as a result are often used as a measure of peak power (Stone et al., 2004). Production of high-velocity movements during sporting tasks, such as kicking a ball, jumping or throwing, requires high power output, in unison with segmental sequential coordination of the spinal musculature (Watkins et al., 1996; Newton and Kraemer, 1994).

Static RFD, or muscular stiffness, is defined as the ability of the vertebral column to maintain spinal alignment, while resisting deformation from external yielding forces (Graham and Brown, 2012; Brown and McGill, 2008). The muscular stiffness created is dependent on the magnitude of contractile forces in the spine, being equal to the rate and direction of force exerted against the spinal column. There are morphological and neurological similarities between static RFD and dynamic RFD (Cormie et al., 2009). However, these appear to be task-orientated. For example, bracing the spinal column against a low-threshold load may bias the neurological system, compared with high-threshold loads, which not only challenge the neurological system, but also require morphological factors, such as cross-sectional area and fiber type, to produce greater levels of stiffness to protect the spine (Cormie et al., 2011; Brown and McGill, 2008).

Clinically, muscle capacity and strength may be measured through specific tests, to record the maximum level of work at a given intensity, for either a specific number of repetitions or for a specific duration. Results from such tests can then be used to provide a baseline, from which specific rehabilitation exercises can be prescribed to target deconditioned tissues. For example, static side-lying plank exercises are often prescribed to produce muscular activation in the spinal tissues and develop endurance and robustness, helping to improve strength, endurance and the cross-sectional area of these muscles (Durall et al., 2009; Danneels et al., 2001).

Case study: more on Patient O

Let's return to Patient O, the young athlete who had developed anterior hip and groin pain and responded to low-threshold motor control exercises. His program was to progress towards developing muscle capacity and strength. His progress was measured with capacity-based tests that involved handheld dynamometry to record MVC strength (pounds) and duration (seconds). A program was created that challenged his muscle capacity and tissue compliance, by working his body at 60–80 percent MVC, at varying degrees of intensity and duration, to mimic the performance demands of his sport (Ratamess et al., 2009; Siff, 2003). This type of exposure to increasing levels of physical activity was aimed at making his tissues clinically robust; exercises for developing this quality are described below.

Clinical gem

When patients reach the late stages of their rehabilitation, they require optimum recovery strategies. I emphasized the benefits of motor control activation over

manipulation earlier in this chapter. Now it is important to understand how the pendulum can swing towards the benefits of soft tissue and joint manipulation for the athlete at this stage. The reason is a simple one: any increase in loading will cause the athlete to develop stiffness, and clearly stiffness is important to make our athlete "bullet-proof." However, as previously discussed, stiffness can influence articular mobility (Campbell et al., 2014; Vad et al., 2004; Lindsay and Horton, 2002) and soft tissue extensibility (Langevin and Sherman, 2007; Sahrmann, 2002), and so manipulation can help to address these effects of late-stage training, allowing the athlete to recover adequately and continue with loading.

Examples of activation techniques for muscle capacity and strength
Hip flexion capacity: standing with TB (Figure 7.40)

- Indications: (1) Developing inner-range muscle capacity, (2) Weakness on hip flexion testing, (3) Positive FADIR symptoms, (4) Recurrent anterior hip or groin symptoms.

- Ensure lateral hip stability is maintained with the contralateral leg.

- Ensure sagittal plane motion is maintained in the hip that is flexed and avoid allowing the patient to drop into frontal plane adduction as they fatigue.

- Arm movements may be exaggerated as in the "running man" drill, to maintain stability and control.

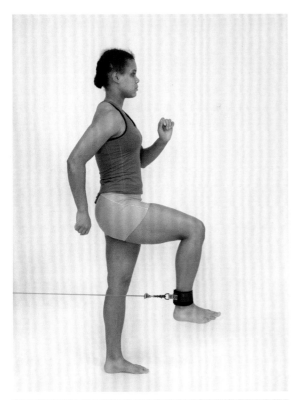

Figure 7.40

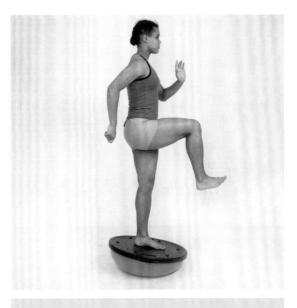

Figure 7.41

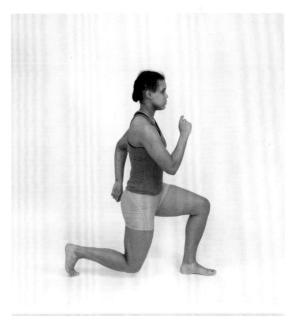

Figure 7.42

- A modification of this exercise is to perform inner-range hip flexion capacity with TB on a BOSU® board (Figure 7.41).

Hip flexion capacity: eccentric hip lunge (Figure 7.42)

- Indications: (1) Developing outer-range eccentric muscle capacity, (2) Weakness on hip flexion testing, (3) Positive FADIR symptoms, (4) Recurrent anterior hip, groin or lower abdominal symptoms, (5) Symptoms specifically aggravated by sprinting activities.

- Specific attention to detail is needed, especially regarding the depth of the lunge, until tissues start to comply with the load.

- Feet should be placed apart, to achieve as wide an area as possible for greater stability, but care should be taken not to overload the adductor muscles and groin region.

- The forward knee should track over the front foot and the thoracolumbar spine should remained aligned over the pelvic girdle.

- Reduce the depth of lunge initially to minimize over-stretching the anterior hip of the rear leg.

- A modification of the exercise is to perform eccentric hip flexion capacity using a Bulgarian split squat (Figure 7.43); however, care must be taken not to over-stretch the anterior hip rear leg. This may be modified by minimizing the depth of lunge or by allowing a forward lean of the trunk.

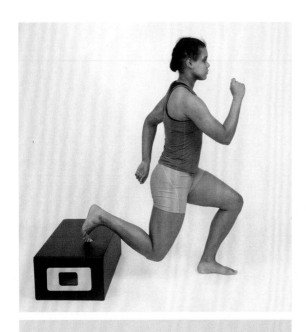

Figure 7.43

Hip abduction capacity: side-lying short-/long-lever plank (Figure 7.44)

- Indications: SIJ, LBP and buttock pain, (2) Lateral gluteal tendon pain, (3) Positive SL stance with loss of lateral hip and trunk control, (4) Positive Trendelenburg sign, (5) ITB syndrome.

- Alignment is maintained to ensure the upper hip is placed in extension.

- Abdominals, particularly emphasizing the oblique muscles, are engaged.

- With the knee bent, a short lever is maintained to ensure a bias in load towards the GMed.

- A modification is to perform this exercise using a TB, or progress to a long-lever plank by extending the knee (Figure 7.45).

Squat with hip abduction capacity: using Pilates ring or TB (Figure 7.46)

- Indications: (1) Precursor to performing a squat, (2) Maintains lateral hip stability and avoids knee valgus,

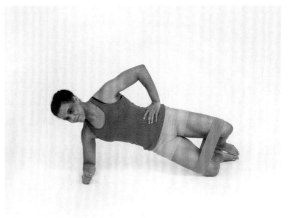

Figure 7.44

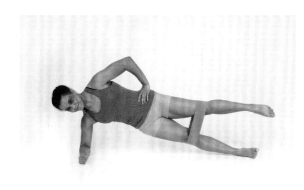

Figure 7.45

(3) Functional progression to address weak links within the kinetic chain.

- Ensure the spinal column is aligned over the pelvis.

- Instruct the patient to sit back into the hips when performing the squat, while abducting against the Pilates ring.

- Specific attention should be paid to ensuring a neutral lumbar spine is maintained and avoiding lumbar kyphosis by squatting too deep.

- Progress to a functional squat.

Sumo squats with lateral walk capacity: TB around feet (Figure 7.47)

- Indications: (1) Targets hip extension in a frontal plane, (2) Precursor to performing a squat.

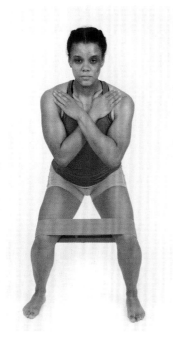

Figure 7.46

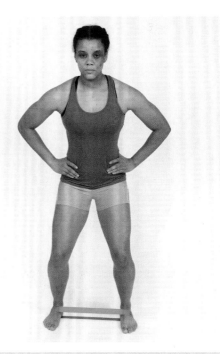

Figure 7.47

- Greater gluteal activation/recruitment is developed with the TB placed around feet.

- Instruct the patient to shoot the foot out and maintain tension in the TB while performing the exercise.

Hip adduction capacity: side-lying isometric plank, short-/long-lever (Figure 7.48)

- Indications: (1) SIJ, symphysis pubis and hip joint pain, (2) Medial knee pain, (3) Recurrent adductor issues.

- Ensure trunk and hip alignment is maintained, engage abdominals, and lift into a side bridge and hold (10–30 seconds).

- Repeat on the opposite side.

- A modification to this exercise is to use a higher step, or move to a long-lever, adductor-capacity, isometric plank (10–30 seconds).

Hip adduction capacity: side-lying isotonic short-/long-lever plank (Figure 7.49)

- The starting position is similar to that for the short-lever isometric adductor plank.

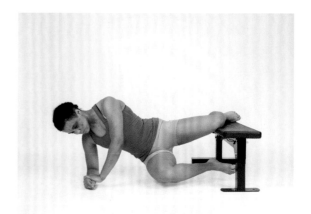

Figure 7.49

- Rather than performing isometric holds, control through the range is developed by performing an isotonic exercise.

- A modification to this exercise is to use a higher step or move to a long-lever, adductor-capacity, isotonic plank.

Squat with hip adduction capacity: with Pilates ring or ball (Figure 7.50)

- Indications: (1) Precursor to performing a squat, (2) Maintains hip stability and maintains knee alignment, (3) Functional progression to address weak links within the kinetic chain.

- Ensure the spinal column is aligned over the pelvis.

- Instruct the patient to sit back into the hips when performing the squat, while squeezing the Pilates ring.

- Specific attention should be paid to ensuring a neutral lumbar spine is maintained and avoiding lumbar kyphosis by squatting too deep.

- A modification to this exercise is the Swiss ball squat, or seated adductor squeeze in the squat position.

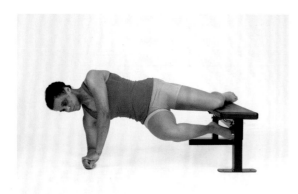

Figure 7.48

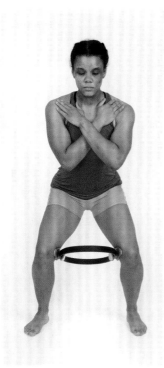

Figure 7.50

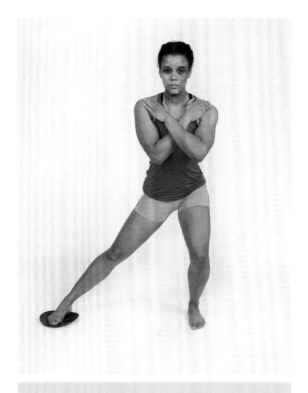

Figure 7.51

Hip adduction capacity: SL slide board (Figure 7.51)

- Indications: (1) Developing outer-range adductor muscle capacity, (2) Recurring adductor-related or pubic-related groin pain.

- The standing leg is stabilized to maintain lateral hip control.

- The patient is instructed to slide the contralateral leg through the range to develop capacity in the adductor muscles.

- Specific attention should be paid to maintaining pelvic alignment, ensuring the range is developed in the hip muscles rather than rotating through the pelvis.

- A modification to this exercise is to use Swiss ball rollouts to develop SL adductor capacity.

Hip adduction/abduction capacity: cable side-steps (Figures 7.52 and 7.53)

- Indications: (1) Develop capacity in the adductor/abductor muscles through the functional range.

- The cable/band is attached around the patient's ankle and they are instructed to take up tension in the cable/band by stepping sideways.

- The patient is instructed to adopt a quarter-squat position and then side-step out or in, to bias the adductor or abductor mechanism.

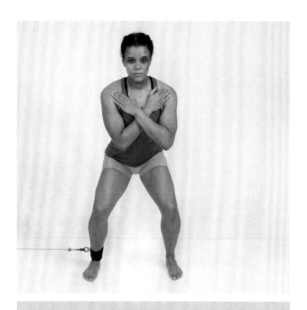

Figure 7.52

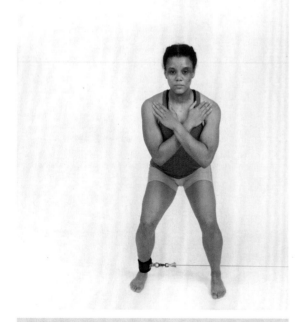

Figure 7.53

Hip extension capacity: high bridge (Figure 7.54)

- Indications: (1) LBP and/or SIJ pain, (2) Gluteal or recurring hamstring pain, (3) Developing posterior chain capacity.

- The patient adopts a DL bridge with the feet placed on a step or bench.

- Abdominal muscles, particularly the obliques, are engaged to prevent the lower ribcage from flaring and the patient is instructed to work through the range.

- A modification of this exercise is progressing to the SL bridge hip extension capacity exercise (Figure 7.55).

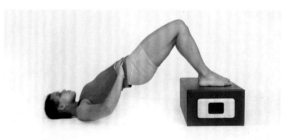

Figure 7.54

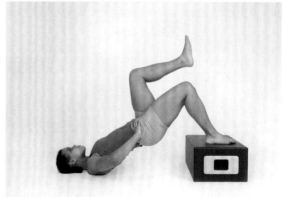

Figure 7.55

- Progression 3: Hip extension capacity on a Swiss ball (Figure 7.56).

- Progression 4: Hip extension capacity on a BOSU board (Figure 7.57).

Hip extension capacity: SL slides (Figure 7.58)

- Indications: (1) Developing outer-range hip extension muscle capacity, (2) Recurring hamstring-related or gluteal-related buttock pain.

- The standing leg is stabilized to maintain lateral control.

- The patient is instructed to slide the contralateral leg through the range to develop capacity in the posterior chain mechanism.

- Specific attention should be paid towards maintaining pelvic alignment, ensuring the range is developed in the hip muscles rather than through the pelvis, by maintaining abdominal contraction.

- A modification to this exercise is the SL hip extension capacity Swiss ball sliders.

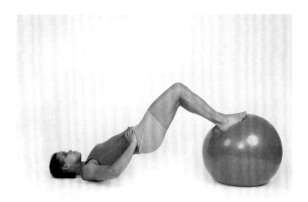

Figure 7.56

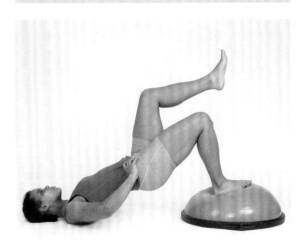

Figure 7.57

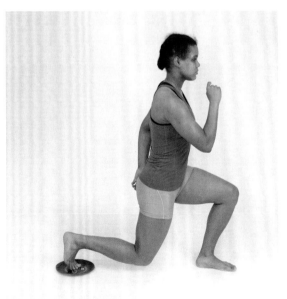

Figure 7.58

Hip extension capacity: SL box steps (Figure 7.59)

- Indications: (1) LBP, SIJ and buttock pain, (2) Developing capacity in the posterior longitudinal sling, (3) Developing capacity in the lateral sling.

- The patient is instructed to place one foot on a step/bench, maintain control through their abdominals and drive up into the step/bench.

- The contralateral knee is raised as high as possible, to ensure maximum gluteal recruitment is achieved on the weight-bearing leg.

Hip extension capacity: Romanian deadlift (RDL) (Figure 7.60)

- Indications: (1) LBP, SIJ, posterior hip pain, (2) Recurring hamstring or posterior longitudinal sling issues.

- The patient is instructed to engage the abdominals and transfer weight on to one leg while maintaining lateral hip stability.

- The non-weight-bearing leg is taken into extension, while the spinal column leans forward.

- Spinal and pelvic alignment is maintained throughout.

- Specific attention should be paid to avoid shifting into frontal or transverse plane motion around the weight-bearing hip.

- A modification to this exercise involves adding weights or using an unstable surface.

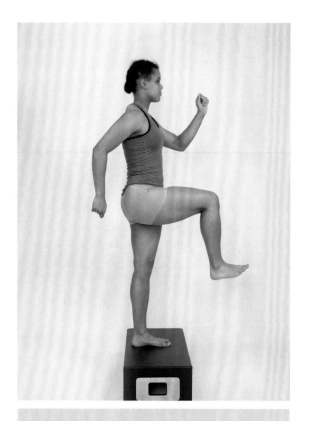

Figure 7.59

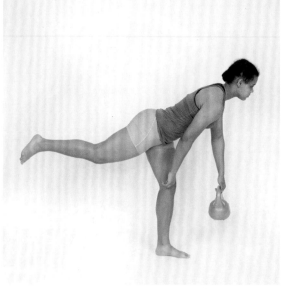

Figure 7.60

Thoracic capacity: segmental rotation with TB (Figure 7.61)

- Indications: (1) Loss of thoracic rotation ROM, (2) Loss of hip joint rotation.

- Encourage sitting back onto the pelvis, if hip and knee joints allow, to minimize lumbar motion.

- One hand is placed behind the head to encourage GHJ external rotation (an alternative position for patients with shoulder pathology is to place one hand behind the back to encourage GHJ internal rotation).

- Active thoracic rotation should be encouraged in an axial plane to increase length through the spine.

Lumbar spine capacity: side-lying lateral flexion, short plank (Figure 7.62)

- Indications: (1) Developing capacity in spinal and abdominal, particularly the oblique, muscles.

- The patient is side lying, resting on their elbow, with knees bent in a short-lever position.

- Abdominal muscles are engaged and the patient is instructed to lift the pelvis off the floor and hold.

- Progression 1: an isometric hold (10–30 seconds).

- Progression 2: an isotonic capacity exercise through the range.

- Progression 3: a long-lever isometric hold (10–30 seconds).

- Progression 4: a long-lever isotonic capacity exercise through the range (Figure 7.63).

- Progression 5: an isometric hold with thoracic arm movement to train spine rotation dissociation (Figure 7.64AB).

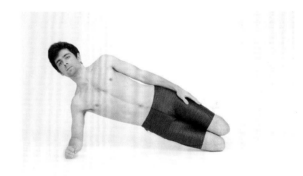

Figure 7.62

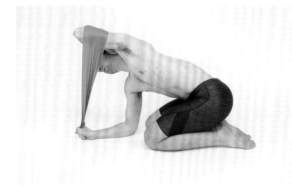

Figure 7.61

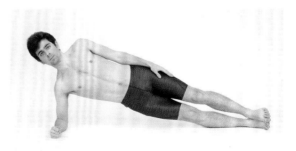

Figure 7.63

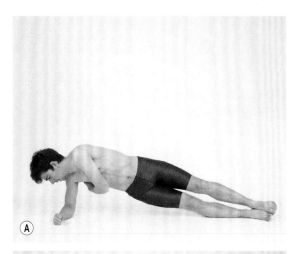

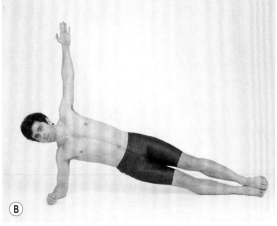

Figure 7.64

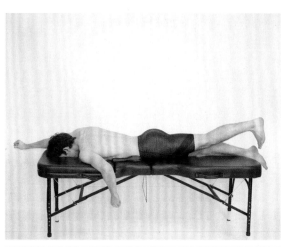

Figure 7.65

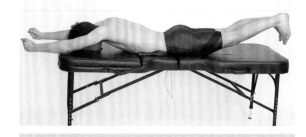

Figure 7.66

Lumbar spine capacity: prone extension (Figure 7.65)

- Indications: (1) Developing capacity in lumbar extensor muscles.

- The patient is prone lying, with a small pillow under the abdominals to reduce lumbar lordosis.

- The patient is instructed to engage the abdominals and raise the opposite arm and leg, holding for 5–10 seconds.

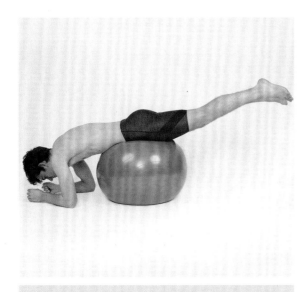

Figure 7.67

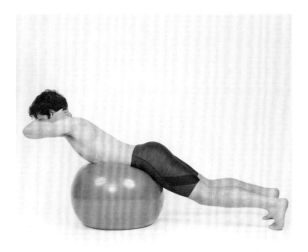

Figure 7.68

- Progression 2: raising both arms and legs (Figure 7.66).

- Progression 3: hip extension capacity over the Swiss ball (Figure 7.67).

- Progression 4: spinal extension capacity over the Swiss ball (Figure 7.68).

Conclusion

In my opinion, having a more in-depth understanding of when and how to use appropriate activation techniques, within the sporting environment and in clinical practice, is a skillful art that should be refined by all clinicians. In my practice, corrective exercises are prescribed to re-establish mobility and to optimize motor control, muscle capacity, and strength in specific muscles, while developing appropriate flexibility in others. The benefit of this approach is that it ensures that the nervous system works more efficiently and effectively, with the correct muscles activating at the correct time and in the correct sequence.

If an athlete can move reasonably well and demonstrates an adequate level of mobility and motor control, but reports fatigue-like symptoms when volume and loading increase, do not waste time attempting to refine their motor control patterns. Instead, challenge their neuromuscular system to develop muscle capacity and, ultimately, strength. Similarly, for any athlete who can demonstrate a reasonable capacity, but reports experiencing pain or symptoms before, during or after exercise, seek to address underlying mobility and motor control deficits, while trying to maintain the capacity to train and compete.

References

Aagaard, P., Simonsen, EB., Andersen, JL. et al., 2002. Increased rate of force development and neural drive of human skeletal muscle following resistance training. *Journal Applied Physiology (1985)*, 93(4), pp. 1318–1326.

Adams, MA. and Dolan, P., 2007. How to use the spine, pelvis, and legs effectively in lifting. In: Vleeming A., Mooney V., Stoeckart R. (eds). *Movement, Stability and Lumbopelvic Pain: Integration of Research and Therapy.* 2nd ed. New York: Churchill Livingstone/Elsevier, pp. 167–183.

Bandy, WD. and Sanders, B., 2001. *Therapeutic Exercise: Techniques for Intervention.* Baltimore: Lippincott Williams & Wilkins.

Billot, M., Martin, A., Paizis, C. et al., 2010. Effects of an electrostimulation training program on strength, jumping and kicking capacities in soccer players. *Journal Strength Conditioning Research*, 24(5), pp. 1407–1413.

Borghuis, J., Hof, AL. and Lemmink, KA., 2008. The importance of sensory motor control in providing core stability: implications for measurement and training. *Sports Medicine*, 38(11), pp. 893–916.

Boyle, M., 2010. *Advances in Functional Training: Training Techniques for Coaches, Personal Trainers and Athletes.* Aptos, CA: On Target Publications, pp. 21–34.

Bradley, H. and Esformes, J., 2014. Breathing pattern disorders and functional movement. *International Journal Sports Physical Therapy*, 9(1), 28–39.

Brown, SH. and McGill, SM., 2008. How the inherent stiffness of the in vivo human trunk varies with changing magnitudes of muscular activation. *Clinical Biomechanics (Bristol, Avon)*, 23(1), pp. 15–22.

Brumagne, S., Lysens, R. and Spaepen, A., 1999. Lumbosacral position sense during pelvic tilting in men and women without low back pain: test development and reliability assessment. *Journal Orthopaedic Sports Physical Therapy*, 29(6), pp. 345–351.

Campbell, A., O'Sullivan, P., Straker, L. et al., 2014. Back pain in tennis players: a link with lumbar serve kinematics and range of motion. *Medicine Science Sports Exercise*, 46(2), pp. 351–357.

Cheung, K., Hume, PA. and Maxwell, L., 2003. Delayed onset muscle soreness. *Sports Medicine*, 33(2), pp. 145–164.

Cholewicki, J. and McGill, SM., 1992. Lumbar posterior ligament involvement during extremely heavy lifts estimated from fluoroscopic measurements. *Journal Biomechanics*, 25(1), pp. 17–28.

Cook, G., Bruton, L., Kiesel, K. et al., 2010. *Movement: Functional Movement Systems. Screening, Assessment, Corrective Strategies.* Aptos, CA: On Target Publications, pp. 26–28.

Cormie, P., McBride, JM. and McCaulley, GO., 2009. Power-time, force-time, and velocity-time curve analysis of the countermovement jump: impact of training. *Journal Strength Conditioning Research*, 23(1), pp. 177–186.

Cormie, P., McGuigan, MR. and Newton, RU., 2011. Developing maximal neuromuscular power: part 1. Biological basis of maximal power production. *Sports Medicine*, 41(1), pp. 17–38.

Croisier, JL., Ganteaume, S., Binet, J. et al., 2008. Strength imbalances and prevention of hamstring injury in professional soccer players: a prospective study. *American Journal Sports Medicine*, 36(8), pp. 1469–1475.

Danneels, LA., Vanderstraeten, GG., Cambier, DC. et al., 2000. CT imaging of trunk muscles in chronic low back pain patients and healthy control subjects. *European Spine Journal*, 9(4), pp. 266–272.

Danneels, LA., Vanderstraeten, GG., Cambier, DC. et al., 2001. Effects of three different training modalities on the cross sectional area of the lumbar multifidus muscle in patients with chronic low back pain. *British Journal Sports Medicine*, 35(3), pp. 186–191.

D'hooge, R., Cagnie, B., Crombez, G. et al., 2012. Increased intramuscular fatty infiltration without differences in lumbar muscle cross-sectional area during remission of unilateral recurrent low back pain. *Manual Therapy*, 17(6), pp. 584–588.

Diedrichsen, J., Shadmehr, R. and Ivry, R., 2010. The coordination of movement: optimal feedback control and beyond. *Trends in Cognitive Sciences*, 14(1), pp. 31–39.

Durall, CJ., Udermann, BE., Johansen, DR. et al., 2009. The effects of preseason trunk muscle training on low-back pain occurrence in women collegiate gymnasts. *Journal Strength Conditioning Research*, 23(1), pp. 86–92.

Falvey, EC., King, E., Kinsella, S. et al., 2016. Athletic groin pain (part 1): a prospective anatomical diagnosis of 382 patients – clinical findings, MRI findings and patient-reported outcome measures at baseline. *British Journal Sports Medicine*, 50, pp. 423–430.

Frost, R., 2002. *Applied Kinesiology: A Training Manual and Reference Book of Basic Principles and Practice.* Berkeley, CA: North Atlantic.

Garland, SJ. and McComas, AJ., 1990. Reflex inhibition of human soleus during fatigue. *Journal Physiology*, 429(1), pp. 17–27.

Gondin, J., Cozzone, PJ. and Bendahan, D., 2011. Is high frequency neuromuscular stimulation a suitable tool for muscle performance improvement in both healthy humans and athletes? *European Journal Applied Physiology*, 111(10), pp. 2473–2487.

Graham, RB. and Brown, SH., 2012. A direct comparison of spine rotational stiffness and dynamic spine stability during repetitive lifting tasks. *Journal Biomechanics*, 45(9), pp. 1593–1600.

Greenman, P., 1996. *Principles of Manual Medicine*. 5th ed. Philadelphia: Lippincott Williams and Wilkins.

Griffin, DR., Dickerson, EJ., O'Donnell, J. et al., 2016. The Warwick Agreement on femoroacetabular impingement syndrome (FAI syndrome): an international consensus statement. *British Journal Sports Medicine*, 50, pp. 1169–1176.

Hides, JA., Boughen, CL., Stanton, WR. et al., 2010. A magnetic resonance imaging investigation of the transversus abdominis muscle during drawing-in of the abdominal wall in elite Australian Football League players with and without low back pain. *Journal Orthopaedic Sports Physical Therapy*, 40(1), pp. 4–10.

Hodges, PW., 2011. Pain and motor control: from the laboratory to rehabilitation. *Journal Electromyography Kinesiology*, 21(2), pp. 220–228.

Hodges, P. and Moseley, G., 2003. Pain and motor control of the lumbopelvic region: effect and possible mechanisms. *Journal Electromyography Kinesiology*, 13(4), pp. 361–370.

Hodges, PW., Eriksson, AE., Shirley, D. et al., 2005. Intra-abdominal pressure increases stiffness of the lumbar spine. *Journal Biomechanics*, 38(9), pp. 1873–1880.

Hodges, P., Sapsford, R., Pengel, L., 2007. Postural and respiratory functions of the pelvic floor muscles. *Neurourology Urodynamics*, 26, pp. 362–371.

Hölmich, P., 2007. Long-standing groin pain in sportspeople falls into three primary patterns, a "clinical entity" approach: a prospective study of 207 patients. *British Journal Sports Medicine*, 41, pp. 247–252.

Iles, JF., 1986. Reciprocal inhibition during agonist and antagonist contraction. *Experimental Brain Research*, 62, pp. 212–214.

Iosia, MF. and Bishop, PA., 2008. Analysis of exercise-to-rest ratios during division 1A televised football competition. *Journal Strength Conditioning Research*, 22(2), pp. 332–340.

Jessen, R.L. and Ebben, WP., 2003. Kinetic analysis of complex training rest interval effect on vertical jump performance. *Journal Strength Conditioning Research*, 17, pp. 345–349.

Jones, P. and Lees, A., 2003. A biomechanical analysis of the acute effects of complex training using lower limb exercises. *Journal Strength Conditioning Research*, 17, pp. 694–700.

Jones, MA., Stratton, G., Reilly, T. et al., 2005. Biological risk indicators for recurrent non-specific low back pain in adolescents. *British Journal Sports Medicine*, 39(3), pp. 137–140.

Kilduff, L., Bevan, H., Kingsley, M. et al., 2007. Postactivation potentiation in professional rugby players: optimal recovery. *Journal Strength and Conditioning Research*, 21(4), pp. 1134–1138.

King, E., Franklyn-Miller, A., Richter, C. et al., 2018. Clinical and biomechanical outcomes of rehabilitation targeting intersegmental control in athletic groin pain: prospective cohort of 205 patients. *British Journal Sports Medicine*, 52, pp. 1054–1062.

Langberg, H., Skovgaard, D., Asp, S. et al., 2000. Time pattern of exercise-induced changes in type I collagen turnover after prolonged endurance exercise in humans. *Calcified Tissue International*, 67(1), pp. 41–44.

Langevin, HM. and Sherman, KJ., 2007. Pathophysiological model for chronic low back pain integrating connective tissue and nervous system mechanisms. *Medical Hypotheses*, 68(1), pp. 74–80.

Lee, D., 2011. *The Pelvic Girdle: An Integration of Clinical Expertise and Research*. 4th ed. Edinburgh: Churchill Livingstone, Elsevier.

Lewit, K., 1994. The functional approach. *Journal Orthopaedic Medicine*, 16(3), pp. 73–74.

Lindsay, M., 2008. *Fascia: Clinical Applications for Health and Human Performance*. Clifton Park, NY: Cengage Learning.

Lindsay, D. and Horton, J., 2002. Comparison of spine motion in elite golfers with and without low back pain. *Journal Sports Science*, 20(8), pp. 599–605.

MacDonald, DA., Moseley, GL. and Hodges, PW., 2006. The lumbar multifidus: does the evidence support clinical beliefs? *Manual Therapy*, 11(4), pp. 254–263.

McGill, S., 2004. *Ultimate Back Fitness and Performance*. Waterloo, Ontario: Wabuno.

"Maximum Voluntary Contraction.," 2012. In: *Medical Dictionary for Health Professions and Nursing*. Huntingdon Valley, PA: Farlex.

Mihata, T., Gates, J., McGarry, MH. et al., 2009. Effect of rotator cuff muscle imbalance on forceful internal impingement and peel-back of the superior labrum. *American Journal Sports Medicine*, 37(11), pp. 2222–2227.

Monnier, A., Heuer, J., Norman, K. et al., 2012. Inter- and intra-observer reliability of clinical movement-control tests for marines. *BMC Musculoskeletal Disorders*, 13, pp. 263.

Naito, H., Yoshihara, T., Kakigi, R. et al., 2012. Heat stress-induced changes in skeletal muscle: heat shock proteins and cell signaling transduction. *Journal Physical Fitness and Sports Medicine*, 1(1), pp. 125–131.

Newton, RU. and Kraemer, WJ., 1994. Developing explosive muscular power: implications for a mixed methods training strategy. *Strength and Conditioning*, 16(5), pp. 20–31.

Oscar, E., 2012. *Corrective Exercise Solutions to Common Hip and Shoulder Dysfunction*. Chichester: Lotus.

Page, P., Frank, CC. and Lardner, R., 2010. Chapter 10 – Restoration of Muscle Balance. In *Assessment and Treatment of Muscle Imbalance: The Janda Approach*. Champaign, IL: Human Kinetics, p. 145.

Panjabi, MM., 2003. Clinical spinal instability and low back pain. *Journal Electromyography Kinesiology*, 13(4), pp. 371–379.

Powers, CM., 2003. The influence of altered lower-extremity kinematics on patellofemoral joint dysfunction: a theoretical perspective. *Journal Orthopaedic Sports Physical Therapy*, 33(11), pp. 639–646.

Ratamess, NA., Alvar, A., Evetoch, TK. et al., 2009. American College of Sports Medicine position stand: progression models in resistance training for healthy adults. *Medicine Science Sports Exercise*, 41(3), pp. 687–708.

Reiman, M. and Lorenz, D., 2011. Integration of strength and conditioning principles into a rehabilitation program. *International Journal Sports Physiotherapy*, 6(3), pp. 241–253.

Rhea, MR., Hunter, RL. and Hunter, TJ., 2006. Competition modeling of American football: observational data and implications for high school, collegiate, and professional player conditioning. *Journal Strength Conditioning Research*, 20(1), pp. 58–61.

Robbins, DW., 2005. Postactivation potentiation and its practical applicability: a brief review. *Journal Strength Conditioning Research*, 19(2), pp. 453–458.

Sahrmann, S., 2002. *Diagnosis and Treatment of Movement Impairment Syndromes*. St Louis: Mosby, pp. 12–15.

Shan, G. and Westerhoff, P., 2005. Soccer. *Sports Biomechanics*, 4(1), pp. 59–72.

Siff, MC., 2003. Strength and fitness. In: Siff, MC. (ed.). *Supertraining*. 6th ed. Denver: Supertraining Institute, pp. 32–33.

Smith, B., Hendrick, P., Smith, T. et al., 2017. Should exercises be painful in the management of chronic musculoskeletal pain? A systematic review and meta-analysis. *British Journal Sports Medicine*, 51, pp. 1679–1687.

Spencer, S., Wolf, A. and, Rushton, A., 2016. Spinal-exercise prescription in sport: classifying physical training and rehabilitation by intention and outcome. *Journal Athletic Training*, 51(8), pp. 613–628.

Stone, MH., Sands, WA., Carlock, J. et al., 2004. The importance of isometric maximum strength and peak rate-of-force development in sprint cycling. *Journal Strength Conditioning Research*, 18(4), pp. 878–884.

Suter, E. and Lindsay, D., 2001. Back muscle fatigability is associated with knee extensor inhibition in subjects with low back pain. *Spine*, 26(16), pp. E361–E366.

Tak, I. and Langhout, R., 2014. Groin injuries in soccer. *Aspetar Journal Sports Medicine*, 3, pp. 272–277.

Thorstensson, A. and Carlson, H., 1987. Fibre types in human lumbar back muscles. *Acta Physiology Scandinavica*, 131(2), pp. 195–202.

Tsao, H. and Hodges, PW., 2007. Immediate changes in feed forward postural adjustments following voluntary motor training. *Experimental Brain Research*, 181(4), pp. 537–546.

Tsao, H. and Hodges, PW., 2008. Persistence of improvements in postural strategies following motor control training in people with recurrent low back pain. *Journal Electromyography Kinesiology*, 18(4), pp. 559–567.

Tsao, H., Druitt, TR., Schollum, TM. et al., 2010. Motor training of the lumbar paraspinal muscles induces immediate changes in motor coordination in patients with recurrent low back pain. *Journal Pain*, 11(11), pp. 1120–1128.

Umphred, D., 2007. *Neurological Rehabilitation*. 5th ed. St Louis: Mosby/Elsevier.

Vad, VB., Bhat, AL., Basrai, D. et al., 2004. Low back pain in professional golfers: the role of associated hip and low back range-of-motion deficits. *American Journal Sports Medicine*, 32(2), pp. 494–497.

Van Cutsem, M., Duchateau, J. and Hainaut, K., 1998. Changes in single motor unit behaviour contribute to the increase in contraction speed after dynamic training in humans. *Journal Physiology*, 513(1), pp. 295–305.

van Dieën, J. and de Looze, M., 1999. Directionality of anticipatory activation of trunk muscles in a lifting task depends on load knowledge. *Experimental Brain Research*, 128(3), pp. 397–404.

Van Dillen, LR., Sahrmann, SA., Norton, BJ. et al., 1998. Reliability of physical examination items used for classification of patients with low back pain. *Physical Therapy*, 78(9), pp. 979–988.

Vickery, R., 2007. *The Effect of Breathing Pattern Retraining on Performance in Competitive Cyclists.* Available at: <https://citeseerx.ist.psu.edu/viewdoc/download?doi=10.1.1.839.9081&rep=rep1&type=pdf> [accessed February 22, 2022].

Walther, DS., 2000. *Applied Kinesiology: Synopsis.* 2nd ed. Pueblo, CO: Systems DC.

Watkins, RG., Uppal, GS., Perry, J. et al., 1996. Dynamic electromyographic analysis of trunk musculature in professional golfers. *American Journal Sports Medicine*, 24(4), pp. 535–538.

Chapter 8 structure

Introduction	253
Lumbar facet-related pain	254
Lumbar disk-related pain	256
Sacroiliac joint-related pain	258
Pubic-related groin pain	261
Hip joint-related pain	264
Adductor-related pain	266
Psoas-related pain	269
Abdominal-related pain	271
Conclusion	273

Introduction

 In this chapter, my goal is to highlight how to *integrATE* the "five 'ATEs" approach for managing the spino-pelvic-hip complex. I am using a simplified structure to manage some of the more common issues affecting this region. I should emphasize that these bullet points are not exhaustive and are aimed at providing a quick "go-to guide" for the more inexperienced clinician. A battery or cluster of clinical and functional tests can be used to *evaluATE* the patient. This helps to inform the clinical reasoning process and promote a deeper understanding to enable the clinician to create a working hypothesis.

 Symptom modification techniques, or mini treatments, can be used to *educATE* individuals on how they may help themselves. These can take the form of either a combination of manual therapy techniques, to *manipulATE* soft tissue or joint restrictions, and/or movement-based exercises to *activATE* dysfunctional tissues.

 Cases that involve patients or athletes who demonstrate signs and have symptoms of movement restrictions may initially respond well to manual techniques to *manipulATE* their restricted tissues. However, we should also consider that patients who present with movement control issues may also respond to an element of manual therapy, if it is used appropriately. Remember, very often movement and control issues coincide (occur together).

 Patients who present specifically with movement control issues can generally perform and demonstrate adequate ROM, but often exhibit "shifting," "catching" or "hinging" actions when they are asked to carry out ROM tests. This is commonly seen in the spinal column during clinical evaluation. This particular subgroup of patients will always respond better to motor control movement strategies to *activATE* their tissues, rather than endless hours of unnecessary manual therapy.

Similarly, the *activATE* approach is beneficial for patients who report increasingly frequent episodes of pain that fail to resolve, despite seeking the expert opinion of numerous manual therapy specialists. In my experience, this subgroup also responds better to appropriate exercises that *activATE* their neuromusculoskeletal system.

The guide in this chapter is presented as a list of bullet points, pertaining to the *evaluATE, educATE, manipulATE and activATE* components of the "five 'ATEs." Clinicians should be aware that there is no one particular starting point that is more important than the others. Remember: in Chapter 1 I stressed that one of the strengths of the "five 'ATEs" was the flexibility it offers clinicians. Furthermore, the ability to select or prioritize one bullet point over another is, in my opinion, down to the discretion of the clinician and the situation that they may be dealing with at that time.

The functional or clinical tests highlighted in the *evaluATE* sections are not the only tests that can be used to examine the eight conditions that I address in this chapter. Similarly, I have only suggested techniques that I find extremely useful to *manipulATE* soft tissue or joint restrictions associated with these musculoskeletal conditions. Other clinicians may use different manipulative approaches that they have become comfortable with over years of practice. Exercises that I have described in the bullet point lists to *activATE* weak or inhibited muscles are by no means exhaustive and I would propose that the present chapter, and this book as a whole, act only as a starting point for further exploring and understanding the management of the spino-pelvic-hip complex.

In my opinion, any exercise, prescribed correctly, should benefit the patient or athlete directly and help reinforce the goals that have been discussed, agreed and set, once the functional and clinical aspects of *evalu-ATE* have been undertaken. This helps to *educATE* the patient and can take many forms, from utilizing manual therapy techniques such as *manipulATE* for pain modification, to using exercise prescription to address movement control deficits to *activATE* deconditioned neuromyofascial tissues.

What follows, then, is a concise "go to guide" to assist the continuum of clinical care of some common conditions associated with the spino-pelvic-hip complex.

Lumbar facet-related pain

EvaluATE

- Lumbar extension motion
- Lumbar quadrant test (Figure 8.1) (Stuber et al., 2014; Laslett et al., 2006)
- Thoracic segmental passive evaluation
- Adapted Thomas test (Reiman et al., 2015)
- Prone knee bend (Anloague et al., 2015)
- Femoral nerve (Figure 8.2) (Butler, 2010; Shacklock, 2005; Tawa et al., 2017).

EducATE

- Thoracic spine self-mobilization and dissociation (Figure 8.3)
- Anterior hip stretches (Figure 8.4) (iliopsoas, rectus femoris, TFL)
- Lumbar spine segmental motor control
- Sitting, driving, sleeping positions.

ManipulATE

- Thoracic spine T4–9 (articular mobilization, MET, HVLA)

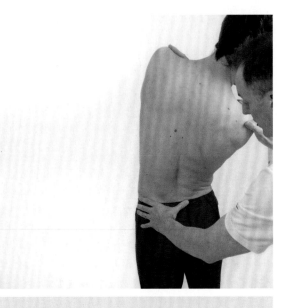

Figure 8.1
Lumbar quadrant test.

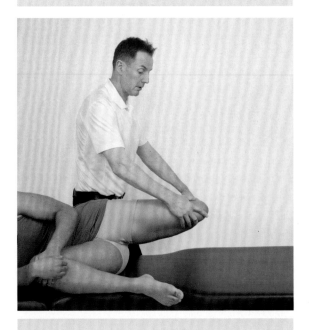

Figure 8.2
Femoral nerve evaluation.

- Thoracolumbar spine dependent on level of hypomobility (articular mobilization, MET, HVLA) (Figure 8.5)

- Anterior hip capsule (mobilization) (Figure 8.6)

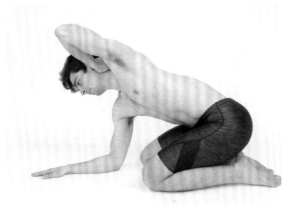

Figure 8.3
Self-mobilization of thoracic spine.

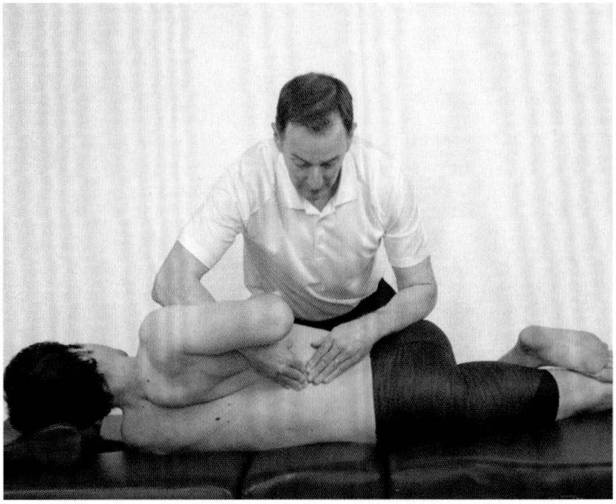

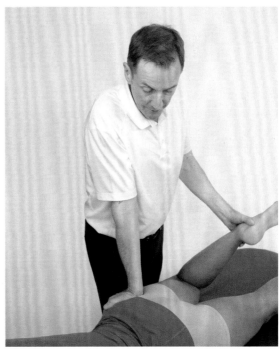

Figure 8.5
HVLA thoracolumbar spine.

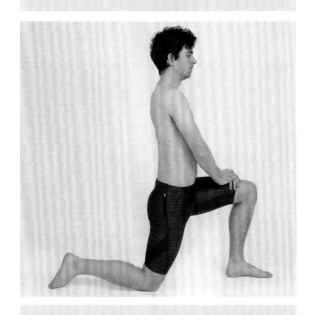

Figure 8.4
Anterior hip stretch.

Figure 8.6
Anterior hip capsule mobilization.

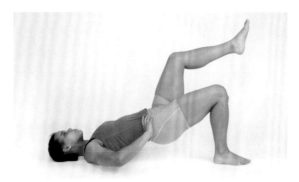

Figure 8.7
Lumbar segmental control (single-leg bridge).

- Iliopsoas, rectus femoris, TFL (soft tissue manipulation, MET)

- Femoral nerve (neural sliders/tensioners).

ActivATE

- Lumbar segmental motor control (DL bridge, SL bridge) (Figure 8.7)

- Thoracic spine dissociation (quadruped heel to pelvis)

- Gluteus maximus (hip hinge, reverse lunge, box step) (Figure 8.8).

Lumbar disk-related pain
EvaluATE

- Lumbar flexion motion

- Spinal segmental passive evaluation (Figure 8.9) (Haneline et al., 2008)

- Squat pattern

- Neurological evaluation – slump sitting (Figure 8.10) (Majlesi et al., 2008), SLR (Majlesi et al., 2008), power, reflexes, two-point discrimination

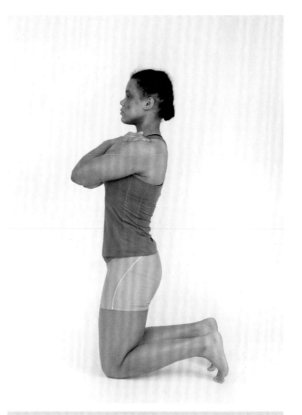

Figure 8.8
Hip hinge.

- Seated and active piriformis evaluation (Martin et al., 2014).

EducATE

- Hip hinge

- Retrain squat pattern (Figure 8.11)

- Lumbar segmental motor control

- Neural mobilization (Figure 8.12)

- Sitting, driving, sleeping positions.

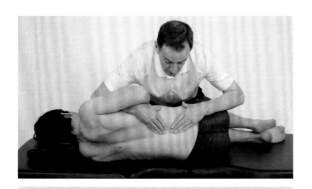

Figure 8.9
Passive physiological segmental evaluation.

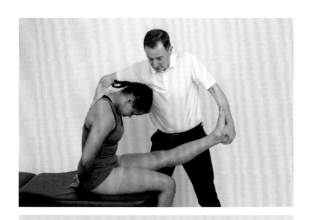

Figure 8.10
Slump sitting evaluation.

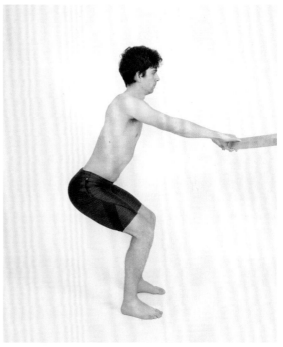

Figure 8.11
Retrain squat pattern.

ManipulATE

- Thoracic spine T4–9 (articular mobilization, MET, HVLA)

- Thoracolumbar spine, dependent on level of hypomobility (articular mobilization, MET, HVLA)

- Piriformis (inhibition techniques, MET) (Figure 8.13)

- Sciatic nerve mobilization (Figure 8.14) (neural sliders or tensioners).

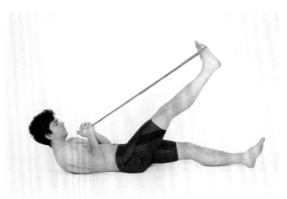

Figure 8.12
Neural mobilization.

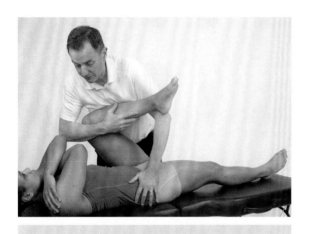

Figure 8.13
Piriformis MET.

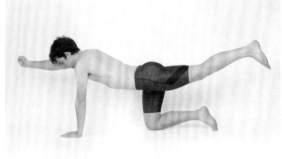

Figure 8.15
Bird dog.

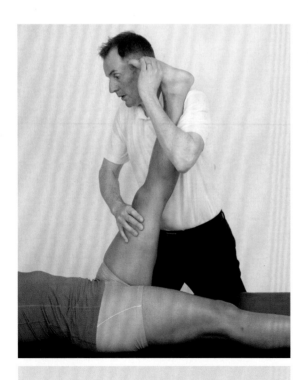

Figure 8.14
Sciatic nerve mobilization.

ActivATE

- Waiter's bow and squat pattern

- Lumbar segmental motor control (DL bridge, side-lying bridge, four-point kneeling, bird dog) (Figure 8.15)

- Posterior chain muscle capacity (lumbar spine lateral flexion short-lever plank, squat, Romanian deadlift, reverse lunge

- Self practice: neural mobilizations (Figure 8.16).

Sacroiliac joint-related pain

EvaluATE

- SL stance test (Figure 8.17) (Lequesne et al., 2008; Hungerford et al., 2007; Youdas et al., 2007)

- ASLR in supine with or without reinforcement (Mens et al., 2006; Vleeming et al., 1990ab)

- Thigh thrust (Figure 8.18) (Laslett et al., 2005)

- Positional and passive pelvic evaluation (Lee, 2011; Laslett et al., 2005; Dreyfuss et al., 1996; 1994)

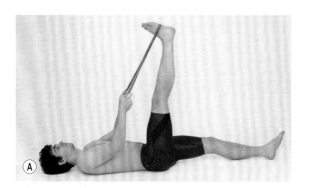
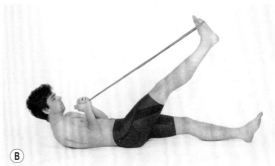

Figure 8.16
Self neural mobilizations similar to 8.12.

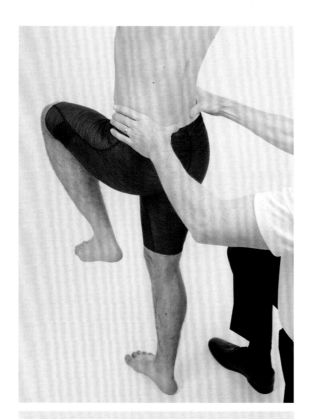

Figure 8.17
Single-leg stance test.

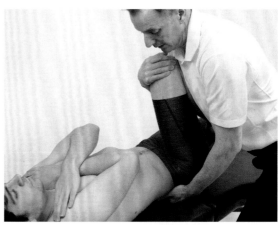

Figure 8.18
Thigh thrust test.

- Spinal segmental passive evaluation (Haneline et al., 2008)

- Adductor passive evaluation (Hölmich et al., 2004)

- Inner-range gluteus medius control

- Seated and active piriformis evaluation (Martin et al., 2014).

EducATE

- Adductor frontal plane mobility (Figure 8.19)
- Abductor frontal plane motor control
- Thoracolumbar spinal mobility (Figure 8.20)
- SL stance load/unload with SKB
- Sitting, driving, sleeping position.

ManipulATE

- Thoracolumbar or SIJ manipulation (Figure 8.21) (HVLA, MET)
- Symphysis pubis (MET)

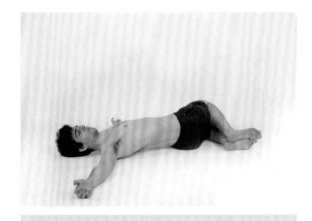

Figure 8.20
Thoracolumbar spinal mobility.

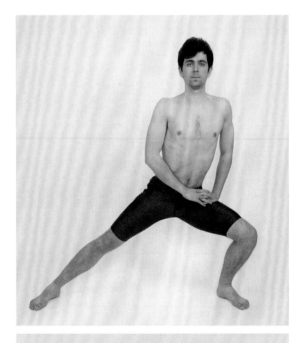

Figure 8.19
Adductor flexibility.

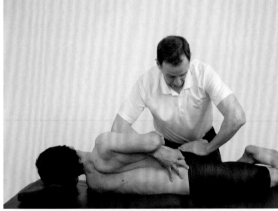

Figure 8.21
Manipulation sacroiliac joint.

- Adductor mechanism (Figure 8.22) (soft tissue manipulation, MET)
- TFL/ITB (soft tissue manipulation, MET).

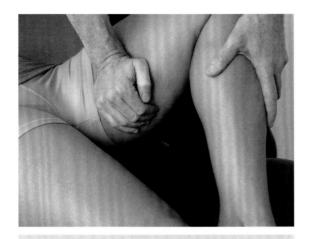

Figure 8.22
STM adductors.

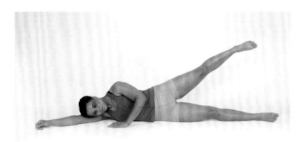

Figure 8.23
Inner-range hip abduction side-lying.

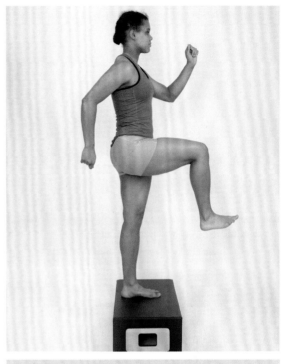

Figure 8.24
Box step.

ActivATE

- Inner-range hip abduction side-lying (Figure 8.23)

- Hip extension with abduction bias (gluteus maximus and medius)

- Box step (Figure 8.24)

- Thoracolumbar rotation (quadruped heel to pelvis).

Pubic-related groin pain

EvaluATE

- SL stance test load/unload (Lequesne et al., 2008; Hungerford et al., 2007; Youdas et al., 2007)

- ASLR in supine with or without reinforcement (Figure 8.25) (Mens et al., 2006; Vleeming et al., 1990ab)

- Adductor strength in straight leg neutral (that is, no rotation) (Figure 8.26) (Mens et al., 2002)

- Positional and passive pelvic evaluation (Lee, 2011; Laslett et al., 2005; Dreyfuss et al., 1996; 1994)

- Hip joint motion.

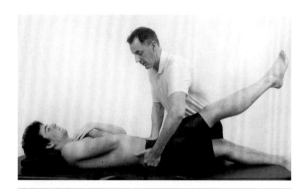

Figure 8.25
ASLR in supine.

EducATE

- Pelvic reinforcement
- Lower abdominal activation (Figure 8.27)

- Psoas activation

- Adductor activation (Figure 8.28).

ManipulATE

- Thoracolumbar or SIJ manipulation (HVLA, MET)

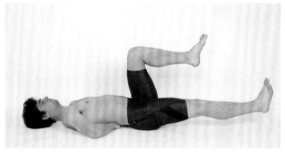

Figure 8.27
Lower abdominal activation.

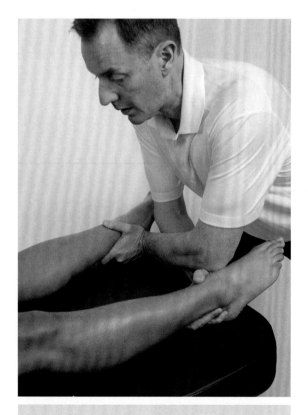

Figure 8.26
Adductor strength.

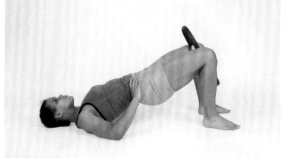

Figure 8.28
Adductor activation.

- Symphysis pubis (MET) (Figure 8.29)

- Hip joint articular mobilization and capsular stretching

- Adductor mechanism (soft tissue manipulation, MET) (Figure 8.30)

- Lower abdominals, obliques and iliacus (soft tissue manipulation)

- TFL/ITB (soft tissue manipulation, MET).

 ActivATE

- Adductors (isometric squeezes with Pilates ring) (Figure 8.31), outer-range adductor sliders, modified short-lever isometric Copenhagen (Figure 8.32)

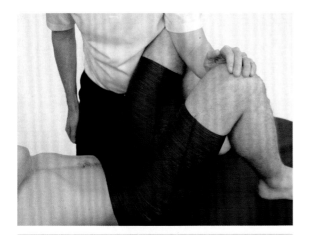

Figure 8.29
MET symphysis pubis.

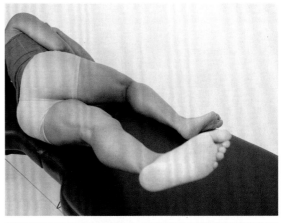

Figure 8.31
Adductor isometric activation.

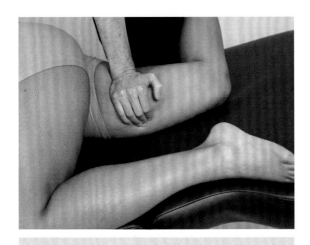

Figure 8.30
STM adductors.

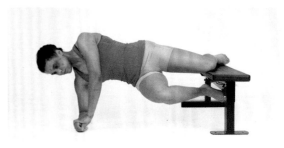

Figure 8.32
Short-lever isometric plank (Copenhagen).

- Lower abdominals (heel slides, modified dead bug, side-lying modified short-lever Sorenson)

- Psoas (thigh bone to socket "suction," progressing to inner-range hip flexion and outer-range eccentric hip control)

- All the above with or without pelvic reinforcement (that is, manual pressure applied by clinician).

Hip joint-related pain

EvaluATE

- Hip joint FADIR evaluation (Figure 8.33) (Reiman et al., 2015)

- Hip joint FABER evaluation (Figure 8.34) (Cibulka et al., 2009)

- SIJ thigh thrust evaluation (Laslett et al., 2005)

- SL stance test (Lequesne et al., 2008; Hungerford et al., 2007; Youdas et al., 2007)

- Spinal segmental passive evaluation (Haneline et al., 2008)

- Positional and passive pelvic evaluation (Lee, 2011; Laslett et al., 2005; Dreyfuss et al., 1996; 1994)

- Seated hip flexion evaluation

- Inner-range hip abduction evaluation.

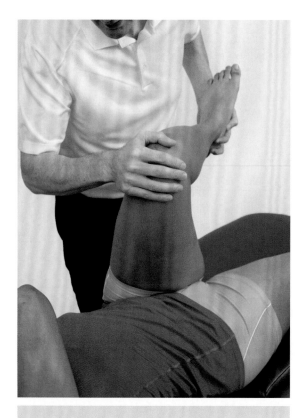

Figure 8.33
Hip joint FADIR.

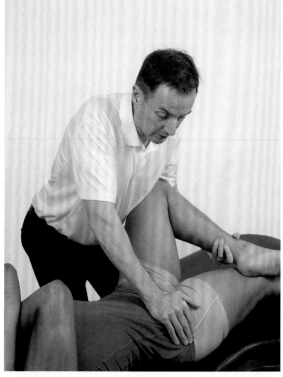

Figure 8.34
Hip joint FABER.

EducATE

- Inner-range hip flexion control (Figure 8.35)
- Inner-range hip abduction control (Figure 8.36)
- Sitting, driving, sleeping positions.

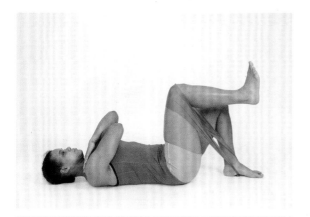

Figure 8.35
Inner-range hip flexion control.

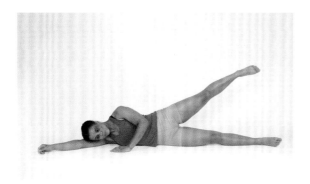

Figure 8.36
Inner-range hip abduction control.

ManipulATE

- TFL/ITB (Figure 8.37), adductors, piriformis (soft tissue mobilization, MET)
- Hip joint capsular mobilizations (anterior/posterior) (Figure 8.38)
- Hip joint articular mobilization, combined with traction or Mulligan mobilization belt.

ActivATE

- Supine inner-range hip flexion control with TB (Figure 8.39), progressing to seated and standing (Figure 8.40)
- Side-lying inner-range hip abduction control
- Retrain squat pattern
- Retrain SL stance in SKB (gym ball against a wall), progressing to box step.

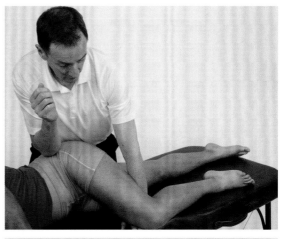

Figure 8.37
STM tensor fasciae latae/iliotibial band.

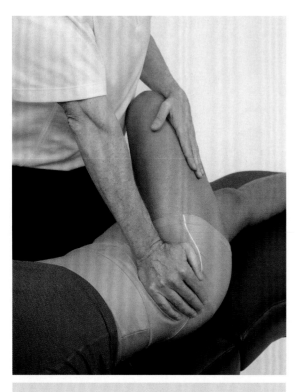

Figure 8.38
Hip joint capsular mobilization.

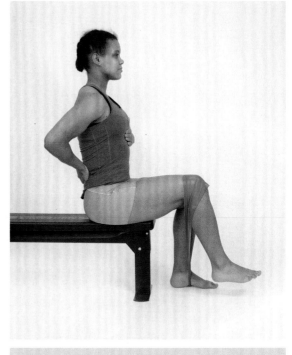

Figure 8.40
Inner-range seated hip flexion with Theraband®.

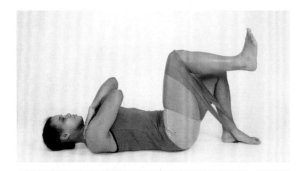

Figure 8.39
Inner-range supine hip flexion with Theraband® similar to Figure 8.35.

Adductor-related pain

EvaluATE

- Adductor mobility evaluation (Figure 8.41) (Hölmich et al., 2004)

- Adductor strength in straight leg squeeze (Figure 8.42) (Mens et al., 2002)

- Adductor strength testing at 45° squeeze (Verrall et al., 2005)

- Adductor strength testing at 90° squeeze (Verrall et al., 2005)

- Adductor SL outer-range strength testing (Verrall et al., 2005)

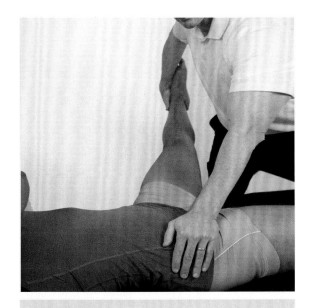

Figure 8.41
Adductor flexibility.

- Adduction palpation evaluation (Serner et al., 2016; Hölmich et al., 2004)

- Adductor side-lying inner-range control in hip neutral and hip internal, external rotation

- Hip joint articular motion (Reiman et al., 2015; Cibulka et al., 2009)

- SIJ thigh thrust (Laslett et al., 2005)

- Thoracolumbar segmental evaluation (Haneline et al., 2008)

- Obturator nerve testing (Butler, 2010; Shacklock, 2005).

 EducATE

- Use of SIJ belt for pelvic reinforcement (Figure 8.43)

- Frontal plane mobility

- Frontal plane stability

- Thoracolumbar mobility (Figure 8.44)

- Active pelvic tilt.

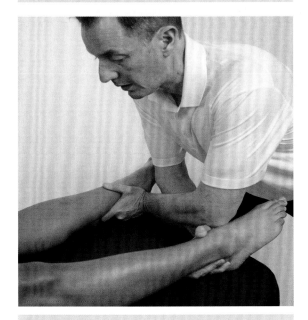

Figure 8.42
Adductor strength in straight leg squeeze.

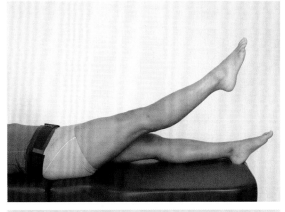

Figure 8.43
Sacroiliac joint belt for pelvic reinforcement.

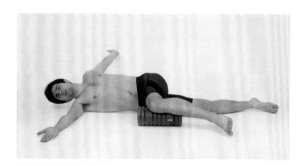

Figure 8.44
Thoracolumbar mobility.

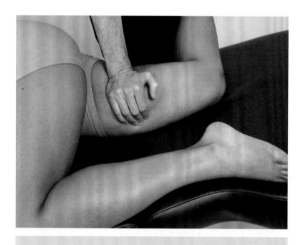

Figure 8.45
STM adductor muscles (side-lying).

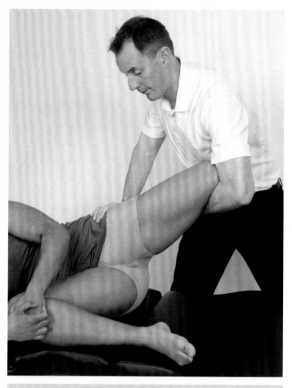

Figure. 8.46
Obturator nerve mobilization.

- Obturator nerve mobilization (Figure 8.46) (neural sliders or tensioners).

 ActivATE

- Adductors (isometric squeezes with Pilates ring in neutral and inner range) (DL bridge) (Figure 8.47)

- Adductor outer-range control through range (floor or Swiss ball sliders)

- Adductor capacity with resistance band/cables/free weights (Figure 8.48)

- Adductor side-lying plank (modified Copenhagen).

 ManipulATE

- Lower thoracic spine T6–9, thoracolumbar spine, SIJ and symphysis pubis (HVLA, MET)

- Hip joint (articular and soft tissue manipulation)

- Adductors (Figure 8.45) (soft tissue mobilization, MET)

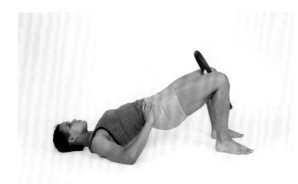

Figure 8.47
Adductor isometric squeeze in hip extension (double-leg bridge).

Psoas-related pain

EvaluATE

- Seated hip flexion evaluation (Figure 8.49)

- ASLR (Vleeming et al., 1990ab)

- Adapted Ober's test (Reese and Bandy, 2003)

- Adapted Thomas test (Reiman et al., 2015)

- Positional and passive evaluation (Lee, 2011; Laslett et al., 2005; Dreyfuss et al., 1996; 1994) (Figure 8.50)

- Respiration control evaluation (Hodges et al., 2005; Lewit, 1994; Greenman, 1990)

- Thoracolumbar segmental evaluation (Haneline et al., 2008)

- Femoral and obturator nerve adverse neural tension.

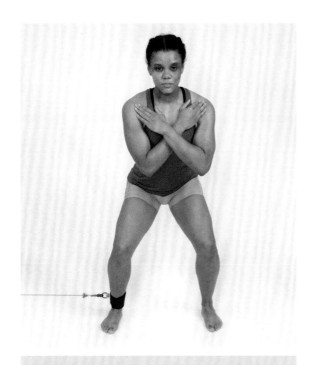

Figure 8.48
Adductor capacity with resistance bands (standing).

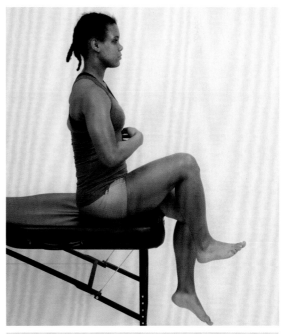

Figure 8.49
Seated hip flexion evaluation.

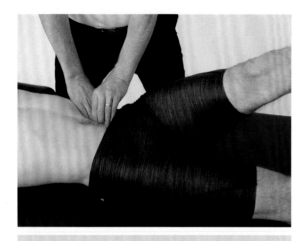

Figure 8.50
Palpation of deep psoas with ASLR.

EducATE

- Rectus femoris and TFL mobility (Figure 8.51)

- Thoracolumbar mobility (quadruped heel to bottom)

- Psoas activation techniques (supine or prone lying) (Figure 8.52)

- Sitting, driving, sleeping positions.

ManipulATE

- TFL/ITB, iliacus and rectus femoris (soft tissue manipulation, MET)

- Femoral nerve and obturator nerve mobilizations (neural sliders and tensioners) (Figure 8.53)

- Lower thoracic T6–9, thoracolumbar junction and SIJ (HVLA, MET) (Figure 8.54).

ActivATE

- Deep fibers of psoas in inner range (hip suction, TB in supine, sitting – Figure 8.55, standing)

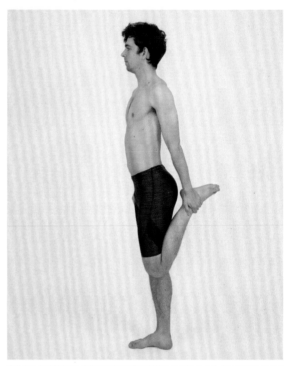

Figure 8.51
Anterior thigh stretching.

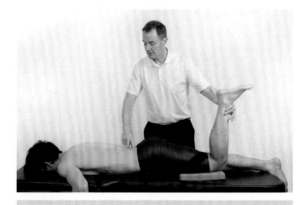

Figure 8.52
Psoas activation techniques.

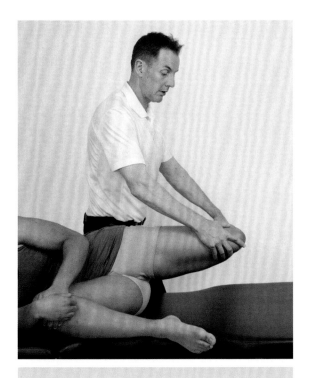

Figure 8.53
Femoral nerve mobilization.

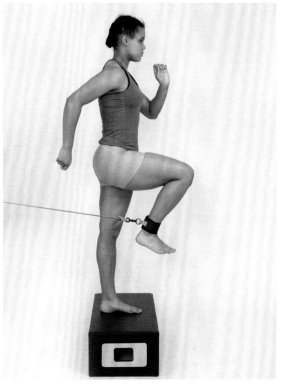

Figure 8.55
Psoas hip flexion activation.

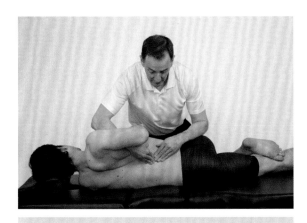

Figure 8.54
HVLA thoracolumbar spine.

- Standing SL heel slides (Figure 8.56)
- High box step
- Reverse lunge
- Bulgarian split squat.

 Abdominal-related pain

EvaluATE

- ASLR in supine with or without pelvic reinforcement (Figure 8.57) (Mens et al., 2006; Vleeming et al., 1990ab)
- Positional and passive pelvic evaluation (Lee, 2011)

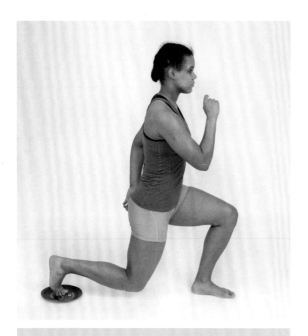

Figure 8.56
Standing single-leg heel slides.

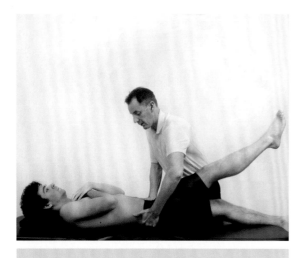

Figure 8.57
ASLR with reinforcement.

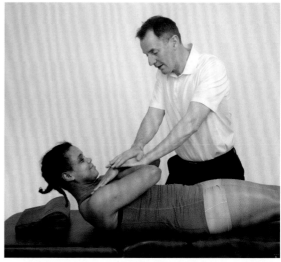

Figure 8.58
Abdominal resisted testing.

- Respiration control evaluation (Hodges et al., 2005; Lewit, 1994; Greenman, 1990)

- Abdominal muscles (Figure 8.58) (Hölmich et al., 2004).

EducATE

- Use of SIJ belt for pelvic reinforcement

- Deep abdominal contraction with pressure biofeedback unit (PBU) (Figures 8.59 and 8.60) (Grooms et al., 2013).

ManipulATE

- Thoracolumbar and SIJ, if required (HVLA or MET)

- Abdominals, particularly the oblique muscles (soft tissue mobilization and inhibition techniques to TrPs or TnPs) (Figure 8.61)

- Lower ribs (HVLA or MET) (Figure 8.62).

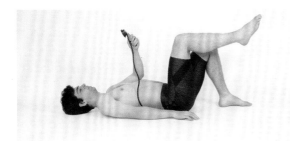

Figure 8.59
Deep abdominal contraction with pressure biofeedback unit supine.

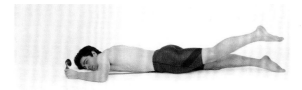

Figure 8.60
Deep abdominal contraction with pressure biofeedback unit prone.

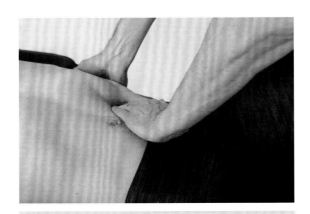

Figure 8.61
Soft tissue mobilization trigger points and tender points in abdominals.

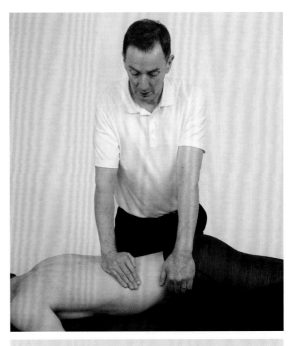

Figure 8.62
Soft tissue mobilization lower ribs and thoracolumbar fascia.

ActivATE

- Diaphragmatic breathing strategies

- Deep fibers of psoas ("suction" thigh bone into socket)

- Deep abdominal system (modified dead bug; Figure 8.63), progressing to abdominal/oblique sit-up)

- Lumbar spine lateral flexion (short-/long-lever plank capacity) (Figure 8.64).

Conclusion

The aim of this chapter was to provide a comprehensive, quick "go-to guide" for clinicians. My intention was to highlight how to *integrATE* the management of some of the more common clinical pathologies pertaining to the

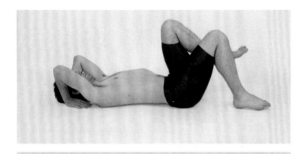

Figure 8.63
Modified dead bug.

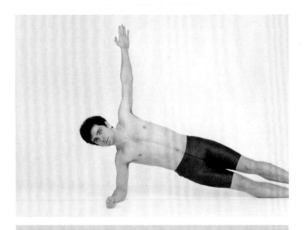

Figure 8.64
Lumbar spine lateral flexion plank.

ego influence our ability to see the bigger picture, when attempting to understand the many complex presentations that arise. Similarly, I would counsel against an approach that classifies every patient into a particular category in order to use a simple protocol to treat and manage them more effectively. While it could be argued that this chapter, with its simplified "go-to guide," is appearing to suggest that we can, in fact, fit patients into categories and follow a "one size fits all" approach to treatment, my response would be a categoric "no"! It isn't about that at all! My intention is to create a better perspective on this subject to facilitate learning.

Protocols very often will not work and the reason for this is straightforward. Everyone is unique. Patients will present with their own story, influenced by many factors, such as injury and compensation patterns that develop from continual loading during training and competitions, habits, preconceived ideas and longstanding beliefs. These factors combine with many others, such as the role of family, friends and relationships, lack of team selection, and social media and financial issues, and all exert their influence on the "story" the clinician is presented with. Our role as a clinician is to manage the person in their entirety, as an individual, not just their musculoskeletal issues or damaged tissues, and we must use the best strategies we can to help them set realistic goals and achieve them.

To conclude, my advice for dealing with patients is simple: always strive to do the best you can. If you do your best and your approach works, then fantastic; even if it fails, you will know that you tried your best, with the best intentions. By picking up this book and going through the case studies and methods it describes, I hope you have learned things that will help extend your practice, make your existing "best" somehow "better." As clinicians, it is a goal we all should strive towards.

spino-pelvic-hip complex. It is important to remind you that my concept for using the "five 'ATEs" was to offer a flexible framework to manage musculoskeletal issues in clinical practice and in elite sport.

Researchers and other experienced clinicians may disagree with some of the ideas and concepts I have suggested, and I welcome discussion and discovery; most importantly, I'm always happy to be proved wrong. Quite simply, my feeling is the more I learn, the more I realize I don't know. I strongly believe that, as clinicians, we should never let our position of responsibility or our

References

Anloague, PA., Chorny, WS., Childs, KE. et al., 2015. The relationship between the femoral nerve tension and hip flexor length. *Journal Novel Physiotherapy*, 5(244), p. 2.

Butler, D., 2010. *The Neurodynamic Techniques*. Melbourne: Noigroup Publications.

Cibulka, MT., White, DM., Woehrle, J. et al., 2009. Hip pain and mobility deficits – hip osteoarthritis: clinical practice guidelines. *Journal Orthopaedic Sports Physical Therapy*, 39(4), pp. A1–A25.

Dreyfuss, P., Dreyer, S, Griffin, J. et al., 1994. Positive sacroiliac screening tests in asymptomatic adults. *Spine*, 10, pp. 1138–1143.

Dreyfuss, P., Michaelsen, M., Pauza, K. et al., 1996. The value of medical history and physical examination in diagnosing sacroiliac pain. *Spine*, 21, pp. 2594–2602.

Greenman, P., 1990. *Principles of Manual Medicine*. 5th ed. Philadelphia: Lippincott Williams & Wilkins.

Grooms, DR., Grindstaff, TL., Croy, T. et al., 2013. Cinimetric analysis of pressure biofeedback and transversus abdominis function in individuals with stabilization classification low back pain. *Journal Orthopaedic Sports Physical Therapy*, 43, pp. 184–193.

Haneline, MT., Cooperstein, R., Young, M. et al., 2008. Spinal motion palpation: a comparison of studies that assessed intersegmental end feel vs excursion. *Journal Manipulative Physiology Therapy*, 31(8), pp. 616–626.

Hodges, PW., Eriksson, AE., Shirley, D. et al., 2005. Intra-abdominal pressure increases stiffness of the lumbar spine. *Journal Biomechanics*, 38(9), pp. 1873–1880.

Hölmich, P., Hölmich, LR. and Bjerg, AM., 2004. Clinical examination of athletes with groin pain: an intraobserver and interobserver reliability study. *British Journal of Sports Medicine*, 38(4), pp. 446–451.

Hungerford, B., Gilleard, W., Moran, M. et al., 2007. Evaluation of the ability of physical therapists to palpate intrapelvic motion with the stork test on the support side. *Physical Therapy*, 87(7), pp. 879–887.

Laslett, M., Aprill, C., McDonald, B. et al., 2005. Diagnosis of sacroiliac joint pain: validity of individual provocation tests and composites of tests. *Manual Therapy*, 10(3), pp. 207–218.

Laslett, M., McDonald, B., Aprill, C. et al., 2006. Clinical predictors of screening lumbar zygapophyseal joint blocks: development of clinical prediction rules. *Spine Journal*, 6(4), pp. 370–379.

Lee, D., 2011. *The Pelvic Girdle. An Integration of Clinical Expertise and Research*. 4th ed. Edinburgh: Churchill Livingstone/Elsevier.

Lequesne, M., Mathieu, P., Vuillemin-Bodaghi, V. et al., 2008. Gluteal tendinopathy in refractory greater trochanter pain syndrome: diagnostic value of two clinical tests. *Arthritis & Rheumatism*, 59(2), pp. 241–246.

Lewit, K., 1994. The functional approach. *Journal Orthopaedic Medicine*, 16(3), pp. 73–74.

Majlesi, J., Togay, H., Unalan, H. et al., 2008. The sensitivity and specificity of the slump and the straight leg raising tests in patients with lumbar disc herniation. *Journal Clinical Rheumatology*, 14(2), pp. 87–91.

Martin HD, Kivlan BR, Palmer IJ et al., 2014. Diagnostic accuracy of clinical tests for sciatic nerve entrapment in the gluteal region. *Knee Surgery Sports Traumatology and Arthroscopy*, 22(4), pp. 882–888.

Mens, J., Vleeming, A., Snijders, C. et al., 2002. Reliability and validity of hip adduction strength to measure disease severity in posterior pelvic pain since pregnancy. *Spine*, 27(15), pp. 1674–1679.

Mens, J., Damen, L., Snijders, C. et al., 2006. The mechanical effect of a pelvic belt in patients with pregnancy-related pelvic pain. *Clinical Biomechanics*, 21(2), pp. 122–127.

Reese, NB. and Bandy, WD. 2003. Use of an inclinometer to measure flexibility of the iliotibial band using the Ober test and the modified Ober test: differences in magnitude and reliability of measurements. *Journal Orthopaedic & Sports Physical Therapy*, 33(6), pp. 326–330.

Reiman, M., Mather, R. and Cook, C., 2015. Physical examination tests for hip dysfunction and injury. *British Journal of Sports Medicine*, 49(6), pp. 357–361.

Serner, A., Weir, A., Tol, J. et al., 2016. Can standardised clinical examination of athletes with acute groin injuries predict the presence and location of MRI findings? *British Journal Sports Medicine*, 50(24), pp. 1541–1547.

Shacklock, M., 2005. *Clinical Neurodynamics. A New System of Musculoskeletal Treatment*. Edinburgh: Butterworth Heinemann/Elsevier.

Stuber, K., Lerede, C., Kristmanson, K. et al., 2014. The diagnostic accuracy of the Kemp's test: a systematic review. *Journal Canadian Chiropractic Association*, 58(3), pp. 258–267.

Tawa, N., Rhoda, A. and Diener, I. 2017. Accuracy of clinical neurological examination in diagnosing lumbo-sacral radiculopathy: a systemic literature review. *BMC Musculoskeletal Disorders*, 18(1), p. 93.

Verrall, G., Slavotinek, J., Barnes, P. et al., 2005. Description of pain provocation tests used for the diagnosis of sports-related chronic groin pain: relationship of tests to defined clinical (pain and tenderness) and MRI (pubic bone marrow oedema). *Scandinavian Journal Medicine & Science in Sports*, 15(1), pp. 36–42.

Vleeming, A., Stoeckart, R., Volkers, A. et al., 1990a. Relation between form and function in the sacroiliac joint. *Spine*, 15(2), pp. 130–132.

Vleeming, A., Volkers, A., Snijders, C. et al., 1990b. Relation between form and function in the sacroiliac joint. *Spine*, 15(2), pp. 133–136.

Youdas, J., Mraz, S., Norstad, B. et al., 2007. Determining meaningful changes in pelvic-on-femoral position during the Trendelenburg test. *Journal of Sport Rehabilitation*, 16(4), pp. 326–335.

The Keele STarT Back Screening Tool

Patient name		Date

Thinking about the **last two weeks,** tick your response to the following questions

		Disagree 0	Agree 1
1	My back pain has **spread down my leg(s)** at some time in the last 2 weeks	☐	☐
2	I have had pain in the **shoulder** or **neck** at some time in the last 2 weeks	☐	☐
3	I have only **walked short distances** because of my back pain	☐	☐
4	In the last 2 weeks, I have **dressed more slowly** than usual because of back pain	☐	☐
5	It's not really safe for a person with a condition like mine to be physically active	☐	☐
6	**Worrying thoughts** have been going through my mind a lot of the time	☐	☐
7	I feel that **my back pain is terrible** and it's never going to get any better	☐	☐
8	In general I have **not enjoyed** all the things I used to enjoy	☐	☐

9 Overall, how **bothersome** has your back pain been in the **last 2 weeks**?

Not at all ☐	Slightly ☐	Moderately ☐	Very much ☐	Extremely ☐
0	0	0	1	1

Total score (all 9) ☐   Sub-score (Q 5–9) ☐

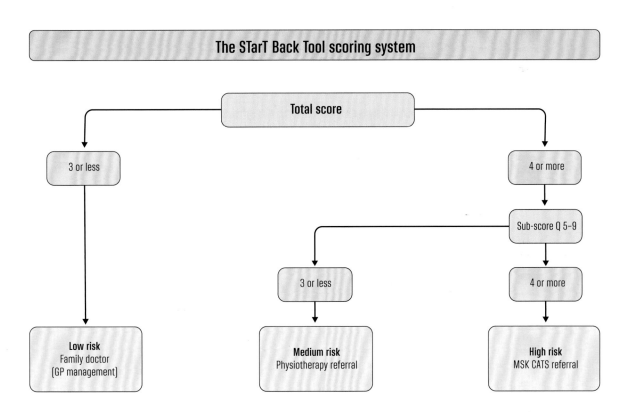

The STarT Back Tool scoring system

Total score

3 or less → **Low risk** Family doctor (GP management)

4 or more → Sub-score Q 5–9

3 or less → **Medium risk** Physiotherapy referral

4 or more → **High risk** MSK CATS referral

MSK CATS: musculoskeletal clinical assessment and treatment service.
The nine-item tool is available to download online at www.keele.ac.uk/sbst/downloadthetool.

Back Pain Functional Scale: overview

Stratford et al. (2000) developed the Back Pain Functional Scale (BPFS) to evaluate functional ability in patients with back pain. The authors are from McMaster University Appalachian Physical Therapy (Georgia) and Virginia Commonwealth University.

Measures

1 Any of your usual work, housework or school activities

2 Your usual hobbies and recreational or sporting activities

3 Performing heavy activities around your home

4 Bending or stooping

5 Putting on your shoes or socks (or stockings or pantyhose)

6 Lifting a box of groceries from the floor

7 Sleeping

8 Standing for 1 hour

9 Walking 1 mile

10 Going up or down 2 flights of stairs (about 20 steps)

11 Sitting for 1 hour

12 Driving for 1 hour

Responses	Points
Unable to perform activity	0
Extreme difficulty	1
Quite a bit of difficulty	2
Moderate difficulty	3
A little bit of difficulty	4
No difficulty	5

Total score = SUM(points for all 12 measures)
Adjusted total score = (total score) / 60

Interpretation

Minimum score	0
Maximum score	0
Maximum adjusted score	1 (100%)

The higher the score, the greater the patient's functional ability

Total score (adjusted)	Interpretation
0 (0%)	Unable to perform any activity
60 (100%)	No difficulty in any activity

Performance

Test-related reliability	0.88
Internal consistency	0.93

The score strongly correlates with the Roland-Morris questionnaire

APPENDIX 3

Copenhagen Hip and Groin Outcome Score (HAGOS) questionnaire

Patient name	Today's date

Date of birth

INSTRUCTIONS This questionnaire asks for your view about your hip and/or groin problem. The questions should be answered considering your hip and/or groin function during the **past week**. This information will help us keep track of how you feel, and how well you are able to do your usual activities.

Answer **every** question by ticking the appropriate box. Tick only one box for each question. If a question does not pertain to you or you have not experienced it in the past week, please make your "best guess" as to which response would be the most accurate.

Symptoms

These questions should be answered considering your hip and/or groin symptoms and difficulties during the **past week**

S1 Do you feel discomfort in your hip and/or groin?

Never ☐　Rarely ☐　Sometimes ☐　Often ☐　Always ☐

S2 Do you hear clicking or any other type of noise from your hip and/or groin?

Never ☐　Rarely ☐　Sometimes ☐　Often ☐　Always ☐

S3 Do you have difficulties stretching your legs far out to the side?

None ☐　Mild ☐　Moderate ☐　Severe ☐　Extreme ☐

S4 Do you have difficulties taking full strides when you walk?

None ☐　Mild ☐　Moderate ☐　Severe ☐　Extreme ☐

S5 Do you experience sudden twinging/stabbing sensations in your hip and/or groin?

Never ☐　Rarely ☐　Sometimes ☐　Often ☐　Always ☐

Stiffness

The following questions concern the amount of stiffness you have experienced during the **past week** in your hip and/or groin. Stiffness is a sensation of restriction or slowness in the ease with which you move your hip and/or groin.

S6 How severe is your hip and/or groin stiffness after first awakening in the morning?

None ☐   Mild ☐   Moderate ☐   Severe ☐   Extreme ☐

S7 How severe is your hip and/or groin stiffness after sitting, lying or resting **later in the day**?

None ☐   Mild ☐   Moderate ☐   Severe ☐   Extreme ☐

Pain

P1 How often is your hip and/or groin painful?

Never ☐   Monthly ☐   Weekly ☐   Daily ☐   Always ☐

P2 How often do you have pain in areas other than your hip and/or groin that you think may be related to your hip and/or groin problem?

Never ☐   Monthly ☐   Weekly ☐   Daily ☐   Always ☐

The following questions concern the amount of pain you have experienced during the **past week** in your hip and/or groin. **What amount of hip and/or groin pain have you experienced during the following activities?**

P3 Straightening your hip fully

None ☐   Mild ☐   Moderate ☐   Severe ☐   Extreme ☐

P4 Bending your hip fully

None ☐   Mild ☐   Moderate ☐   Severe ☐   Extreme ☐

P5 Walking up or down stairs

None ☐   Mild ☐   Moderate ☐   Severe ☐   Extreme ☐

P6 At night while in bed (pain that disturbs your sleep)

None ☐   Mild ☐   Moderate ☐   Severe ☐   Extreme ☐

P7 Sitting or lying

None ☐   Mild ☐   Moderate ☐   Severe ☐   Extreme ☐

> The following questions concern the amount of pain you have experienced during the **past week** in your hip and/or groin. **What amount of hip and/or groin pain have you experienced during the following activities?**

P8 Standing upright

None ☐   Mild ☐   Moderate ☐   Severe ☐   Extreme ☐

P9 Walking on a hard surface (asphalt, concrete, etc.)

None ☐   Mild ☐   Moderate ☐   Severe ☐   Extreme ☐

P10 Walking on an uneven surface

None ☐   Mild ☐   Moderate ☐   Severe ☐   Extreme ☐

Physical function, daily living

> The following questions concern your physical function. **For each of the following activities, please indicate the degree of difficulty you have experienced in the past week due to your hip and/or groin problem.**

A1 Walking up stairs

None ☐   Mild ☐   Moderate ☐   Severe ☐   Extreme ☐

A2 Bending down, e.g., to pick something up from the floor

None ☐   Mild ☐   Moderate ☐   Severe ☐   Extreme ☐

A3 Getting in/out of the car

None ☐   Mild ☐   Moderate ☐   Severe ☐   Extreme ☐

A4 Lying in bed (turning over or maintaining the same hip position for a long time)

None ☐   Mild ☐   Moderate ☐   Severe ☐   Extreme ☐

A5 Heavy domestic duties (scrubbing floors, vacuuming, moving heavy boxes, etc.)

None ☐   Mild ☐   Moderate ☐   Severe ☐   Extreme ☐

Function, sports and recreational activities

The following questions concern your physical function when participating in higher-level activities. Answer **every** question by ticking the appropriate box. If a question does not pertain to you or you have not experienced it in the past week, please make your "best guess" as to which response would be the most accurate. **The questions should be answered considering what degree of difficulty you have experienced during the following activities in the past week due to problems with your hip and/or groin.**

SP1 Squatting

None ☐   Mild ☐   Moderate ☐   Severe ☐   Extreme ☐

SP2 Running

None ☐   Mild ☐   Moderate ☐   Severe ☐   Extreme ☐

SP3 Twisting/pivoting on a weight-bearing leg

None ☐   Mild ☐   Moderate ☐   Severe ☐   Extreme ☐

SP4 Walking on an uneven surface

None ☐   Mild ☐   Moderate ☐   Severe ☐   Extreme ☐

SP5 Running as fast as you can

None ☐   Mild ☐   Moderate ☐   Severe ☐   Extreme ☐

SP6 Bringing the leg forcefully forward and/or out to the side, such as in kicking, skating, etc.

None ☐   Mild ☐   Moderate ☐   Severe ☐   Extreme ☐

SP7 Sudden explosive movements that involve quick footwork, such as accelerations, decelerations, changes of direction, etc.

None ☐   Mild ☐   Moderate ☐   Severe ☐   Extreme ☐

SP8 Situations where the leg is stretched into an outer position (such as when the leg is placed as far away from the body as possible)

| None | | Mild | | Moderate | | Severe | | Extreme | |

Participation in physical activities

The following questions are about your ability to participate in your preferred physical activities. Physical activities include sporting activities as well as all other forms of activity where you become slightly out of breath. **When you answer these questions consider to what degree your ability to participate in physical activities during the past week has been affected by your hip and/or groin problem.**

PA1 Are you able to participate in your preferred physical activities for as long as you would like?

| Always | | Often | | Sometimes | | Rarely | | Never | |

PA2 Are you able to participate in your preferred physical activities at your normal performance level?

| Always | | Often | | Sometimes | | Rarely | | Never | |

Quality of life

Q1 How often are you aware of your hip and/or groin problem?

| Never | | Monthly | | Weekly | | Daily | | Constantly | |

Q2 Have you modified your lifestyle to avoid activities potentially damaging to your hip and/or groin?

| Not at all | | Mildly | | Moderately | | Severely | | Totally | |

Q3 In general, how much difficulty do you have with your hip and/or groin?

| None | | Mild | | Moderate | | Severe | | Extreme | |

Q4 Does your hip and/or groin problem affect your mood in a negative way?

| Not at all | | Rarely | | Sometimes | | Often | | All the time | |

Q5 Do you feel restricted due to your hip and/or groin problem?

| Not at all | | Rarely | | Sometimes | | Often | | All the time | |

Thank you very much for completing all the questions in this questionnaire.

HAGOS: HAGOS is a patient-reported outcome measure employing 5-item Likert scales. HAGOS covers 6 dimensions (subscales): Symptoms, Pain, Function in daily living (ADL), Function in sport and recreation (Sports/Rec), Participation in Physical Activities (PA) and Hip and/or groin-related Quality of Life (QOL).

Missing data: If a mark is placed outside a box, the closest box is used. If 2 boxes are marked, the box indicating the more severe problems is chosen. Missing data are treated as such; 1 or 2 missing values are substituted with the average value for the dimension. If more than 2 items are omitted for the subscales Symptoms, Pain, ADL, Sport/Rec and QOL, the response is considered invalid. If more than 1 item is omitted for the subscale PA, the response is considered invalid.

Score calculation: The 6 HAGOS subscales are scored separately: Symptoms (7 items); Pain (10 items); ADL (5 items); Sport/Rec (8 items); PA (2 items) and QOL (5 items). The past week is taken into consideration when answering the questions. Standardized answer options are given (5 Likert boxes) and each question gets a score from 0 to 4, where zero indicates no problem. The 6 scores are calculated as the sum of the items included, in accordance with score calculations of the HOOS score. Raw scores are then transformed to a 0–100 scale, with zero representing extreme hip and/or groin problems and 100 representing no hip and/or groin problems, as common in orthopedic scales. Scores between 0 and 100 represent the percentage of total possible score achieved. An aggregate score is not calculated since it is regarded desirable to analyze and interpret the different dimensions separately.

HAGOS instructions manual scoring sheet

Assign the following scores to the boxes:

None	Mild	Moderate	Severe	Extreme
0	1	2	3	4

Missing data: If a mark is placed outside a box, the closest box is chosen. If 2 boxes are marked, the box indicating the more severe problems is chosen. Missing data are treated as such; 1 or 2 missing values are substituted with the average value for that subscale. If more than 2 items for the subscales PAIN, SYMPTOMS, ADL, SPORT/REC and QOL are omitted, the response is considered invalid and no score is calculated. If more than 1 item for the subscale PA is omitted, the response is considered invalid and no score is calculated. Sum up the total score of each subscale and divide by the possible maximum score for the scale. Traditionally in orthopedics, 100 indicates no problems and 0 indicates extreme problems. The normalized score is transformed to meet this standard. Please use the formulas provided for each subscale:

1. PAIN

$$100 - \frac{\text{Total score P1–P10} \times 100}{40} \qquad = 100 - \frac{}{40} = \underline{\hspace{2cm}}$$

2. SYMPTOMS

$$100 - \frac{\text{Total score S1–S7} \times 100}{28} \qquad = 100 - \frac{}{28} = \underline{\hspace{2cm}}$$

3. ADL

$$100 - \frac{\text{Total score A1–A5} \times 100}{20} \qquad = 100 - \frac{}{20} = \underline{\hspace{2cm}}$$

4. SPORT/REC

$$100 - \frac{\text{Total score SP1–SP8} \times 100}{32} \qquad = 100 - \frac{}{32} = \underline{\hspace{2cm}}$$

5. PA

$$100 - \frac{\text{Total score PA1–PA2} \times 100}{8} \qquad = 100 - \frac{}{8} = \underline{\hspace{2cm}}$$

6. QOL

$$100 - \frac{\text{Total score Q1–Q5} \times 100}{20} \qquad = 100 - \frac{}{20} = \underline{\hspace{2cm}}$$

Profile

To visualize differences in the 6 different HAGOS subscores and change between different administrations of the HAGOS (e.g., pre-treatment to post-treatment), HAGOS Profiles can be plotted, as illustrated in the example below.

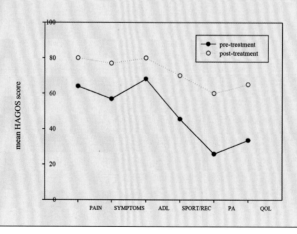

INDEX

Note: Page numbers followed by italics denotes figures and bold denotes tables respectively.

A

Abdominal muscles, *39,* 39–40
Abdominal-related pain, 271–273
Accuracy, clinical evaluation, 18
ActivATE approach, 253
Activation techniques, 211, 214
    case study, 214–215, 225–226, 226–234, 236
    clinical progression, *211*
    for motor control, 226–234
    muscle capacity, 234–235
    muscular strength, 236
    theory, 214
Active straight leg raise (ASLR), 38, *38,* 112, *113*
    case study, 38–39
    in prone, 136–137, *137*
    in prone with pelvic reinforcement, 137
    in supine, 136, *136*
    in supine with pelvic reinforcement, 136, *136*
Acute low back pain, 87–90
    case study, 88–89
    differential diagnosis, **88**
    loss of range of movement (ROM), 87
    manual therapy techniques, 89
    pain relief medication and NSAIDs, 89
    reactive phase, 87–89
    regeneration or subacute phase, 89–90
    remodeling phase, 90
    signs or symptoms, 88
    sleep disturbance in, 88
Adapted Thomas test, *40,* 40–41
    case study, 40–41
Adductor evaluation, 36, *37*
    case study, 36–38
Adductor exercises, *114*
Adductor muscles, 69–70, *70,* 131
    clinical implications, 70–71
    functional connections between abdominal and, 70
Adductor-related pain, 266–268
Adductor stretch, 219, *219*
Alignment, 13. *see also* functional alignment
Anatomy slings, 68
Anterior fascicles, innervation to, 62
Anterior hip
    capsule mobilization, *255*
    stretch, *255*
Anterior oblique sling, 69, *69*

Anterior superior iliac spine (ASIS), 79
Articular evaluation, 142–143
    gold standard, 143
    hip joint passive flexion, abduction and external rotation (FABER), 145–146, *146*
    hip joint passive flexion, adduction and internal rotation (FADIR), 145, *146*
    lumbar segmental passive evaluation, *143,* 143–144
    normal and abnormal barriers, 142
    physiological barrier, 142
    thoracic segmental extension/flexion passive evaluation, 144
    thoracic segmental lateral flexion passive evaluation, 144, *145*
    thoracic segmental rotation passive evaluation, 144–145, *145*
Articular mobility, 217
Athletes, low back pain, 92–96
    age differences, 94
    case study, 94–95
    due to spinal radiological abnormality, 93
    incorrect posture, 93
    movement and control dysfunctions, 95, *95*
    pelvic parameters, 93
    from poor athlete training techniques, 93
    repetitive micro- or acute macro-trauma, 94
    spinal curvatures, 93
    in young athletes, 94
Autogenic inhibition, 12

B

Back Pain Functional Scale (BPFS), 18, 124
Barrier concept, *142,* 179
Biceps femoris, 75–77
    clinical implications, 77–78
Bio-psychosocial (BPS) model, 8–9, 48
Bio-psychosocial non-specific LBP, 97–98

C

Cam-type FAI impingement, 106–107
    prevalence of, 107
Cauda equina syndrome, 88
Central nervous system (CNS), 10, 97
Central sensitization, 99

Cervical lordosis, 55
Chronic low back pain (LBP), 90–92
    case study, 91
    healthcare management of, 99–100
    movement and control impairments, 90
    sensitization in, 98–99
Clinical evaluation, 16–19, 33–34
    abdominal muscles, *39,* 39–40
    accuracy, 18
    active straight leg raise (ASLR), 38–39
    adapted Thomas test, *40,* 40–41
    adductor evaluation, 36–38
    case study, 34–35
    considerations, *34*
    for hip joint FADIR testing, 46
    hip joint passive flexion, adduction and internal rotation (FADIR), 35, *35,* 35–36
    lumbar segmental passive evaluation, *42,* 42–43
    principles, *17*
    red flags, **17**
    reliability, 18
    respiratory control, 41, *41*
    sensitivity, 18–19
    specificity, 18–19
    validity, 18
    yellow flags, **17**
Clinical reasoning, 5–8, 125–126
    approaches, 5–8
    diagnostic reasoning, 44–47
    drawbacks, 6
    hypothetical deductive reasoning, 44
    interpretative reasoning, 47
    knowledge and practitioner insight, 44
    pattern recognition, 43
Coccygeus, 67
Connective tissue, 175
Control system, 10
Copenhagen Hip and Groin Outcome Score (HAGOS), 18, 124
    questionnaire, *280–284*
Critical thinking, 5
C sign, 107
"Cytoskeleton" of cell, 173

D

Davis's law, 173
Decision-making, 5
Deep erector spinae group, 75, *76*

Deep gluteal muscles, *80*

Delayed-onset muscle soreness (DOMS), 213

Descending pain mechanism, 172, *172*

Diagnostic reasoning, 6–7, 44–47

Diaphragm, 62

Diaphragmatic breathing, 62

Dysfunction, defined, 9

E

Elastic zone, 13

Erector spinae, 74–75
    extension self-mobilization, 220, *221*
    flexion stretch, 220, *220*
    supine rotation stretch, 220, *221*

External oblique, 66

Extra-cellular matrix (ECM), 173

F

Fascia, role as passive structure, 10

Fast high-threshold motor units, 12

Femoral nerve test, 159, *159*

Femoroacetabular impingement (FAI), 15, 102, 106–107, *107*, 110
    diagnosis, 107
    reliability of clinical tests for, 107
    syndrome, 23, 142

Femoroacetabular impingement (FAI) syndrome, 217

Five 'ATEs framework, 3, *3*, 123, 163–164. *see also* low back pain
    ActivATE, 5
    aim, 4
    EducATE, 5, 126–127
    EvaluATE, 5
    IntegrATE, 5
    management strategy, **4, 49**
    ManipulATE, 5

Flexion, abduction, external rotation, 107

Flexion, adduction, internal rotation, 107

Force closure, 13–14, *14*, 111
    clinical implications of increased or reduced, 112

Form closure, 13, *14*, 111

Functional alignment, 13–14

Functional evaluation, 9–13, 127–128
    active straight leg raise, 136–137, *136–137*
    active system, 11–12
    of an athlete or patient, 9–10

control system, 10

influence of psoas on spinal control, 137, *137*

kinetic chain and, *11*

motor units, 12

muscle fibers, 12

of muscle fibers, 12

muscle stiffness, 12

of muscle stiffness, 12–13

passive system, 10–11

pelvis and hip, 27–30

principles, 10, *10*

seated flexion, 135–136

seated hamstring test, 138, *138*

seated hip flexion test, 137–138, *138*

single-leg (SL) stance test, 132–134, *134*

single-leg stance test with small knee bend, 109, *109*

single-leg stance with small knee bend, 134, *135*

spinal, 25–27

spinal extension, 129–130, *129–130*

spinal flexion, 128, 128–129

spinal lateral flexion, *130*, 130–131

spinal rotation, 131, *131*

squat, 131–132, *132*

standing, 128

thoracic spine rotation in heel-sit position, 134–135, *135*

Functional movement, 15

Functional slings, 68–69

Functional spinal unit, 54

Functional squat, 28, *28*

G

Gluteus maximus, 72, 73, 80, 111

Gluteus maximus stretch, 219, *220*

Gluteus medius (GMed), 72, 78, 80, 81

Gluteus minimus, 78, 80

Golgi tendon organs (GTOs), 12

Gracovetsky's "spinal engine" theory, 68

Groin, 71, *71*

H

Hamstring stretch, 219, *219*

Handheld dynamometer (HHD), 160

High-velocity, low-amplitude thrust (HVLA) technique, 171

Hip flexion capacity, 237

Hip flexor strength training, 110

Hip functional evaluation, 27–30

Hip joint, 59–60, *60*
    architecture of, *60*
    micro-instability, 59
    movements, 59
    passive flexion, abduction and external rotation, 145–146, *146*
    passive flexion, adduction and internal rotation, 35, *35*, 35–36, 145, *146*
    stability, 59–60

Hip joint and groin injuries in young athletes, 104–107
    assessment of risk factors, 104
    case study, 110–111
    clinical implications, 109–110
    diagnosis, 104–105
    extra-articular overload injuries, 105–106
    hip-joint related pain, 106–107
    hip-related pubic pain, 106, *106*
    loss of ROM and flexibility of soft tissues, 104
    management of extra-/intra-articular hip and groin-related pain, 107–110

Hip joint-related pain, 264–266

Hip joint techniques, 195–202
    anterior hip capsule stretch, 196, *197*
    HVLA hip joint prone, 195, *196*
    HVLA hip joint supine, 195, *196*
    MET adductors, 200, *201*
    MET hamstrings, 202, *202*
    MET psoas and rectus femoris, 201, *202*
    posterior hip capsule stretch, 197, *197*
    STM adductors in supine, 199, *200*
    STM deep hip external rotators, 198, *199*
    STM obturator membrane, 199, *199*
    STM tensor fasciae latae, 197, *198*

Hip-related intra-articular overload injuries, 106–107

Hip-related pubic pain, 106, *106*

Human soleus, 12

HVLA techniques, 174, 177, 179

HVLA thoracolumbar spine., *255*

Hypoalgesia, 173

Hypothetical deductive reasoning, 6–7, 44

I

Iliacus, 62, 65
    innervation of, 65

Iliococcygeus, 66–67

Iliopsoas tendon, 110

Increased muscle extensibility, 174
Inexperienced clinicians, 6
Inferential thinking, 5
Internal oblique, 64, 66
Interpretative reasoning, 6, 8, 47
Inter-tester reliability analysis, 18
Intervertebral disk, 54, 87
Intra-class correlation coefficient (ICC), 18
Intra-tester reliability analysis, 18
Intrinsic muscle stiffness, 12–13
Ipsilateral quadratus lumborum muscle, 128
Isometric contractions, 215

J

Joint capsule, 59–60
Joint centration and dissociation, 15–16, 16
Joint manipulation, 170, 171, 174
  neurophysiology, 171
Judgment, 5

K

Knowledge and practitioner insight, 6–7, 44

L

Lateral sling, 78, 79
Latissimus dorsi, 72–73
Levator ani muscles, 66–67
Ligamentous suspension, 111
Low back pain (LBP), 23–24, 90–91, 96
  acute, 87–90
  case study, 102–104, 104
  as a cause of disability, 87
  chronic, 90–92
  diagnosis, 87
  evidence-based medicine, 91
  factors influencing, 100–104
  initial hypotheses, 23–24
  of length-tension relationships of
    musculoskeletal system, 24
  lifestyle changes and, 98
  management, flowchart, 96
  neuropathic, 92
  nociceptive, 92
  non-specific, 90, 96–98
  over-emphasis on a pathoanatomical
    diagnosis, 100–101
  over-medicalization of, 87
  over-use of surgery, 101–104

in patient/athlete management strategy,
  101
  performance of tasks and activities, 24
  positional alignment palpation, 24, 25
  prolonged bed rest, 101
  specific, 92–96
  spine, functional evaluation of, 25–27
  spino-pelvic complex, 24
  in sporting environments, 91, 92
  standing compensatory non-functional
    alignment, 25, 25
  of standing functional alignment, 24
  understanding, 97–98
Lumbar anomaly, 87
Lumbar disk herniation, 92
Lumbar disk-related pain, 256
Lumbar facet joint syndrome pain, 92
Lumbar facet-related pain, 254
Lumbar flexion movement, 13
Lumbar lordosis, 55
Lumbar multifidus muscles, 13
Lumbar segmental passive evaluation, 42,
  42–43
  case study, 42–43
Lumbar spine techniques, 188–191
  HVLA innominate supine, 192, 193
  HVLA side-lying, 189, 189
  MET erector spinae, 190, 191
  MET quadratus lumborum, 190, 190
  STM quadratus lumborum and lateral
    sling, 190, 190

M

Magnetic resonance imaging (MRI), 215
Manipulation therapy, 169, 172
  action response, 170
  adverse reactions, 177
  case study, 169–170, 175–170, 176
  complications, 177
  contra-indications, 177, 178
  joint, 170
  mechanical response, 170
  red flags, 178, 178
  side effects, 177
  soft tissue, 170
  suitability of, 176
Manual therapy, 204
Maximum voluntary contraction (MVC), 212
Mechanoreceptors, 10
Mechanotherapy, 170

Medical Dictionary for Health Professions and
  Nursing, 212
Mobility, 216, 217
Motor
  control, 15, 224
  neuron, 12
  programming, 174
  strategies, 224
  units, 12
Movement
  functional, 15
  joint centration and dissociation, 15–16,
    16
  motor control, 15
  patterns, 9
Multifidus, 75, 77
Muscle activation techniques, 170–171, 174
  capacity, 234–235
  effects of, 175
  energy techniques, 170
  inhibition, 211
  neurophysiology, 173–174
Muscle energy technique (MET), 144
Muscle fibers, 12
Muscle spindles, 12
Muscle stiffness, 12–13
  intrinsic, 12–13
  reflex-mediated, 13
Muscle strength and capacity evaluation,
  108, 160
  case study, 160–161
  HHD testing hip abductors, 162, 162
  HHD testing hip adductors, 161
  HHD testing hip extensors, 161, 162
  HHD testing hip flexors, 161, 161
  modified Sorenson's side-lying short-
    lever plank, 163, 163
  short-lever capacity test: isometric
    adductor plank, 162–163, 163
  sit-to-stand squat, 163, 164
Muscle tone, 147
Muscular evaluation, 146–147
  abdominal strength testing, 152, 154
  abdominals with pelvic reinforcement,
    154
  active side-lying piriformis evaluation,
    154, 155
  adapted Thomas test, 149, 151
  adductors, 149, 150–151
  case studies, 148–149
  contractile capability of a muscle,
    147–148

electromyography (EMG), 147
functional efficiency, *148*
hamstring strength testing, 152
HHD testing, 155
inner-range hip abduction side-lying, 154–155, *155*
physiological and mechanical insufficiency, *148*
prone knee bend (PKB), 151–152, *152*
psoas and rectus femoris, 149–151
psoas strength testing, 152, *153*
seated piriformis evaluation, 154
tensor fasciae latae (TFL)/iliotibial band (ITB) evaluation, 155, *156*
tonic and phasic muscles, 147, **147**
trigger point (TrP), 147
viscoelastic properties, 147
Muscular strength, 235
Musculoskeletal evaluation, phases of, *127*
Myofascial slings, 68
Myofascial stretch technique, 144
Myotactic reflex, 12

N

Neural dynamic techniques, 203–204
femoral nerve, 203, *204*
obturator nerve, 204, *204*
sciatic nerve straight leg raise, 203
Neural sensitivity evaluation, 155–157
femoral nerve test, 159, *159*
obturator nerve test, 159, *159*
refining or sensitizing neural testing, 158
slump sitting test, *158,* 158–159
straight leg raise (SLR), 157–158, *158*
Neural tension dysfunction, 157
Neuromuscular-controlled movement of articulation, 15
Neuropathic LBP, 92
Neurotransmitters, 173
Neutral zone, 13
Non-specific LBP, 96–98

O

Ober's test, 16
Obturator internus, 67
Obturator muscle strain, 71
Obturator nerve test, 159, *159*
Optimal function, 13
Optimal functional alignment, 14, *14*

Optimal mobility, 217
Osteoarthritis, 87
Oxford Manual Muscle Grading Scale, 36, **38**

P

Pain gate mechanism, 171, *171*
Pain modulation, 173–174
Panjabi's stability system, 10, *11*
Passive accessory intervertebral motion palpation (PAIVM), 144
Passive physiological intervertebral motion (PPIVM), 143
Passive segmental evaluation, 144
Passive system, 10–12
Pattern recognition, 5–6, 43
Pelvic floor
dysfunction, clinical implications of, 68
muscles of, *65,* 66
Pelvic girdle techniques, 55, *57–58,* 191–195
HVLA innominate prone, 191
HVLA innominate side-lying, 192, *192, 193*
HVLA innominate supine, 191, *192*
HVLA sacroiliac joint (SIJ) supine, 193, *193*
MET innominate anterior restriction in side-lying, 194, *195*
MET innominate posterior restriction in side lying, 194, *195*
MET SIJ supine, 193, *194*
physiology and dysfunction, 111–112, 113–114
Pelvic incidence, 56–58
Pelvic tilt, 56, 58
Pelvis functional evaluation, 27–30
intra-articular hip pain, 28
pelvic movement, 28
pelvic tilt and girdle, 28–29
range of motion (ROM), 27–28
sacroiliac joints (SIJs), 27–28
single-leg (SL) stance test, *29,* 29–30
tri-planar motion, 28
Peripheral sensitization, 98
Physiological movement, 10
Pincer-type FAI, 106
Piriformis stretch, 67, 219, *220*
Positional alignment, 31–32
case study, 33
palpation of PSIS, 32
prone, *33*
soft tissue tension and tone, 32
supine, *32*

Positional and passive evaluation, 138–139, **139**
prone spino-pelvic alignment, 139
respiration control supine, 141
supine SIJ evaluation, 139–140
supine spino-pelvic alignment, 139
thigh thrust test, 140
Positional release technique, 170
Post-activation potentiation (PAP), 215
Posterior fascicles, innervation to, 62
Posterior longitudinal sling, 74, *75*
Posterior oblique sling, 71–72
Posterior superior iliac spine (PSIS), 67, 128–129, 133
palpation of, 130
Pre-manipulation provocative testing, 177, 178–180
clinical implications, 179
Problem-solving, 5
Program design, 212
Proprioceptive neuromuscular facilitation (PNF), 170
Proprioceptive system, 10
Psoas, 40
influence on spinal control, 137, *137*
major, 15, 62, *63*
minor, 62
muscle, 15, 65, 68
related pain, 269–271
as stabilizer, 68
Pubic-related groin pain, 261–264
Pubic symphysis, 27–28, 55, *57, 59*
Pubococcygeus, 66

Q

Quadratus lumborum (QL), 65

R

Range of motion (ROM), 27–28, 31, 49, 55, 59–60, 74, 87, 90–91, 96, 100, 103–104, 106–108, *108,* 110, 111, 124, 126, 128, 132, 138, 142, *142,* 144, 146, 157
testing, 108, *108*
Range of movement, 169
Rectus abdominis, 66
Rectus femoris stretch, 217, *218*
Refining or sensitizing neural testing, 158
Reflex-mediated muscle stiffness, 13
Rehabilitation programs, 212

Reliability, clinical evaluation, 18
Respiratory control, 41, *41*
Retrain squat pattern, *257*
Return to play (RTP) plan, 91
Rib techniques
    HVLA ribs 2-10, 185, *186*
    HVLA ribs 3-10, 187, *187*
    HVLA ribs 6-10, 184, *185*
    MET ribs 3-10, 188, *188*
    MET ribs 6-9, 185, *186*
    STM diaphragm, 186, *187*

S

Sacral slope (SS), 56, 58–59
Sacroiliac joint-related pain, 258–261
Sacroiliac joints (SIJs), 27–28, 55, *59*, 67, 72
    pain, 92
Sagittal spinal balance, 55
Seated flexion, 135–136
Seated hamstring test, 138, *138*
Seated hip flexion test, 137–138, *138*
Segmental motion, 144
Sensitivity, clinical evaluation, 18–19
Sensitization in chronic LBP
    central sensitization, 99
    peripheral sensitization, 98
Shoulder assessment, 8
Single-leg (SL) stance test, 25, 132–134, *134*
    with small knee bend (SKB), 134, *135*
Skeletal muscle
    fibers, 12
    tissue, 215
Slow low-threshold motor units, 12
Slump sitting
    evaluation, 180, *257*
    test, *158*, 158–159
Soft tissue injuries, 23
Soft tissue manipulation technique, 170,
    171, 215
    muscle activation, 175–176
    neurophysiology of, 173
Soft tissues distribute strain, 10
Specificity, clinical evaluation, 18–19
Spinal alignment, 55
Spinal column, 53
    anterior and posterior pillars, 55
    cranial and caudal lordotic curves, 53
    curvatures, 53, *53*, 55, *56*
    functional spinal unit, 54
    intervertebral disk, 54

pelvic girdle, 55, *57*
pelvic parameters, 56–59, *60*
sacroiliac joints, 55, *59*
vertebra-disk-vertebra, 54
Spinal extension, 129–130, *129–130*
Spinal flexion, *128*, 128–129
Spinal functional evaluation, 25–27
    in frontal plane, 26
    limitations, 31
    optimal spinal extension, 26
    optimal spinal flexion, 26
    optimal spinal lateral flexion, 27
    optimal spinal rotation, 27, *27*
    posterior superior iliac spines, 26
    spinal extension and spinal flexion,
        30
    standing extension quadrant test,
        30
Spinal lateral flexion, *130*, 130–131
Spinal rotation, 131, *131*
    with glenohumeral joint (GHJ) internal/
        external rotation, 131, 132
Spino-pelvic-hip complex, 96
Spondylolisthesis, 93
Spondylolysis, 93
Squat, 131–132, *132*
    with arms overhead, 132, *133*
    depth, 131
Stabilization/control and dissociation,
    15
Standing, 128
    sagittal spino-pelvic alignments of
        athletes, 93
STarT Back Screening Tool, 18, 124
    scoring system, *277*
Straight leg raise test, 18, 92, 157–158,
    158, 180
Strength and capacity testing, 108–109,
    109
Stretch reflex, 12
Symptom modification techniques (SMTs),
    8, 44–45, *45*, 94, 113–114, 126, 253
    deep hip flexor function, evaluation of,
        46, *46*
    distal positioning of TFL's anatomical
        attachment, evaluation of, 46
    influence of thoracic mobility on
        symptoms, evaluation of, 45, *45*
System-based integrated approach, *6*

T

Tensor fasciae latae (TFL) muscle, 16,
    79–80, *81*, 131, 211
    clinical implications, 80–81
    tender points, 81
    trigger points, 81
Test-retest analysis, 18
Thoracic extension: supine self-mobilization
    with towel, 222
Thoracic kyphosis, 55
Thoracic segmental passive evaluation
    extension/flexion, 144
    lateral flexion, 144, *145*
Thoracic segmental rotation passive
    evaluation, 144–145, *145*
Thoracic spine and rib techniques, 181–188
Thoracic spine rotation in heel-sit position,
    134–135, *135*
Thoracic spine techniques
    HVLA (butterfly), 183, *184*
    HVLA T2-12, 184, *184*
    MET - extension, 182, *182*
    MET - rotation, 182, *182*
    STM active release - flexion/extension,
        183, *183*
Thoracolumbar fascia (TLF), *73*, 73–74
    clinical implications, 74
Thoracopelvic canister, 60–62, 60–67, *61*
    clinical implications, 67–68
    consequences of progressive changes, 67
    functional roles, 61
    muscles essential for maintaining, 62,
        63–64
Tissue extensibility, 217
Transversus abdominis (TA), 65–66
    function of, 66
Tri-planar motion, 28
Type 2 fast-twitch fibers, 12
Type 1 slow-twitch fibers, 12

V

Validity, clinical evaluation, 18
Vertebra-disk-vertebra, 54
Vertebral column, 53, *53*
    functions of, 54
Vertebral motion segment, *54*
Visual Analogue Scale (VAS), 213
Visualization, 215